Thieme

Awake Spine Surgery

Muhammad M. Abd-El-Barr, MD, PhD, FAANS
Professor
Vice-Chair, International Affairs
Chief, Endoscopic Spine Surgery
Spine Fellowship Co-Director
Department of Neurosurgery
Duke University Medical Center
Durham, North Carolina, USA

Alok Sharan, MD, MHCDS
Orthopedic Spine Surgeon
President, Spine and Performance Institute
Edison, New Jersey, USA

Kingsley Abode-Iyamah, MD
Neurosurgeon
Department of Neurological Surgery
Mayo Clinic
Jacksonville, Florida, USA

Bhavuk Garg, MBBS, MS
Orthopedic Surgeon
Associate Professor
Department of Neurosurgery
All India Institute of Medical Sciences (AIIMS)
New Delhi, Delhi, India

Ernest E. Braxton Jr., MD, MBA, FAANS
US Ski Team Physician
Spine and Neurological Surgery
Minimally Invasive Spine Surgery
Vail Summit Orthopaedics and Neurosurgery
Vail, Colorado, USA

76 Illustrations

Thieme
New York • Stuttgart • Delhi • Rio de Janeiro

Library of Congress Cataloging-in-Publication Data
is available from the publisher.

Thieme Publishers New York
333 Seventh Avenue, 18th Floor,
New York, NY 10001, USA
www.thieme.com
+1 800 782 3488,
customerservice@thieme.com

Cover design: ©Thieme
Cover Image source: ©Thieme/Ayşe Heisdorf. Photograph by Ayşe Heisdorf.
Typesetting by Thomson Digital, Noida, India

Printed in India by Replika Press Pvt. Ltd. 6 5 4 3 2 1

DOI: 10.1055/b000001052

ISBN: 978-1-68420-673-5

Also available as an e-book:
eISBN (PDF): 978-1-68420-674-2
eISBN (epub): 978-1-68420-676-6

Important note: Medicine is an ever-changing science undergoing continual development. Research and clinical experience are continually expanding our knowledge, in particular our knowledge of proper treatment and drug therapy. Insofar as this book mentions any dosage or application, readers may rest assured that the authors, editors, and publishers have made every effort to ensure that such references are in accordance with **the state of knowledge at the time of production of the book.**

Nevertheless, this does not involve, imply, or express any guarantee or responsibility on the part of the publishers in respect to any dosage instructions and forms of applications stated in the book. **Every user is requested to examine carefully** the manufacturers' leaflets accompanying each drug and to check, if necessary in consultation with a physician or specialist, whether the dosage schedules mentioned therein or the contraindications stated by the manufacturers differ from the statements made in the present book. Such examination is particularly important with drugs that are either rarely used or have been newly released on the market. Every dosage schedule or every form of application used is entirely at the user's own risk and responsibility. The authors and publishers request every user to report to the publishers any discrepancies or inaccuracies noticed. If errors in this work are found after publication, errata will be posted at www.thieme.com on the product description page.

Some of the product names, patents, and registered designs referred to in this book are in fact registered trademarks or proprietary names even though specific reference to this fact is not always made in the text. Therefore, the appearance of a name without designation as proprietary is not to be construed as a representation by the publisher that it is in the public domain.

Thieme addresses people of all gender identities equally. We encourage our authors to use gender-neutral or gender-equal expressions wherever the context allows.

MIX
Paper | Supporting responsible forestry
FSC
www.fsc.org
FSC™ C016779

To the Almighty, who gave us the opportunity to take care of patients.
To my wife, Mai, and children, Mariam, Sarra, and Mostafa,
who are a source of strength and light. To my parents who instilled in me
the love for knowledge and helping others. To my mentors, who trusted me.
To our patients, who have trusted us with their care.

Muhammad M. Abd-El-Barr, MD, PhD, FAANS

This book is dedicated to my fellow pioneers—those whose vision, courage,
and unwavering commitment continue to redefine what is possible in spine surgery.

Alok Sharan, MD, MHCDS

To my family and their sacrifices that allow me to care for others.
To our patients, for the trust you put in us every day.
To my team, who work tirelessly to provide exceptional care.

Kingsley Abode-Iyamah, MD

To all my patients for allowing me to be a part of their journey,
for reminding me the purpose behind every procedure, and for proving
that hope and healing go hand in hand.

Bhavuk Garg, MBBS, MS

To my wife, Molly, whom I love and adore, and my Spine Team family in Vail.

Ernest E. Braxton Jr., MD, MBA, FAANS

Contents

Videos

Foreword

Spine surgery is an inherently evolving subspeciality. Our understanding of the pathology, biomechanics, and natural history of spine disease coupled with technical and technological innovations is enabling us to achieve better and safer outcomes for our patients. At the forefront of this revolution is awake spine surgery! The ability to surgically treat spinal conditions without the added morbidity of general anesthesia is a bold and necessary step as we collectively aspire to minimize perioperative complications in our aging population undergoing spine surgery. In this new and unique text, Dr. Abd-El-Barr and co-editors brilliantly cover this innovative and emerging topic. This text is appropriately divided into pre-, intra-, and postoperative considerations. Ample content on regional anesthesia and spinal blocks is presented, and innovative techniques like endoscopy, robotics, and minimally invasive lateral spine approaches are also thoroughly covered. This comprehensive text on awake spine surgery will undoubtedly serve as an iconic text on this subject matter and will be the go-to guide for all clinicians interested in this new and exciting space. Congratulations to all the editors and contributors on this great work!

Ali A. Baaj, MD
Professor and Vice-Chair
Department of Neurological Surgery
Northwestern University Feinberg School of Medicine
Chicago, Illinois, USA

Foreword

The emergence of "awake spine surgery" represents a transformational paradigm in spine care. At its core, this textbook, *Awake Spine Surgery*, is a product of collaboration, innovation, and a passionate pursuit to better serve patients by minimizing surgical and anesthetic burdens. It signals not just an evolution but also, perhaps, the beginning of a new era in surgery where general anesthesia becomes the exception, not the rule.

Edited by Muhammad M. Abd-El-Barr, Alok Sharan, Kingsley Abode-Iyamah, Bhavuk Garg, and Ernest E. Braxton Jr., this book tells the compelling story of necessity-driven innovation. During the COVID-19 pandemic, as elective surgeries came to a halt and hospital resources were reallocated, a group of dedicated spine surgeons formed the "Awake Spine Surgery Group." Their mission was simple yet profound: to continue delivering essential spinal care without relying on general anesthesia. What began as virtual meetings and informal discussions quickly evolved into a comprehensive philosophy aimed at minimizing the necessity and burden of general anesthesia, blending surgical precision with anesthetic finesse.

This book thoughtfully details the multidimensional aspects of awake surgery, organized into preoperative, intraoperative, and postoperative considerations. Topics range from ultrasound-guided regional blocks to minimally invasive techniques and outpatient program development. The goal is clear: to empower surgeons to achieve optimal patient outcomes while eliminating the risks and recovery challenges associated with general anesthesia.

The editors and contributors emphasize that awake spine surgery is about more than just avoiding intubation; it is about embracing a holistic approach to patient wellness. By choosing techniques that reduce physiological stress, expedite recovery, and lessen overall morbidity, they are attempting to define a new gold standard for spinal care. This movement aligns closely with Hippocrates' guiding principle to "choose the least troublesome" method whenever possible.

Awake Spine Surgery is more than a textbook. It is a blueprint for the future. It stands as a testament to how adversity can spark remarkable innovation, offering surgeons practical tools, comprehensive protocols, and inspiring case studies to integrate into their practice today. Moreover, it challenges the next generation of surgeons to think critically about traditional norms and to continuously strive for safer, more compassionate surgical solutions.

As you turn these pages, you are not only gaining knowledge but also participating in the birth of a revolutionary movement in surgery. The work of Abd-El-Barr, Sharan, Abode-Iyamah, Garg, and Braxton will undoubtedly leave an indelible mark on the practice of spine surgery for years to come.

The future is awake.

Alexander R. Vaccaro, MD, PhD, MBA
Richard H. Rothman Professor and Chairman,
Department of Orthopaedic Surgery
Professor of Neurosurgery
Sidney Kimmel Medical Center of Thomas
Jefferson University
Co-Director, Delaware Valley Spinal Cord Injury Center
President, Rothman Orthopaedics
Philadelphia, Pennsylvania, USA

Preface

Necessity is the mother of all inventions.

–Plato, Republic, 1894

In 2020, a perfect storm occurred when the world was hit with the COVID-19 pandemic. The fear of spreading the virus during intubation and extubation resulted in hospitals canceling any type of elective surgery. Ventilators were being used mainly for COVID patients in the ICU. This resulted in the halting of all elective spine surgery. During this time, patients who suffered from a foot drop due to a lumbar herniated disk were put on waiting lists for surgery. Disabling back pain from a lumbar spondylolisthesis meant prolonged bed rest till elective surgery resumed.

Fortunately, during this time, once busy spine surgeons were able to pursue academic endeavors. The editors of this book came together to form an informal "Awake Spine Surgery Group." With the desire to proceed with elective spine surgery without the use of general anesthesia, the editors came together to meet virtually and compare notes. Initially, the meetings centered around the use of spinal/epidural anesthesia for elective spine surgery (Awake Spine Surgery). Soon it became clear that there were other aspects of Awake Spine Surgery that resulted in Rapid Recovery after Spine Surgery. The culmination of these notes was the inspiration for this book.

In this book, we attempt to cover all the aspects of awake spine surgery—from preoperative considerations such as patient selection, to intraoperative considerations such as new minimally invasive techniques, to postoperative considerations such as postoperative delirium. As can be seen by the content of the book, awake spine surgery is more than just the avoidance of general anesthesia—it stems from a philosophy of minimizing our "footprint" on our patients. That footprint can be surgical and anesthetic.

As Hippocrates said, "What you should put first in all the practice of our art is how to make the patient well; and if he can be made well in many ways, one should choose the least troublesome."

Our goal is to help the practicing spine surgeon with information to provide the safest, least troublesome treatment.

Muhammad M. Abd-El-Barr, MD, PhD, FAANS
Alok Sharan, MD, MHCDS
Kingsley Abode-Iyamah, MD
Bhavuk Garg, MBBS, MS
Ernest E. Braxton Jr., MD, MBA, FAANS

Acknowledgments

The Editors would like to acknowledge Karen Edmonson and Judith Tomat for their tireless efforts in seeing this project to completion.

Muhammad M. Abd-El-Barr, MD, PhD, FAANS
Alok Sharan, MD, MHCDS
Kingsley Abode-Iyamah, MD
Bhavuk Garg, MBBS, MS
Ernest E. Braxton Jr., MD, MBA, FAANS

Contributors

Muhammad M. Abd-El-Barr, MD, PhD, FAANS
Professor
Vice-Chair, International Affairs
Chief, Endoscopic Spine Surgery
Spine Fellowship Co-Director
Department of Neurosurgery
Duke University Medical Center
Durham, North Carolina, USA

Kingsley Abode-Iyamah, MD
Neurosurgeon
Department of Neurological Surgery
Mayo Clinic
Jacksonville, Florida, USA

Chakib Maurice Ayoub, MD, MBA
Professor
Department of Anesthesiology
Duke University School of Medicine
Durham, North Carolina, USA

Georgios Bakaloudis, MD
Spine Surgeon
Humanitas San Pio X
Milan, Italy

Emily Zoe Barney Hall, MD
Fellow, Regional Anesthesia and Acute Pain Management
Department of Anesthesiology
Duke University Health System
Durham, North Carolina, USA

Alice Baroncini, MD
Spine Fellow
Department of Orthopedics
Starship Hospital
Grafton, Auckland, New Zealand

Alyssa M. Bartlett, MPH
Medical Student
Department of Neurosurgery
Duke University School of Medicine
Durham, North Carolina, USA

Debesh Bhoi, MBBS, MD
Professor
Department of Anesthesiology, Pain Medicine and Critical Care
All India Institute of Medical Sciences
New Delhi, India

Maya Blasingame, BS
Medical Student
Department of Neurosurgery
Duke University School of Medicine
Durham, North Carolina, USA

Michele Bochicchio, MD
Spine Surgeon
Poliambulatorio Labormed
Potenza, Italy

Elird Bojaxhi, MD
Assistant Professor
Department of Anesthesiology
Mayo Clinic
Jacksonville, Florida, USA

Ernest E. Braxton Jr., MD, MBA, FAANS
US Ski Team Physician
Spine and Neurological Surgery
Minimally Invasive Spine Surgery
Vail Summit Orthopaedics and Neurosurgery
Vail, Colorado, USA

W. Michael Bullock, MD, PhD
Assistant Professor
Department of Anesthesiology
Division of Orthopaedic, Plastics, and Regional Anesthesiology
Duke North Site Director, Regional Anesthesiology and Acute Pain Medicine Fellowship
Director, Senior Resident Education for Regional Anesthesiology
Durham, North Carolina, USA

Lorenzo D'Apice, MD
Neurosurgery Resident
Fondazione Policlinico Universitario Agostino Gemelli IRCCS
Rome, Italy

Stephen Davies, MD
Fellow, Regional Anesthesiology and Acute Pain Management
Department of Anesthesiology
Duke University Hospital
Durham, North Carolina, USA

Marie De Ruyter, MD
Anesthesiologist
Department of Anesthesiology and Preoperative Medicine
Mayo Clinic
Jacksonville, Florida, USA

Peter N. Drossopoulos, MD
Department of Neurosurgery
Duke University School of Medicine
Durham, North Carolina, USA

Jeffrey C. Gadsden, MD
Anesthesiologist
Department of Anesthesiology
Duke University Hospital
Durham, North Carolina, USA

Bhavuk Garg, MBBS, MS
Orthopedic Surgeon
Associate Professor
Department of Neurosurgery
All India Institute of Medical Sciences
New Delhi, South Delhi, India

Raymond Gardocki, MD, FAAOS
Associate Professor
Department of Minimally Invasive and Endoscopic Spine Surgery
Vanderbilt University Medical Center
Franklin, Tennessee, USA

Colin Gold, MD
Neurosurgeon
Department of Neurosurgery
Swedish Medical Center Cherry Hill Campus
Seattle, Washington D.C., USA

Benjamin Frederick Gruenbaum, MD, PhD
Associate Professor
Anesthesiology and Perioperative Medicine
Mayo Clinic
Jacksonville, Florida, USA

Shaun E. Gruenbaum, MD, PhD
Anesthesiologist
Department of Anesthesiology and Perioperative Medicine
Mayo Clinic-Florida
Jacksonville, Florida, USA

Alessandra Isidori, MD
Neurosurgeon
Humanitas San Pio X
Milan, Italy

Sukriti Jha, MD, MBBS
Senior Resident
Department of Anesthesiology, Pain Medicine and Critical Care
All India Institute of Medical Sciences
New Delhi, India

Anjaleekrishna K., MBBS
Department of Anesthesiology, Pain Medicine and Critical Care
All India Institute of Medical Sciences
New Delhi, India

Bhavana Kayarat, MD
Department of Anesthesiology, Pain Medicine and Critical Care
All India Institute of Medical Sciences
New Delhi, India

Punit Khanna, MD
Department of Anesthesiology, Pain Medicine and Critical Care
All India Institute of Medical Sciences
New Delhi, India

Mohamed Fawzy Khattab, MD
Professor of Orthopaedic and Spine Surgery
Ain Shams University
Cairo, Egypt

Shahenda Khedr, BA
Medical Student
Department of Neurosurgery
Duke University School of Medicine
Durham, North Carolina, USA

Amanda H. Kumar, MD
Assistant Professor
Department of Anesthesiology
Duke University Medical Center
Durham, North Carolina, USA

Andrew Lucic, MD
Director of Acute Pain Service
Anesthesia Partners of Colorado
Vail, Colorado, USA

Ashwin M., MD
Department of Anesthesiology
All India Institute of Medical Sciences
New Delhi, India

Nabil Matmati, PhD
Clinical Research Director
Department of Neurosurgery
Ayer Neuroscience Institute, Hartford HealthCare
Bridgeport, Connecticut, USA

Angelo Mazzarino, MD
Department of Anesthesiology
Clinica Villa Pia
Rome, Italy

Basma Mohamed, MBChB
Associate Professor of Anesthesiology
Department of Anesthesiology
Duke University School of Medicine
Chapel Hill, North Carolina, USA

Favour C. Ononogbu-Uche, BS
Medical Student
College of Medicine
SUNY Downstate Health Sciences University
Brooklyn, New York, USA

Armaan R. Patel, BS
Student
Department of Biology
Tufts University
Medford, Massachusetts, USA

Bikash Ranjan Ray, MD
Professor
Department of Anesthesiology, Pain Medicine, and Critical Care
All India Institute of Medical Sciences
New Delhi, India

Abdullah Wael Saleh, BS
Clinical Research Assistant
Duke University School of Medicine
Durham, North Carolina, USA

Alok Sharan, MD, MHCDS
Orthopedic Spine Surgeon
President, Spine and Performance Institute
Edison, New Jersey, USA

Arnav Sharma, BS
MD Candidate
Duke University School of Medicine
Durham, North Carolina, USA

Devin St. Clair, MD
Orthopedic Spine Fellow
Department of Orthopedic Surgery
Vanderbilt University
Nashville, Tennessee, USA

Felix Toussaint, BS
Medical Student
Department of Neurosurgery
American University of the Caribbean School of Medicine
Miramar, Florida, USA

Taylor Wallace, BS
Medical Student
Duke University Health System
Durham, North Carolina, USA

Vijay Yanamadala, MD, FAANS
Neurosurgeon
Hartford HealthCare
The Ayer Neuroscience Institute
Milford, Connecticut, USA

Part I

Preoperative Considerations

I

1 Relevant Spine Anatomy for Regional Anesthesia

Ernest E. Braxton Jr. and Colin Gold

Abstract

Spine surgery, particularly for conditions like degenerative spondylolisthesis, spinal stenosis, and lumbar disk herniations, requires a thorough understanding of the relevant spinal anatomy to ensure the safe and effective administration of regional anesthesia. Regional anesthetic techniques, such as neuraxial blocks and peripheral nerve blocks, are increasingly being utilized in awake spine surgeries to provide intraoperative anesthesia and postoperative analgesia. Knowledge of the relevant anatomy of the lumbar spine can be a powerful tool in successfully implementing an anesthetic strategy to perform awake spine surgery. Perhaps the key question when deciding on anesthetic for any surgery is: How much is enough? Understanding the anatomy and innervation of the lumbar spine can help choose an anesthetic that will accomplish the goal of keeping the patient comfortable during the procedure without causing unintended morbidity. In this chapter, we will review the anatomy of the thoracolumbar spine and how that anatomy relates to the variety of regional blocks that can be utilized in awake spine surgery.

Keywords: spine anatomy, regional anesthesia, erector spinae plane block, spinal, epidural

Key Points

- Anatomical structures relevant to lumbar spine anesthesia.
- Detailed description of bones, ligaments, muscles, vasculature, and nerves.
- Techniques and considerations for spinal, epidural, and erector spinae plane blocks.

1.1 Introduction

As Tyrell Gray said in 1909, with a spinal anesthetic, his pediatric patients were comfortable enough to "eat cake throughout the duration of the surgical procedure."[2] The field of anesthesiology has come a long way since 1909, but perhaps what Dr. Gray had observed in the early 20th century has been overshadowed by the power of inhalational anesthetic. The principle that a patient can be fully conscious and not feel any pain during surgery remains true today. Moreover, the choice of regional anesthetic can be even further tailored based on how invasive the surgery will be and what anatomical structures will be disturbed. To choose the appropriate block, an understanding of the three-dimensional, computed tomography, and ultrasound anatomy of the lumbar spine is necessary. Additionally, the risks of each type of block, drugs that can be used, and necessary equipment will be covered in this chapter.

1.2 Lumbar Spine Anatomy

- The anatomy of the lumbar spine can be broken down into the components of bones, ligaments, muscles, vasculature, and nerves (▶ Fig. 1.1).

1.2.1 Bones and Disks

- The bones of the lumbar spine or vertebrae are five individual units that each articulate with the adjacent vertebra.
- Each lumbar vertebra consists of multiple components:
  - A vertebral body.
  - Bilateral pedicles.
  - Bilateral superior articular processes.
  - Bilateral inferior articular processes.
  - Bilateral transverse processes.
  - Bilateral pars interarticularis.
  - Bilateral laminae.
  - Midline spinous process.
- The zygapophyseal joints (facet joints) are composed of the superior articular process of the corresponding vertebra and the inferior articular process of the level above.
- Facet joints in the lumbar spine are sagittally oriented to allow for flexion and extension except at L5–S1 where they tend to have more of a coronal orientation.
- Vertebral bodies of adjacent levels are separated by an intervertebral disk composed of an inner gelatinous nucleus pulposus and bounded by the fibrous annulus fibrosus.

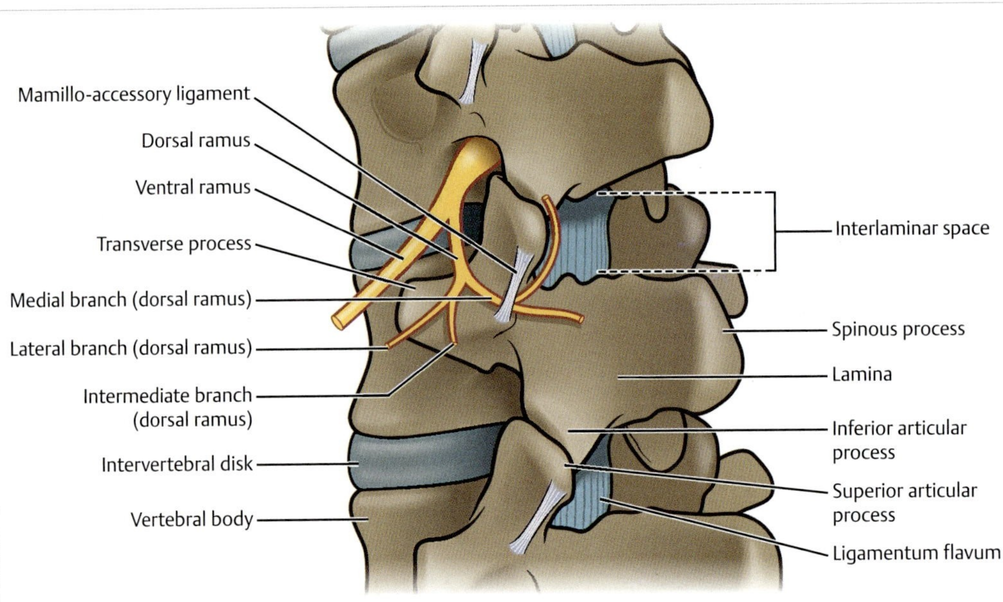

Fig. 1.1 Overview of relevant regional anatomy. (Illustration created by Graeme Chambers at Illumina Medical Illustration Ltd.© Thieme)

1.2.2 Ligaments

- Running along the ventral surface of the vertebral bodies and disks is the robust anterior longitudinal ligament, which resists translation, extension, and rotation.
- Running along the dorsal surface of the vertebral bodies is the posterior longitudinal ligament (PLL), which resists flexion.
- The ligamentum flavum (yellow ligament) is a segmental ligament just dorsal to the epidural space and ventral to the lamina.
  - The ligamentum flavum attaches at the superior aspect of the lamina below, covers the interspinous space, and extends two-thirds of the way up the lamina.
- The interspinous ligament spans between spinous processes of adjacent levels, and the supraspinous ligament runs dorsally to the tips of the spinous processes.
  - Both ligaments resist lumbar flexion.[3]

1.2.3 Nerves

- The thecal sac, which is composed of the dura mater and arachnoid membrane.
  - The arachnoid contains cerebrospinal fluid (CSF).
- The spinal cord terminates in the conus medullaris, which is most often found at the L1 level in adults.
- The cauda equina is the bundle of intrathecal nerve roots that will eventually become the spinal nerves.
- Spinal nerves are mixed sensory and motor nerves that exit the spinal canal via the neural foramen.
  - Each nerve is named for its related vertebra and exits below the pedicle of its corresponding vertebra.
- The neural foramen is bounded by the intervertebral disk anteriorly, facet joint posteriorly, and pedicles of the adjacent vertebrae superiorly and inferiorly.
- After exiting the neural foramen, a spinal nerve forms four branches:
  - The ventral ramus:
    - It supplies sensory and motor innervation to the lower extremities.
  - The dorsal ramus:
    - It supplies motor innervation to the erector spinae muscles and sensation to the skin on the dorsal trunk.
    - From L1 to L4, the dorsal ramus branches from the spinal nerve at a 90-degree angle and traverses the neural foramen. The

dorsal ramus then branches at the superior border of the transverse process into a medial, an intermediate, and a lateral branch.[3]
  - The lateral branch innervates the iliocostalis.
  - The intermediate branch innervates the longissimus.
  - The medial branch innervates the multifidus, the facet joint, and structures medial to the facet joints.
  - After the branch point, the medial branch wraps around the superior articular process and passes through a notch created by the mamillo-accessory ligament and traverses the lamina.[4]
  - The medial branch subsequently divides into the cutaneous, muscular, and articular segments. These branches innervate the facet joint, multifidus muscles, supraspinous ligament, and interspinous ligament.
  - There is discrepancy in the literature about how many facet joints a particular medial branch of the dorsal ramus will innervate, but due to a complex network of communicating branches, it is thought to be between one and three.
  - The L5 dorsal ramus is unique because it has a longer course than the other levels' dorsal rami. It originates at the junction of the superior sacral ala and the S1 superior articular process.[3]
- The communicating branch.
- The meningeal branch (sinuvertebral nerve):
  - It is formed by the joining of a somatic nerve from the ventral ramus and an autonomic nerve from the gray ramus communicans.
  - It innervates the ventral dura, blood vessels, the PLL, and posterior annulus fibrosis.

- Each spinal nerve contributes to sensation in a stereotyped pattern called a dermatome.
- Spinal nerves are organized into myotomes to describe the muscles to which they contribute innervation.
- The dorsal dura has no innervation.
- The anterior and lateral aspects of the annulus fibrosis are innervated by nerves from the ventral rami and sympathetic nerves.[4]

1.2.4 Muscles

- The muscles related to the lumbar spine can be broken down into groups by function.
- The extensor group includes the erector spinae muscles and the multifidus.
  - The erector spinae group is composed of the iliocostalis lumborum and longissimus in the lumbar spine.
  - In the thoracic spine, there is an additional erector spinae muscle referred to as the spinalis.[5]
- Each of the muscles is bounded by a retinacular fascial sheath.
- The ventral portion of the combined fascial sheath has many perforations.
- The erector spinae sheath is tethered to each spinous process and transverse process.[6]
- The psoas muscles lie ventral to the spine and allow for flexion.
  - The psoas major originates from the transverse processes of T12–L4 and becomes the iliopsoas muscle in the thigh after joining with the iliacus muscle.[7]

1.3 Types of Blocks

1.3.1 Spinal

- The most potent form of anesthetic used in awake spine surgery is spinal anesthesia (▶ Fig. 1.2).
- This neuraxial anesthesia involves puncturing the intrathecal space.
- The spinal anesthetic may be placed in the preoperative area or on the operating table.
- Spinal anesthetic is most effective when placed above the level of intervention.
- An anatomical consideration to spinal anesthetics is that the intrathecal space is continuous from the injection site in the lumbar spine up to the thoracic and cervical cord and even the brain.
- The most dreaded complication of spinal anesthesia is complete neuraxial anesthesia with loss of pulmonary function.
- There are a number of drugs available for use as a spinal anesthetic. The most widely used is bupivacaine 0.75%.

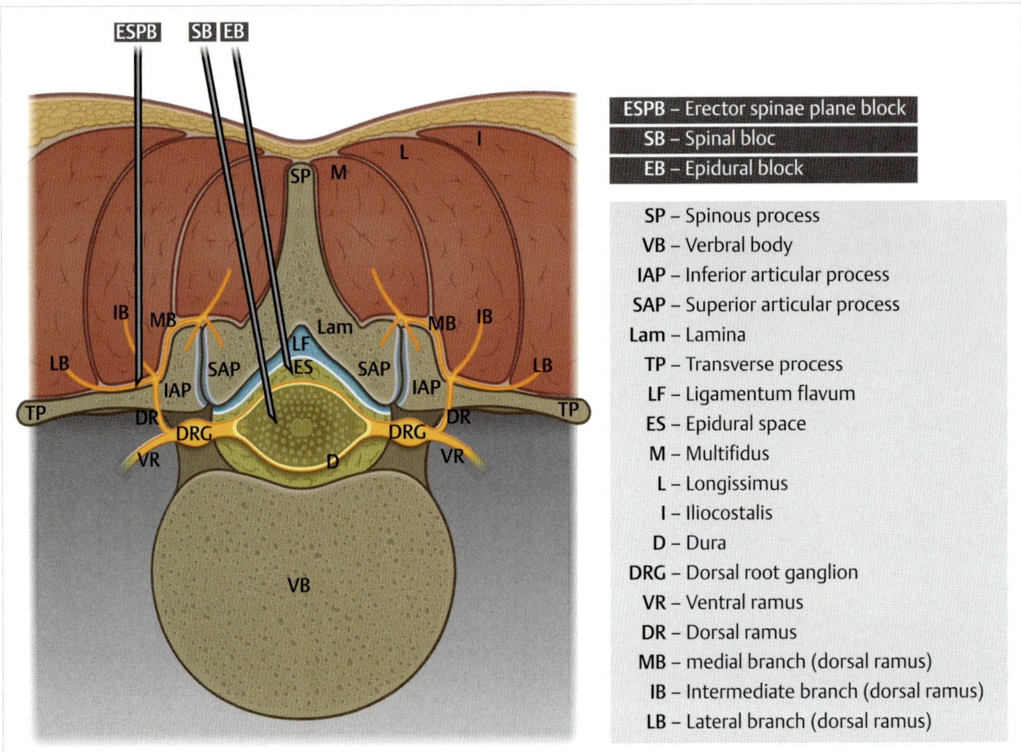

Fig. 1.2 Anatomical sites for regional anesthesia. (Illustration created by Graeme Chambers at Illumina Medical Illustration Ltd.© Thieme)

Expert Tip

After the spinal anesthetic has taken effect, the patient should not feel any pain. If the surgery begins and the patient is moving due to pain, the surgeon should pause the surgery and place a new spinal anesthetic at a higher level. Fluoroscopy can help localize the level more precisely. The technique employed at our institution involves using a combination needle. This needle has a larger Tuohy needle to first enter the epidural space and a smaller gauge telescoping needle to enter the thecal sac. We prefer to use mepivacaine 1.5% due to its shorter duration of action. The surgeon should inform the anesthesiologist that the spinal anesthetic is being re-dosed, especially at a higher level so the anesthesiologist can monitor for hypotension. The primary consideration for dosage is height. At our institution, we primarily use 3 to 4 mL of 1.5% mepivacaine for procedures with an expected duration of about 120 minutes.

- A spinal can be placed by either a midline or a paramedian approach (▶ Fig. 1.3, ▶ Fig. 1.4, ▶ Fig. 1.5).
  - For the midline approach, the needle entry point should be in the midline in the area palpated to be between the tips of two spinous processes.
    - After skin and adipose tissue are passed, the needle will pass into the supraspinous and interspinous ligaments, which will feel like an increase in resistance.
    - The needle will next puncture the ligamentum flavum, which will feel like a pop and sudden loss of resistance. CSF egress should be seen either immediately after this pop or with slightly more advancement.
  - The paramedian approach entry point should be 1 to 2 cm lateral to the midline.
    - The needle is then advanced toward the midline and into the interlaminar space.
    - The spinous processes and lamina may be palpated with the needle tip after insertion if midline localization is challenging.

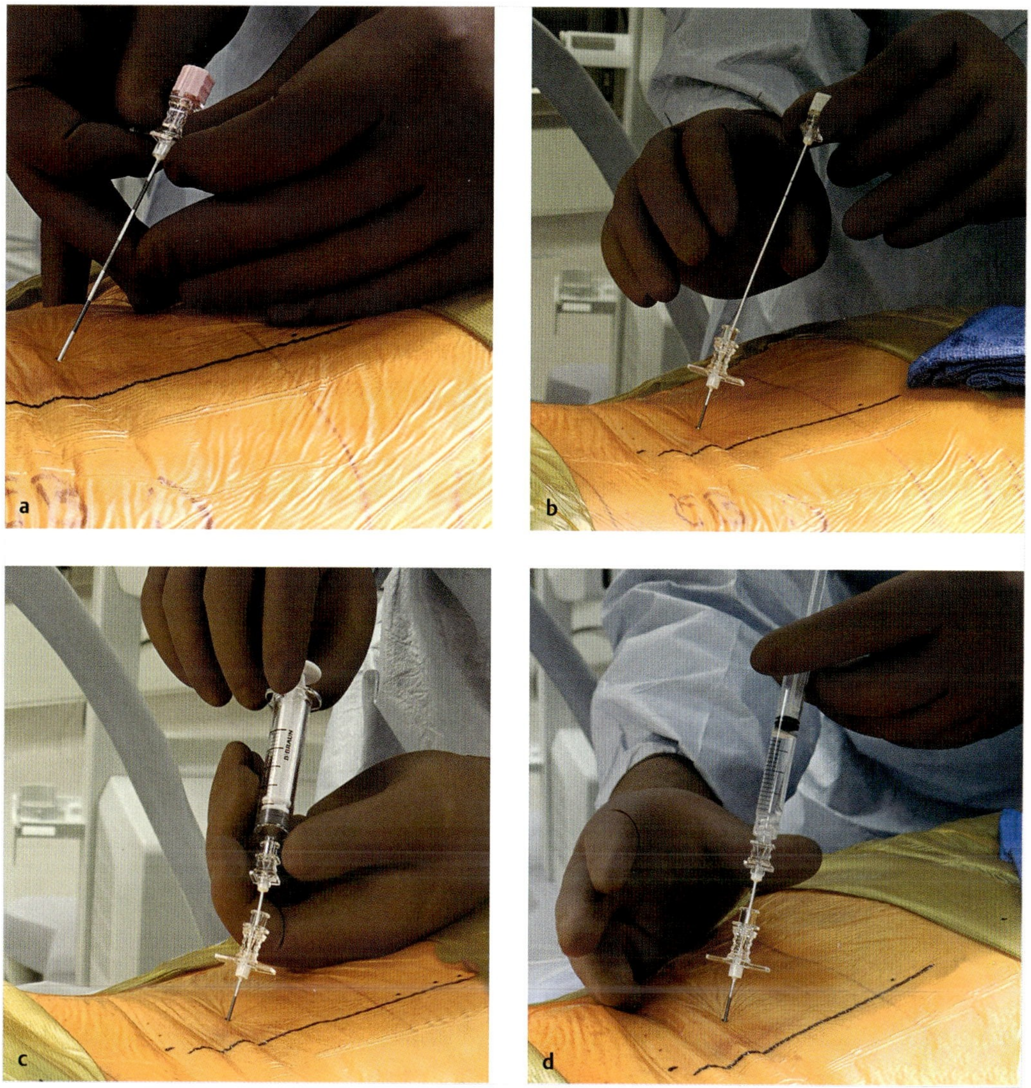

Fig. 1.3 Paramedian approach for spinal anesthesia with ESPOCAN combined spinal and epidural anesthesia set with docking system from B Braun, Bethlehem, PA. **(a)** The ESPOCAN 18-gauge Tuohy epidural needle is introduced one to two segments above the surgical side. **(b)** The PENCAN 27-gauge spinal needle is placed intrathecally via the 18-gauge Tuohy epidural needle. **(c)** A small amount of cerebrospinal fluid (CSF) is aspirated to confirm intrathecal placement with 5-mL plastic Luer slip procedural syringe. **(d)** Three to 4 mL of 1.5% Polocaine methylparaben free (MPF; mepivacaine HCL injection) is injected intrathecally in a single shot.

1.3.2 Epidural

- An epidural is a less potent form of neuraxial anesthesia in which the anesthetic is placed in the epidural space rather than the intrathecal space.
- The contents of the spinal epidural space include lymphatics, blood vessels, fat, and venous plexuses.
- The epidural space is divided into three compartments: anterior (ventral), posterior (dorsal), and lateral (inter-root).

- These compartments normally communicate with one another.
- The dorsal epidural space is the usual site of epidural anesthetic injection.
- There is no communication of the epidural space in the lumbar spine to that around the brain due to the thick attachment of the external layer of the cranial dura to the foramen magnum.

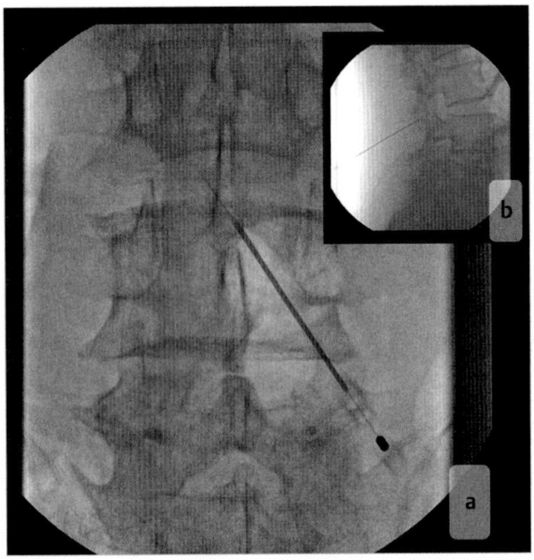

Fig. 1.4 Spinal anesthesia needle trajectory on **(a)** anteroposterior and **(b)** lateral views.

- The dura overlying the spinal cord is derived from the inner layer of the cranial dura and is not firmly tethered to bony structures as nerve roots exit the thecal sac.
  - The dura here is continuous with the epineural and perineural connective tissues.
  - This loose junction is thought to be the location of medication spread from the epidural space to the subarachnoid space.
  - Additionally, there are intercellular pores in these locations that allow passage of small water-soluble particles into the CSF.[8]
  - There is also an endothelial lining of arachnoid villi that creates lipid pores for penetration of lipid-soluble molecules.[9]
- When an epidural injection is performed, the pressure in the epidural space transiently rises above the CSF pressure, forcing flow into the subarachnoid space.[10]
- With normal aging, the arachnoid villi increase in number and depth, further increasing the permeability into the subarachnoid space.
  - Additionally, the neural foramina are occluded by fibrous tissue, preventing any paravertebral escape of fluid injected into the epidural space. This likely provides an explanation for the higher risk of spinal headaches in the younger population compared to the elderly as well as faster onset time and increased dermatomal spread in the elderly.[11]

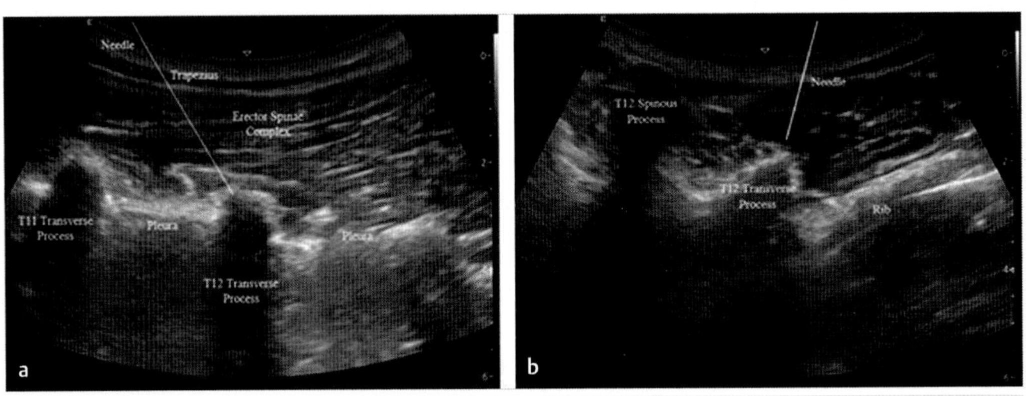

Fig. 1.5 **(a)** Bilateral erector spinae plane (ESP) block technique in the sagittal orientation and **(b)** coronal orientation. The ultrasound probe is placed in the parasagittal orientation over the posterior aspect of the T12 transverse process. The needle with catheter is inserted to the caudal aspect of the T12 transverse process. Correct needle tip position is confirmed by hydrodissection to visualize linear fluid spread under the erector spinae complex.

- *Epidurography:* Our technique for lumbar epidural placement involves the use of epidurography for radiographic confirmation of successful entrance into the epidural space.
  - The epidural anesthetic injection is performed in the operating room with the patient prone on the operating table.
  - Fluoroscopy is used to localize the level just above the most rostral level to be included in surgical intervention.
  - The entry point on the skin is identified using anteroposterior (AP) fluoroscopy as the inferolateral corner of the vertebral body just caudal to the target interlaminar space. This is typically 1 to 2 cm lateral to the midline.
  - An 18-gauge Tuohy needle is advanced to the ligamentum flavum. Once resistance is felt at the ligamentum flavum, a loss of resistance syringe is attached to the Tuohy needle and slowly advanced.
  - When the epidural space is entered, there should no longer be resistance against the syringe plunger.
  - Epidural contrast is then injected through the Tuohy needle and AP fluoroscopy is used to confirm epidural spread.[12]
  - We use Isovue-M 200 (Bracco Diagnostics, Monroe Township, NJ) to ensure safety in the case of accidental intrathecal injection.
  - The epidural anesthetic can be safely injected after radiographic confirmation.
- There are many different combinations of drugs that can be used for epidural anesthetic.
  - We use 400 mg of 2% lidocaine and 100 µg of fentanyl. This combination has a relatively short duration (about 1 hour) and is used for decompression surgeries but may not provide adequate time for an instrumentation surgery.

1.3.3 Erector Spinae Plane Block

- The erector spinae plane block is performed by injecting local anesthetic into the fascial plane between the erector spinae muscles and the tips of the transverse processes.[13]
- Medication spread occurs along the fascial plane as well as laterally and ventrally.
- The injected drug has been found to spread by one dermatomal level per 3.4 mL of injected liquid.[14]
- The mechanism of action for the block is not yet fully understood, but it is proposed that the posterior ramus of the spinal nerve is blocked.[15,16]
- The injection will spread cranially and caudally if it is injected within the erector spinae sheath compartment.
- The injection can also spread ventrally via perforations in the anterior erector spinae sheath to the paravertebral space.
- If the injection is performed anterior to the erector sheath, it will not successfully spread cranially and caudally beyond one interspace due to the intermittent tethering of the sheath to the transverse processes.[16]

1.4 Technique

The injection is generally performed in the preoperative area under ultrasonic guidance (see ▶ Fig. 1.5). A 10-cm-long 21-gauge needle is inserted through the skin 2 to 3 cm lateral to the midline at the target level. The needle tip is docked on the transverse process under ultrasound guidance and then retracted slightly. Location in the correct plane is confirmed by injecting normal saline. Local anesthetic is then injected. The injection is often performed bilaterally[13,17] (see ▶ Fig. 1.6).

1.5 Conclusions

Understanding the intricate anatomy of the lumbar spine is essential for effectively implementing regional anesthesia techniques in awake spine surgery. The lumbar spine is composed of complex structures including bones, ligaments, muscles, and nerves, each playing a crucial role in the overall function and innervation of the spine. Key anatomical features such as the vertebral bodies, intervertebral disks, facet joints, and the cauda equina must be thoroughly understood to select the appropriate anesthetic approach.

The chapter reviewed several types of blocks, including spinal, epidural, and erector spinae plane blocks, each with distinct anatomical and technical considerations. Spinal anesthesia, involving the intrathecal space, provides potent analgesia but requires careful placement to avoid complications such as complete neuraxial blockade. Epidural anesthesia, placed in the epidural space, offers a safer alternative with a lower risk of severe complications, though it requires precise radiographic confirmation to ensure

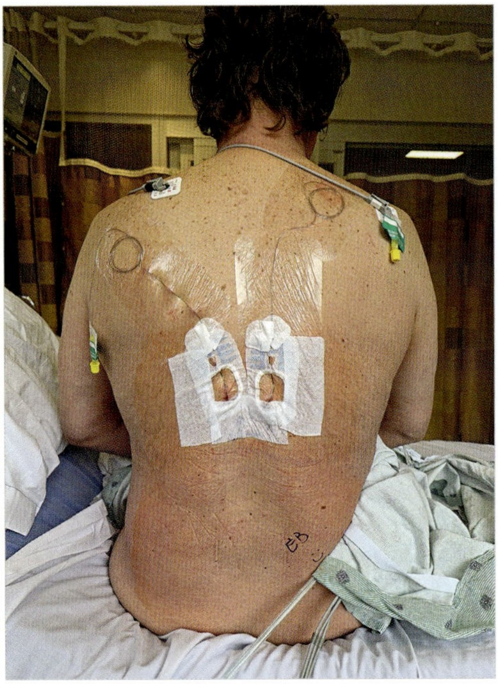

Fig. 1.6 Erector spinae catheters are placed prior to elective revision spine surgery. The erector spinae plane block is performed by injecting local anesthetic into the fascial plane between the erector spinae muscles and the tips of the transverse processes for post op pain control. (Contiplex®Continous Nerve Block Set B. Braun Bethehem, PA).

proper spread of the anesthetic. The erector spinae plane block, a newer technique, involves injecting anesthetic into the fascial plane of the erector spinae muscles, providing effective pain relief by targeting the posterior ramus of the spinal nerve.

By leveraging detailed anatomical knowledge and appropriate imaging techniques, anesthesiologists can tailor their anesthetic approach to the specific surgical procedure and patient needs. This ensures that patients remain comfortable and pain free during awake spine surgeries, minimizing the risk of unintended morbidity and optimizing surgical outcomes.

References

[1] Brown TC. History of pediatric regional anesthesia. Paediatr Anaesth. 2012; 22(1):3–9

[2] Quiroga O, Matozzi F, Beranger M, Nazarian S, Gambarelli J, Salamon G. Normal CT anatomy of the spine. Anatomo-radiological correlations. Neuroradiology. 1982; 24(1):1–6

[3] Kapetanakis S, Gkantsinikoudis N. Anatomy of lumbar facet joint: a comprehensive review. Folia Morphol (Warsz). 2021; 80(4):799–805

[4] Bogduk N. The innervation of the lumbar spine. Spine. 1983; 8(3):286–293

[5] Bogduk N. A reappraisal of the anatomy of the human lumbar erector spinae. J Anat. 1980; 131(Pt 3):525–540

[6] Willard FH, Vleeming A, Schuenke MD, Danneels L, Schleip R. The thoracolumbar fascia: anatomy, function and clinical considerations. J Anat. 2012; 221(6):507–536

[7] Gilchrist RV, Frey ME, Nadler SF. Muscular control of the lumbar spine. Pain Physician. 2003; 6(3):361–368

[8] Shanthaveerappa TR, Bourne GH. The perineural epithelium of sympathetic nerves and ganglia and its relation to the pia arachnoid of the central nervous system and perineural epithelium of the peripheral nervous system. Z Zellforsch Mikrosk Anat. 1964; 61(5):742–753

[9] Mayer SE, Maickel RP, Brodie BB. Disappearance of various drugs from the cerebrospinal fluid. J Pharmacol Exp Ther. 1960; 128(1):41–43

[10] Usubiaga JE, Wikinski JA, Usubiaga LE. Epidural pressure and its relation to spread of anesthetic solutions in epidural space. Anesth Analg. 1967; 46(4):440–446

[11] Shantha TR, Evans JA. The relationship of epidural anesthesia to neural membranes and arachnoid villi. Anesthesiology. 1972; 37(5):543–557

[12] Johnson BA, Schellhas KP, Pollei SR. Epidurography and therapeutic epidural injections: technical considerations and experience with 5334 cases. AJNR Am J Neuroradiol. 1999; 20(4):697–705

[13] Forero M, Adhikary SD, Lopez H, Tsui C, Chin KJ. The erector spinae plane block: a novel analgesic technique in thoracic neuropathic pain. Reg Anesth Pain Med. 2016; 41(5):621–627

[14] De Cassai A, Andreatta G, Bonvicini D, Boscolo A, Munari M, Navalesi P. Injectate spread in ESP block: a review of anatomical investigations. J Clin Anesth. 2020; 61:109669

[15] Elsharkawy H, Pawa A, Mariano ER. Interfascial plane blocks: back to basics. Reg Anesth Pain Med. 2018; 43(4): 341–346

[16] Hamilton DL, Manickam BP. Is the erector spinae plane (ESP) block a sheath block? Anaesthesia. 2017; 72(7):915–916

[17] Braxton EE, Brena KR, Spears H, Conrad E, Heinze JD. Ultrasound-guided bilateral erector spinae plane nerve blocks: a novel application for the management of acute postoperative pain in awake spine surgery. Illustrative case. J Neurosurg Case Lessons. 2022; 3(18):CASE21633

2 Basics of Ultrasound

Bhavuk Garg, Punit Khanna, and Bhavana Kayarat

Abstract

Ultrasound imaging, a cornerstone of diagnostic and interventional medicine, is based on the propagation of high-frequency sound waves (2–15 MHz) through biological tissues. At its core, ultrasound physics integrates principles of wave mechanics and acoustics to create real-time anatomical and functional images. Piezoelectric transducers generate and detect these sound waves, exploiting differences in acoustic impedance at tissue interfaces to produce echoes that form the basis of image construction. Key factors influencing image quality include resolution, penetration, and artifact mitigation; each is dependent on wave frequency and tissue properties. Higher frequencies enhance spatial resolution but compromise penetration due to increased attenuation, while lower frequencies allow deeper tissue visualization at the cost of detail. Doppler ultrasound leverages frequency shifts to quantify blood flow dynamics, while emerging techniques like shear wave elastography and harmonic imaging provide detailed tissue characterization and enhanced image clarity through nonlinear wave interactions. Clinicians must master these foundational concepts to optimize imaging protocols, interpret subtle findings, and address artifacts effectively. A good understanding of ultrasound physics not only enhances diagnostic precision but also enables the integration of cutting-edge technologies, reinforcing the pivotal role of ultrasonography in modern medicine.

Keywords: piezoelectric crystals, transducer, Doppler

Key Points

- Generation of ultrasound waves:
  - Ultrasound is generated using piezoelectric crystals within a transducer, which converts electrical energy into mechanical vibrations, producing sound waves at frequencies between 2 and 15 MHz.
- Propagation of sound waves:
  - Ultrasound waves travel through tissues as longitudinal waves, with velocity determined by the medium's density and stiffness (~1,540 m/s in soft tissue). Key interactions include reflection, refraction, scattering, and absorption.
- Image formation:
  - Image creation relies on the reflection of sound waves at interfaces with different acoustic impedances. Echoes are detected by the transducer and processed to create grayscale or color images based on amplitude, timing, and frequency shifts.
- Resolution and frequency:
  - Higher frequencies provide better axial and lateral resolution but reduce penetration due to greater attenuation. Lower frequencies enable deeper imaging but compromise detail.
- Doppler and advanced techniques:
  - Doppler ultrasound analyses frequency shifts to assess blood flow velocity and direction. Advanced modalities like harmonic imaging and elastography enhance tissue characterization and diagnostic accuracy by utilizing nonlinear acoustic phenomena.

2.1 Sound Wave: General Physical Principles

- Sound travels through a medium in the form of a propagating wave, typically represented graphically as a sine wave (▶ Fig. 2.1). Typically, ultrasound used in medical practice employs sound waves at frequencies ranging from 1 to 20 MHz.
- **Amplitude (A)** refers to the maximal compression of particles above the baseline and is quantified in decibels (dB). Variations in amplitude are responsible for generating the grayscale, two-dimensional (2D) echocardiographic images.
- **Intensity (I)** refers to the level of sound energy within a specific area of tissue. Intensity (W/cm^2) = Power (W)/beam area (cm^2). Intensity is proportional to the amplitude of the ultrasound wave squared. A higher ultrasound

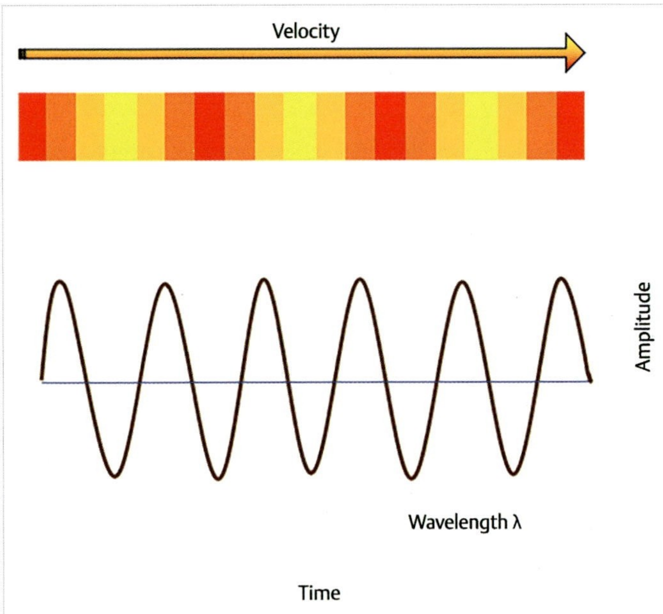

Fig. 2.1 Sound wave. Vibrations from the transducer causes cycles of compression and rarefaction in the adjacent tissue. An ultrasound wave is characterized by amplitude, frequency, wavelength, and propagation velocity. (Based on Perino AC, Reeves ST. A Practical Approach to Transesophageal Echocardiography. 3rd ed. Philadelphia, PA: Lippincott Williams & Wilkins; 2014.)

wave amplitude will cause greater intensity and thus a greater chance of tissue injury.

- The distance the wave travels through one cycle is called **wavelength (λ)**. It is the distance between one peak of the wave to the next peak. The number of waves that pass in a given unit time is referred to as the frequency of the wave (f). The product of wavelength (λ) and frequency (f) gives us the propagation velocity of the wave. Since the propagation velocity of sound waves in human cardiac tissues is a constant (i.e., 1,540 m/s), we can say that the wavelength is related inversely to the frequency.

2.2 Interaction of Ultrasound Waves with Tissues

- **Acoustic impedance** refers to the resistance a medium offers to the propagation of sound. It is the product of the velocity of the sound and the density of the medium it passes through. When sound traverses a homogeneous medium, it follows a linear path. However, when the sound wave encounters an interface, that is, when it passes between two tissues with two different densities (acoustic impedances), a part of the sound beam gets reflected back to the source. The extent to which this reflection occurs is determined by the disparity in their acoustic impedances. A greater difference in acoustic impedance between the two tissues results in a higher proportion of the ultrasound wave being reflected. The magnitude of the reflected beam received by the transducer is contingent upon the angle between the ultrasound beam and the tissue interface. Optimal reflection, or the maximum return of the reflected ultrasound, is achieved when the angle of incidence is 90 degrees (perpendicular) to the interface.
- **Scattering** refers to the phenomenon where ultrasound waves encounter irregularly shaped or small structures (e.g., red blood cells) and this results in the reflection of waves in multiple directions. These scattered reflections are considerably weaker compared to specular reflections (► Fig. 2.2).
- **Attenuation** refers to the reduction in the strength of the ultrasound wave as it traverses through various tissues. This decrease in signal strength occurs primarily due to the absorption of ultrasound energy, which is converted to heat. Attenuation is influenced by both frequency and wavelength. Additionally, attenuation is also affected by acoustic impedance. Air exhibits very high acoustic impedance. This explains the attenuation of signal we observe when imaging through lung tissue, especially appreciated in cases of emphysema. Conversely, the presence of fluid in the pleural space enhances ultrasound imaging.

2.3 Generation of Ultrasound Beam

2.3.1 Piezoelectric Effect

- Ultrasound is produced through the piezoelectric effect. When an electric charge is applied to a piezoelectric crystal, the dipoles within the crystal realign with the electric field, resulting in distortion and vibration of the crystal. These vibrations generate ultrasonic waves that propagate into the body.
- The ultrasound transducer also functions as a receiver; the reflected ultrasonic waves cause slight movements in the crystal's dipoles, inducing an electric field. This electric field is detected by electrodes, subsequently amplified, and processed for display by the ultrasound machine.

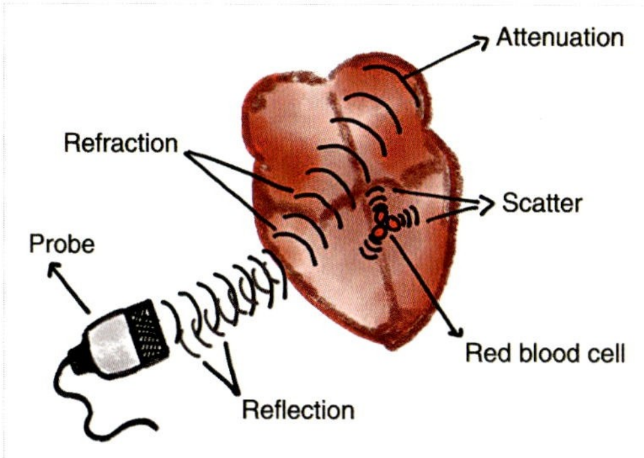

Fig. 2.2 Interaction of ultrasound waves and tissues. (Based on Perino AC, Reeves ST. A Practical Approach to Transesophageal Echocardiography. 3rd ed. Philadelphia, PA: Lippincott Williams & Wilkins; 2014.)

2.3.2 Transducers

The structure of a transducer includes the following (▶ Fig. 2.3): acoustic insulation, backing layer, piezoelectric crystals, matching layer, and acoustic lens.

- The **acoustic insulation** in the transducer ensures that no other sound waves interfere or affect the transducer. The **backing layer** suppresses vibrations of the crystals. By doing so, it allows sound waves to be sent in shorter pulses. This improves the resolution of the image. The **matching layer** reduces the difference in acoustic impedance between the tissue under interest and the crystals. This minimizes the unwanted reflection of the sound

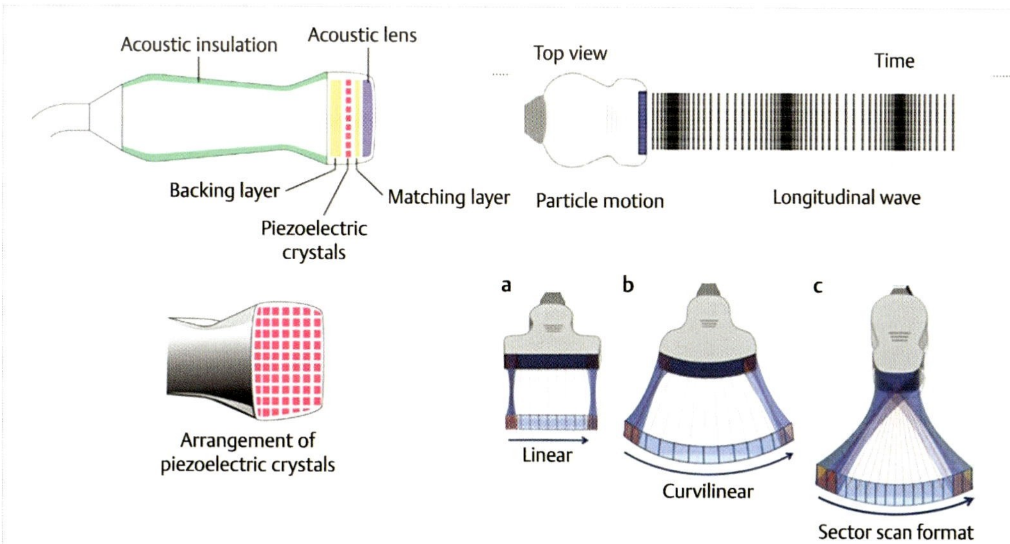

Fig. 2.3 The linear-array transducer activates a subgroup of transducer elements to produce an ultrasound beam directed perpendicular to the array. (a) A rectangular field of view is produced. (b) The convex arrangement in the curvilinear probe produces a trapezoidal field of view. (c) A phased-array transducer produces a beam from the near-simultaneous excitation of all array elements. The beam is electronically steered and a sector scan format is produced.

waves and ensures sound waves penetrate the tissues.

- The simplest ultrasound transducer has a single **piezoelectric crystal** and is employed in M-mode recordings. Creating a 2D image requires mechanical or electronic systems to move the ultrasound beam across the desired plane. Typically, the transducer is composed of multiple crystals (or elements) arranged in a linear array. The sound waves from each crystal combine to form a unified wave front that can be more effectively focused and directed than a single crystal. Additionally, by adjusting the timing of the electrical activation of each crystal in the array, known as a phased array, the beam can be steered without moving the transducer itself. The advantages of an electronic system over a mechanical one include the absence of moving parts and the ability to easily manipulate the ultrasound beam in terms of steering, focusing, and narrowing.
- **Resolution:** The ability of an imaging system to discern two points in space is referred to as resolution. Frequency and wavelength are mathematically related to the velocity of the ultrasound beam within the tissue (~1,540,000 mm/s for human tissue) as follows:
  - Velocity of blood = Wavelength (mm) × frequency (Hz).
  - Wavelength (mm) = 1,540,000 mm/s/ frequency (Hz).
  - Wavelength (mm) = 1.54/frequency (MHz).
- The resolution of a recording, that is, the ability to distinguish two objects that are spatially close together, varies directly with the frequency and inversely with the wavelength. High-frequency, short-wavelength ultrasound can differentiate between objects less than 1 mm apart.
- **Axial resolution:**
  - Axial resolution refers to the ability to distinguish between two structures aligned with the direction of the ultrasound beam (▶ Fig. 2.4).
  - It is influenced by the transducer frequency, transducer bandwidth, and the duration/ length of the ultrasound pulse.
- **Lateral resolution**:
  - Lateral resolution is the minimum distance at which two side-by-side structures can be separated and still produce distinct echoes (▶ Fig. 2.4).

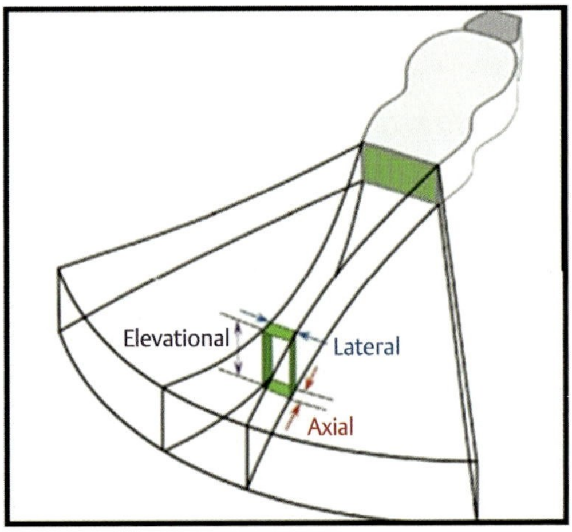

Fig. 2.4 Axial and lateral resolution.

  - It refers to the ability to distinguish closely spaced objects perpendicular to the direction of the ultrasound beam, within the imaging plane.
  - It is approximately equal to the beam diameter.
  - As the beam diameter varies with depth, lateral resolution also varies with depth. Lateral resolution is optimal at the focus, where the beam is narrowest.
- **Temporal resolution**:
  - Temporal resolution pertains to time and is the ability to accurately locate moving structures at a specific moment.
  - Higher frame rates (more images per unit of time) improve temporal resolution.
  - Temporal resolution (particularly in color Doppler) varies with the number of pulses per scan line, line density, imaging depth, and sector size.

Types of Transducers

Transducers are of four types:

- Linear.
- Curvilinear.
- Phased array.
- Intracavitary.

The elements in linear-array transducer fire in sequence to produce a series of parallel beams, thereby generating a rectangular image format, whereas phased-array transducer elements fire sequentially in different directions, producing diverging beams that generate a pie-shaped image format.

Linear transducers: Linear-array transducers are ideal for evaluating superficial structures, including eyes, blood vessels, muscles, nerves, and joints, and for performing ultrasound-guided procedures. Linear transducers generate high-frequency (5–10 MHz) and shorter-wavelength sound waves giving good axial and lateral resolution.

Curvilinear transducers: Curvilinear transducers are named so owing to their curvilinear or convex arrangement of crystals. Curvilinear transducers utilize lower frequencies (2–5 MHz) with longer wavelengths and penetrate deep structures with relatively less attenuation,. They have a greater slice thickness than linear transducers. The ultrasound beam is broad with a wide field of view, but resolution is not as good as linear transducers.

Phased-array transducers consist of multiple ultrasound crystals arranged to allow electronic steering without moving parts. These transducers are the most commonly used type for clinical echocardiography. By precisely timing the activation of individual transducer elements, the ultrasound beam can be swept in an arc across a designated area of interest. Activating the transducer elements in various sequences enables easy narrowing, steering, and focusing of the ultrasound beam in the phased-array system. This electronic beam steering over an arced sector allows for a smaller transducer interface, as used in transthoracic and transesophageal echocardiography (▶ Fig. 2.3).

Higher-frequency (and lower-wavelength) transducers provide enhanced spatial resolution for imaging. However, due to attenuation, the depth of tissue penetration is directly related to wavelength and inversely related to transducer frequency. Consequently, higher-frequency transducers offer reduced tissue penetration. The balance between tissue resolution and penetration influences the choice of transducer frequency for clinical imaging.

2.4 Ultrasound Imaging Modalities

- Ultrasound imaging modalities include one-dimensional (A-mode, B-mode, and M-mode) and 2D imaging (▶ Fig. 2.5).

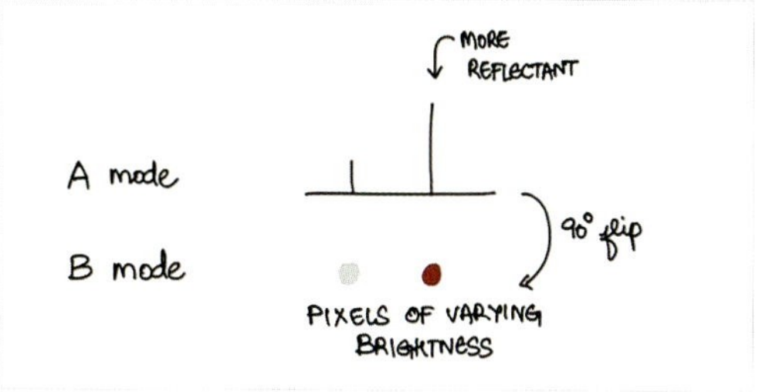

Fig. 2.5 A-mode (amplitude) display in which the intensity of the reflected ultrasound wave is displayed as a vertical deflection along the baseline. Reflected ultrasound signals are displayed as spots of varying brightness in B (brightness) mode proportional to the intensity of the reflected signal.

- **Amplitude mode (A-mode):** In A-mode, the amplitudes of returning signals are displayed as a series of horizontal spikes along the vertical axis of the display. These horizontal spikes correspond to the distance of the reflecting tissue and the strength of the returning echoes.
- **Brightness mode (B-mode):** In B-mode, the amplitudes of returning echoes are displayed as pixels of varying brightness along the vertical axis. The brightness of each pixel correlates with the strength of the returning signal, providing a visual representation of tissue structures.
- **Motion mode (M-mode):** M-mode enhances B-mode imaging, that is, it adds temporal information to B-mode through the sequential display of collected B-mode images. M-mode echocardiography provides a one-dimensional representation of structures and updates B-mode images at a significantly high frequency. This allows for dynamic, real-time imaging. The transducer element captures the reflected energy of the previous pulse before emitting the next one. The frame rate, which is calculated as the reciprocal of the round-trip travel time of the ultrasound pulse, is exceptionally high in M-mode imaging (exceeding 2,000 frames per second). This results in superior visualization of dynamic motion compared to other imaging modalities. However, M-mode is limited to displaying only axial motion.

2.4.1 Doppler Effect

A moving target backscatters an ultrasound beam to the transducer. The frequency observed when the target is moving toward the transducer will be higher and the frequency observed when the target is moving away from the transducer will be lower than the original transmitter frequency. This difference in frequency between the transmitted frequency (*F*[*t*]) and received frequency (*F*[*r*]) is the Doppler shift:

$$\text{Doppler shift } (F[d]) = F[r] - F[t].$$

When ultrasound waves are transmitted into the bloodstream, it is scattered by red blood cells. A portion of this scattered signal reflected back to the transducer. The strength of these returning echoes is proportional to the number of red blood cells reflecting the ultrasound. An increased hematocrit results in more reflecting interfaces and a stronger signal. However, if the hematocrit exceeds 30%, the reflected signal strength may decrease due to destructive interference. Modern echocardiographic systems are now designed to detect Doppler signals across a wide range of hematocrit levels. If red blood cells are stationary, the reflected signal frequency matches the transmitted frequency, resulting in no Doppler shift and a display similar to that of 2D echocardiography (▶ Fig. 2.6).

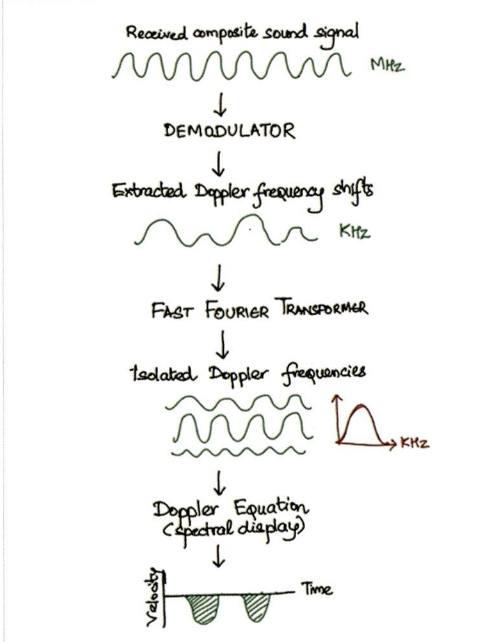

Fig. 2.6 Spectral Doppler display. Fourier analysis is done using an algorithm (FFT) that uses a mathematical tool to extract frequency information from signals. The display thereby generated is called spectral analysis.

Expert Tip

- *Ultrasound refers to any sound waves with frequencies greater than 20 kHz, generated using piezoelectric effect within a transducer.*
- *In clinical scanning, even a thin layer of air in between the transducer and skin could hinder penetration of ultrasound beam into the tissue. Therefore, usage of a coupling medium is of utmost importance.*
- *The choice of transducer depends on the required depth, resolution, and field of view. Therefore, a basic understanding of the physical principles of ultrasound is essential.*
- *Each ultrasound mode serves a specific diagnostic function, from anatomical visualization (B-mode) to blood flow assessment (Doppler) and advanced tissue characterization (elastography, contrast-enhanced ultrasound). Understanding these modes enhances the accuracy and utility of ultrasonography in clinical practice.*

2.5 Conclusion

Ultrasound remains an indispensable imaging modality in modern radiology, offering real-time, nonionizing, and cost-effective evaluation of a wide range of pathologies. Its applications extend across multiple organ systems, including abdominal, vascular, musculoskeletal, obstetric, and interventional imaging. A thorough understanding of ultrasound physics—encompassing principles of wave propagation, acoustic impedance, attenuation, and Doppler effect—is fundamental to optimizing image acquisition and interpretation.

Proficiency in selecting the appropriate transducer, recognizing normal and pathological echogenic patterns, and differentiating true findings from artifacts is essential for accurate diagnosis. Doppler imaging further enhances the assessment of hemodynamics, playing a crucial role in vascular and cardiac evaluations. Despite its operator dependency, ultrasound's dynamic capabilities make it invaluable in both diagnostic and interventional settings. With ongoing advancements such as elastography and contrast-enhanced ultrasound, the diagnostic scope of sonography continues to expand. Mastery of ultrasound principles, combined with continuous skill development, remains paramount to maximize its clinical utility and improve patient outcomes.

Suggested Readings

Khanna P. Ultrasound in Critical Care. New Delhi: Jaypee Brothers Medical Publishers (P) Ltd.; 2018

Soni NJ, Arntfield R, Korry P. Point of Care Ultrasound. New York: Elsevier; 2019

Perino AC, Reeves ST. A Practical Approach to Transesophageal Echocardiography. 3rd ed. Philadelphia, PA: Lippincott Williams & Wilkins; 2014

Tole NM. Basic Principles of Ultrasonic Imaging. Geneva: World Health Organization; 2005

3 Overview of Regional Anesthesia

Stephen Davies, Emily Zoe Barney Hall, Jeffrey C. Gadsden, and W. Michael Bullock

Abstract
Spine surgery is complex. From surgical procedures to analgesia to patient factors, spine surgery warrants special consideration to improve the patient experience and outcomes. Patient-centered protocols offer a better path to success by improving surgical and anesthetic techniques, developing analgesic modalities, and hastening functional outcomes. Awake spine surgery touts many patient-centered benefits and is a novel approach to these procedures. Given the unique needs of both patient and surgeon in this setting, regional anesthesia is the cornerstone of intraoperative success and postoperative pain management. A wide array of regional anesthesia techniques addresses the need for intraoperative analgesia while concurrently forming a strong foundation for a multimodal approach to postoperative pain control.

Keywords: regional anesthesia, postoperative pain control, spinal anesthesia, epidural, paravertebral blocks, erector spinae plane blocks, quadratus lumborum blocks, classical transversus abdominis plane blocks

Key Points

- Spine surgery is reported to be among the most painful surgical procedures and poses significant challenges for pain management. Adverse outcomes associated with poorly controlled pain are well documented, as are the positive effects of multimodal pain control.[1,2]
- Awake approaches to spine surgery demonstrate a clear potential for improved patient outcomes and rely largely on regional anesthesia techniques.
- The most relevant regional anesthesia techniques for spine surgery include spinal anesthesia, epidural anesthesia, paravertebral blocks, erector spinae plane blocks, quadratus lumborum blocks, and anterior transversus abdominis plane blocks.
- Regional anesthesia techniques are imperative for both intraoperative analgesia and postoperative pain management, expanding the population who are eligible to undergo spine procedures and demonstrating a variety of improved outcomes.

3.1 Introduction

When examining the current literature, it becomes highly evident that spine surgery is painful. Severe and diffuse pain has been reported in the postoperative time frame, with median pain scores (using the 0–10 numerical rating scale [NRS]) on the first postoperative day ranging from 5 (spinal decompression) to 7 (spinal fusion).[3,4] Additionally, the negative consequences of poorly controlled postoperative pain are significant, ranging from delayed mobilization or pulmonary and thromboembolic events to prolonged hospital stays and the development of chronic pain syndromes.[5] Conversely, patients who experience effective postoperative pain management report increased satisfaction, as well as earlier mobilization and prevention of pulmonary and thromboembolic complications, leading to reduced postoperative mortality and morbidity.[6] Based on these findings, steps must be taken to ensure the best possible postoperative analgesia for spine surgery patients by utilizing a multimodal approach.

Expert Tip

Enhanced recovery after surgery (ERAS) protocols are multidisciplinary approaches that have been developed for almost every type of surgery to improve patient outcomes. They incorporate early function, diet and fluid balance, and analgesia. If protocols need to be developed, consult primary stakeholders (surgery, anesthesia, nursing, physical therapy, etc.).

Regional anesthesia (RA) proves particularly useful among the array of options for multimodal analgesia, specifically in the growing field of awake spine surgery. These techniques offer a unique combination of intraoperative anesthesia and analgesia and prolonged postoperative pain control. Awake techniques for spine surgery have been used for various spine procedures, including, but not limited to, laminectomy, diskectomy, anterior cervical diskectomy and fusion, lumbar fusion, and dorsal column stimulator placement.[7] This chapter will introduce various RA techniques that are beneficial and relevant to both "asleep" and "awake" spine procedures.

Expert Tip

"Awake" spine surgery can be a misnomer, as the anesthesia given can range from no anesthesia to minimal sedation to deeper levels of sedation. Essentially, these procedures are performed without general anesthesia. The decision to perform an "awake" spine case is made jointly by the surgeon and anesthesiologist based on patient factors.

3.2 Blocks for Spine Surgery

This chapter provides an overview of many of the available and beneficial methods to implement RA in spine surgery.

3.2.1 Spinal

- The goal of spinal anesthesia is the deposition of local anesthetic, with or without opioid in the intrathecal space, resulting in surgical anesthesia up to approximately the T6 level.
- This technique is the cornerstone of anesthesia and analgesia required for awake spine surgery, as it ensures that the patient is insensate and comfortable throughout the operation. Neuraxial placement technique and duration are primarily up to the provider's comfort and local anesthetic choice.[8]
- The choice of local anesthetic for spinal in awake spine surgery is multifactorial. It is mainly based on the spinal level(s) and duration of surgery.

Expert Tip

Spinals are best performed in the operating room. Immediately after spinal placement, patients can help position themselves on the operating room (OR) table. Any additional RA techniques for post-op analgesia can be done before the spinal is placed or after the patient is positioned on the OR table.

Expert Tip

If the spinal anesthesia is wearing off (i.e., the patient begins to feel the operative area during surgery), the surgeon can re-dose using a spinal needle as the dura is in their sterile field.

3.2.2 Epidural

- Epidural administration of local anesthetic and/or opiates provides profound and durable analgesia, the level of which is dictated by the site of placement and volume of injectate.
- While epidural analgesia has demonstrated clear benefit in multiple types of abdominal surgeries, there have been inconsistent data regarding its benefit in posterior spinal fusions.[9]
- Patients cannot be discharged with an epidural catheter, so other RA techniques have been developed to provide adequate analgesia while maintaining functionality (see below).

Expert Tip

Epidural analgesia is mainly performed for asleep spine surgery and more significant spine cases. If an epidural is warranted, it is generally best performed by the surgeon at the conclusion of surgery if an epidural space is present or at the next best location with an existing epidural space.

3.2.3 Paravertebral Blocks

- Currently widely employed in chest and abdominal surgery, paravertebral blocks (PVBs) provide reliable somatic and visceral coverage. They can anesthetize both the ventral and dorsal rami of the spinal nerve as it exits the intervertebral foramen and the sympathetic ganglia at that level of the spine (► Fig. 3.1).
- These can be performed as a single shot block, or a catheter can be placed.
- Data regarding PVB usage in spine surgery are sparse and inconclusive. Small prospective trials showed initial benefits, albeit brief, and more data are needed to establish their role in analgesia for spine surgery.[10]

3.2.4 Erector Spinae Plane Block

- Previously used for abdominal, thoracic, and breast procedures, the erector spinae plane (ESP) block aims to deliver local anesthetic between the transverse process and erector spinae muscles (see Chapter 4 for further discussion). This targets the dorsal rami of the corresponding spinal nerves as they exit at this level.
- These can be performed as a single shot block, or a catheter can be placed.
- The use of the ESP block in spine surgery is well demonstrated in the literature to decrease opioid consumption, increase patient satisfaction, decrease patient-reported pain, decrease length of stay, and decrease the rate of postoperative complications.[11]

3.2.5 Quadratus Lumborum Block

- Originally described as a variation of the transversus abdominis plane (TAP) block, the quadratus lumborum (QL) block, in every variation, aims to deposit local anesthesia in a manner that allows spread around the QL muscle and into the thoracolumbar fascia (see Chapter 9 for further discussion). At this point, both anterior divisions of spinal nerves and sympathetic ganglia within the thoracolumbar fascia are anesthetized, providing somatic and visceral analgesia.
- This block typically provides analgesia in the T7–L1 dermatomes, with additional spread into the thoracolumbar fascia and possibly paravertebral space. This spread allows for the blockade of sympathetic fibers as well as visceral analgesia, a notable and unique aspect of this truncal block.[12]
- These can be performed as a single shot block, or a catheter can be placed.

3.2.6 Classical Transversus Abdominis Plane Block

- Currently used in ERAS protocols for many different types of abdominal and gynecologic surgeries, the TAP block has proven safe and efficacious in reducing pain and opiate consumption postoperatively.
- Local anesthetic deposited in the TAP plane reliably anesthetizes anterior divisions of spinal nerves T6–L1, providing analgesia to the anterior abdominal wall inferior to the umbilicus.[13]
- These can be performed as a single shot block, or a catheter can be placed.

Expert Tip

Ultrasound guidance is instrumental in ensuring RA success and enhancing safety when performing PVB, ESP, QL, and TAP blocks. It can also assist the provider in identifying important landmarks when performing spinal and epidural techniques. It is difficult to perform neuraxial techniques under real-time guidance and should only be attempted by providers adept at both neuraxial and ultrasound techniques.

3.3 Benefits of Regional Anesthesia for Awake Spine Surgery

- The aforementioned truncal blocks have already been implemented in spine surgeries performed under general anesthesia (GA). For example, studies examining the outcomes of the addition of ESP blocks in "asleep" spine surgeries tout decreased opioid use, prolonged time to the first rescue analgesic, reduced number of patients who required rescue analgesia, lowered incidence of postoperative nausea and vomiting (PONV), and increased patient satisfaction.[14,15,16]

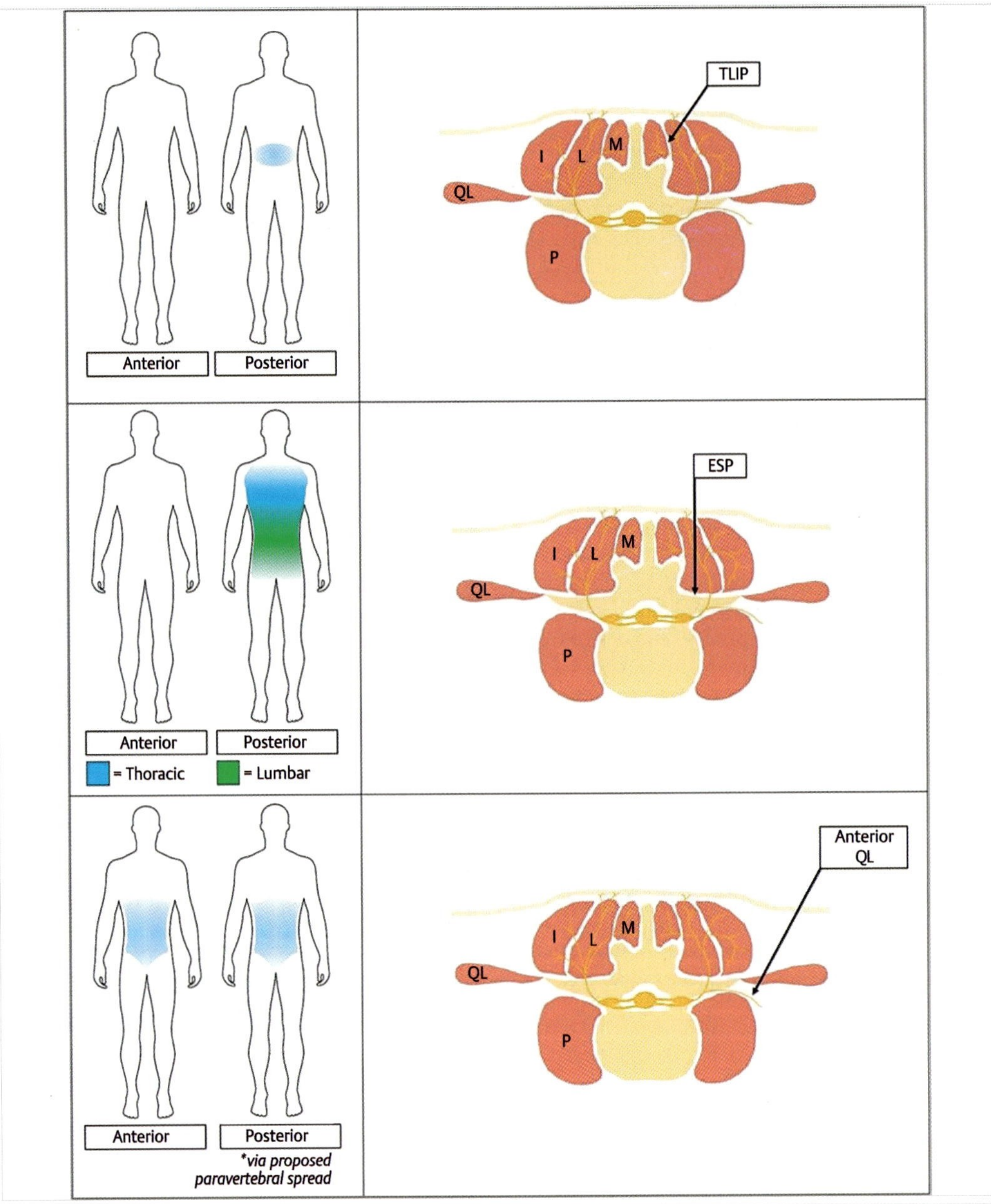

Fig. 3.1 Schematic showing the anatomy of the injection site and area of coverage associated with TLIP, erector spinae plane (ESP), and quadratus lumborum (QL) blocks. A TLIP block placed between the multifidus and longissimus will anesthetize the area two to three levels above and below the injection site. In ESP blocks, injected local anesthetic spreads between the transverse process and erector spinae. Both thoracic and lumbar ESP blocks are used, producing anesthesia of the dorsal rami. Local anesthetic is deposited along the QL in QL blocks, anesthetizing the ventral rami for anterior coverage, while proposed paravertebral anesthetic spread allows for posterior coverage. ESP, erector spinae plane; QL, quaratus lumborum; TLIP, thoracolumbar interfascial plane. (Reproduced from Salven DS, Sykes DAW, Erickson MM, et al. Regional anesthesia in spine surgery: a narrative review. J Spine Pract 2023;2:40–50. Open access article distributed under the terms of the Creative Commons Attribution License (CC BY 4.0).)

- There are significantly fewer studies examining the use and outcomes of RA for awake spine surgery, but early findings suggest similar benefits and improvement in patient outcomes. That said, current evidence provides a promising outlook on these techniques:
  - By meta-analysis, spine surgeries utilizing a spinal anesthetic have been associated with a reduced incidence of PONV, shorter length of hospital stay, and lower intraoperative blood loss.[8,17] The addition of the ESP to a spinal anesthetic revealed a further reduction in opioid use.[18]
  - Compared to a general anesthetic approach, cases that utilized a spinal anesthetic demonstrated decreased rates of PONV, decreased total operative time, improved positioning, increased efficiency, decreased OR cost, decreased blood loss, and decreased length of time in postanesthesia care unit.[19]
  - RA has been associated with less need for intravenous vasoactive agents given a decrease in intraoperative cardiopulmonary lability.[20]
- Additionally, RA provides an alternative anesthetic option for those patients who would be considered at high risk of an adverse event secondary to their comorbidities should they undergo a general anesthetic.[21]
  - One of the ultimate achievements of employing a RA technique for awake spine surgery is sparing the patient exposure to GA.
  - As a blossoming field of research, current data indicate that there are fewer adverse effects to a regional anesthetic compared to a general anesthetic, especially as it relates to the aged brain; in these patients, GA can be a risk of long-lasting cognitive functional impairments.[22]
  - Investigations into the role of GA as a causal mechanism involved in perioperative cognitive disorders implicate alterations to tau protein, inflammation, calcium dysregulation, and mitochondrial dysfunction.[23]
  - Further research continues to examine whether reduced *depth* of anesthesia using spinal anesthesia reduces the incidence of delirium.[24]

3.4 Conclusion

- Many RA techniques are relevant and beneficial for intraoperative and postoperative analgesia in patients undergoing awake spine surgery.
- Each technique has nuanced differences that require thoughtful preparation and discussion between anesthesia and surgical colleagues to develop an appropriate and patient-specific plan.
- While data regarding the improved outcomes for awake spine surgery when utilizing RA techniques are still limited, early signals indicate an array of benefits, including an increased cohort of surgical candidates, reduced length of hospital stay, reduced opioid use, earlier ambulation, reduced PONV, and decreased intraoperative blood loss.

References

[1] Bajwa SJ, Haldar R. Pain management following spinal surgeries: an appraisal of the available options. J Craniovertebr Junction Spine. 2015; 6(3):105–110

[2] Yoo JS, Ahn J, Buvanendran A, Singh K. Multimodal analgesia in pain management after spine surgery. J Spine Surg. 2019; 5 Suppl 2:S154–S159

[3] Gerbershagen HJ, Aduckathil S, van Wijck AJ, Peelen LM, Kalkman CJ, Meissner W. Pain intensity on the first day after surgery: a prospective cohort study comparing 179 surgical procedures. Anesthesiology. 2013; 118(4):934–944

[4] Mathiesen O, Dahl B, Thomsen BA, et al. A comprehensive multimodal pain treatment reduces opioid consumption after multilevel spine surgery. Eur Spine J. 2013; 22(9): 2089–2096

[5] Gottschalk A, Durieux ME, Nemergut EC. Intraoperative methadone improves postoperative pain control in patients undergoing complex spine surgery. Anesth Analg. 2011; 112 (1):218–223

[6] Rodgers A, Walker N, Schug S, et al. Reduction of postoperative mortality and morbidity with epidural or spinal anaesthesia: results from overview of randomised trials. BMJ. 2000; 321(7275):1493

[7] Fiani B, Reardon T, Selvage J, et al. Awake spine surgery: an eye-opening movement. Surg Neurol Int. 2021; 12:222

[8] Garg B, Ahuja K, Sharan AD. Regional anesthesia for spine surgery. J Am Acad Orthop Surg. 2022; 30(17):809–819

[9] O'Hara JF, Jr, Cywinski JB, Tetzlaff JE, Xu M, Gurd AR, Andrish JT. The effect of epidural vs intravenous analgesia for posterior spinal fusion surgery. Paediatr Anaesth. 2004; 14(12): 1009–1015

[10] Lee B, Kim EJ, Park JH, Park KB, Choi YS. Effect of surgeon-performed thoracic paravertebral block on postoperative pain in adolescent idiopathic scoliosis surgery: a prospective randomized controlled trial. J Pers Med. 2024; 14(6): 659

[11] Sachdev D, Mamikunian G, Kia C, Zhou H. Narrative review: erector spinae block in spine surgery. J Spine Surg. 2023; 9 (4):454–462

[12] Elsharkawy H, El-Boghdadly K, Barrington M. Quadratus lumborum block: anatomical concepts, mechanisms, and techniques. Anesthesiology. 2019; 130(2):322–335

[13] Young MJ, Gorlin AW, Modest VE, Quraishi SA. Clinical implications of the transversus abdominis plane block in adults. Anesthesiol Res Pract. 2012; 2012:731645

[14] Kendall MC, Alves L, Traill LL, De Oliveira GS. The effect of ultrasound-guided erector spinae plane block on postsurgical pain: a meta-analysis of randomized controlled trials. BMC Anesthesiol. 2020; 20(1):99

[15] Liang X, Zhou W, Fan Y. Erector spinae plane block for spinal surgery: a systematic review and meta-analysis. Korean J Pain. 2021; 34(4):487–500

[16] Ueshima H, Inagaki M, Toyone T, Otake H. Efficacy of the erector spinae plane block for lumbar spinal surgery: a retrospective study. Asian Spine J. 2019; 13(2):254–257

[17] Xie Q, Zhang J, Lu F, Wu H, Chen Z, Jian F. Minimally invasive versus open transforaminal lumbar interbody fusion in obese patients: a meta-analysis. BMC Musculoskelet Disord. 2018; 19(1):15

[18] Sykes DAW, Tabarestani TQ, Chaudhry NS, et al. Awake spinal fusion is associated with reduced length of stay, opioid use, and time to ambulation compared to general anesthesia: a matched cohort study. World Neurosurg. 2023; 176: e91–e100

[19] Urick D, Sciavolino B, Wang TY, Gupta DK, Sharan A, Abd-El-Barr MM. Perioperative outcomes of general versus spinal anesthesia in the lumbar spine surgery population: a systematic review and meta-analysis of data from 2005 through 2021. J Clin Orthop Trauma. 2022; 30:101923

[20] Chan AK, Gnaedinger A, Ayoub C, Gupta DK, Abd-El-Barr MM. The "in-parallel" technique for awake, bilateral simultaneous minimally invasive transforaminal lumbar interbody fusion and multilevel lumbar decompression. Oper Neurosurg (Hagerstown). 2023; 24(3):e160–e169

[21] Sykes DAW, Tabarestani TQ, Salven DS, et al. Awake spinal anesthesia facilitates spine surgery in poor surgical candidates: a case series. Neurochirurgie. 2023; 69(3): 101444

[22] Wu L, Zhao H, Weng H, Ma D. Lasting effects of general anesthetics on the brain in the young and elderly: "mixed picture" of neurotoxicity, neuroprotection and cognitive impairment. J Anesth. 2019; 33(2):321–335

[23] Belrose JC, Noppens RR. Anesthesiology and cognitive impairment: a narrative review of current clinical literature. BMC Anesthesiol. 2019; 19(1):241

[24] Brown CH , IV, Jones EL, Lin C, et al. Shaping anesthetic techniques to reduce post-operative delirium (SHARP) study: a protocol for a prospective pragmatic randomized controlled trial to evaluate spinal anesthesia with targeted sedation compared with general anesthesia in older adults undergoing lumbar spine fusion surgery. BMC Anesthesiol. 2019; 19(1):192

4 Erector Spinae Plane Blocks

Emily Zoe Barney Hall and W. Michael Bullock

Abstract
The erector spinae plane (ESP) block is a fascial plane block that targets the dorsal spinal nerve roots (rami) prior to traveling through the paraspinal muscles toward more superficial structures. Given that these nerves innervate the posterior spinal structures that are violated in spine surgeries, they are safe, easy, and efficient targets for depositing local anesthetics to achieve intraoperative and postoperative analgesia for posterior spine procedures. While current literature is blossoming with examples of improved patient outcomes when the ESP block is added to traditional anesthetics for lumbar spine surgery, significantly less data exist regarding the same regional anesthetic technique as it applies to awake spine surgery.

Keywords: erector spinae, ESP, regional anesthesia, awake spine surgery, postoperative pain control, truncal blocks

Key Points

- ESP blocks intend to anesthetize the dorsal rami of the spinal nerves by depositing local anesthetic between the deep fascia of the erector spinae muscles and the vertebral transverse process.
- This paraspinal fascial plane block has a bony landmark as an endpoint, making it safe and easy to teach.
- This technique should be performed bilaterally to achieve optimal analgesia.
- Multiple lumbar levels are anesthetized with higher volumes of dilute local anesthetics with one injection.
- A growing body of data demonstrates that the addition of the ESP block to a general anesthetic will decrease postoperative opioid use, lower rates of postoperative nausea and vomiting, increase patient satisfaction, reduce patient-reported pain scores, and decrease length of stay.[1]

4.1 Introduction

The erector spinae plane (ESP) block was first described by Forero et al in 2016 as a means of treating thoracic neuropathic pain.[2] Since then, this paraspinal interfacial plane block has become popular among regional anesthesiologists for various indications. The increase in utilization of the ESP block is likely multifactorial, but, in the era of ultrasonographical guided procedures, it is tied closely to the ease of application, low complication rates, effective postoperative analgesia, and reduction of opioid consumption seen with other fascial plane blocks.[3] Similar findings have been echoed in the literature surrounding the addition of the ESP block to traditional general anesthetics for lumbar spine surgery.[1] This chapter will discuss the relevant anatomy, block performance, function, and current data supporting the use of the ESP block for awake spine surgery.

4.2 Erector Spinae Plane Block

4.2.1 Relevant Anatomy

- The erector spinae muscles are a group of paraspinal muscles that run vertically in the groove lateral to the vertebral column from the base of the skull to the pelvis. This group consists of iliocostalis, longissimus, and spinalis from lateral to medial and lies deep to the thoracolumbar fascia.
- The erector spinae muscles are innervated by the dorsal rami of corresponding spinal nerves and aid with back and head extension.
- The dorsal rami of the spinal nerves, which are also responsible for innervating the posterior spinal structures and their associated tissues, can be found close to where they exit the vertebral foramina. They will then travel posteriorly through the intertransverse connective tissues and paraspinal muscles to reach more superficial layers[4] (▸ Fig. 4.1).

4.2.2 Block Function

- Pain after spine surgery can arise from any violated layer, ranging from skin, muscle, and

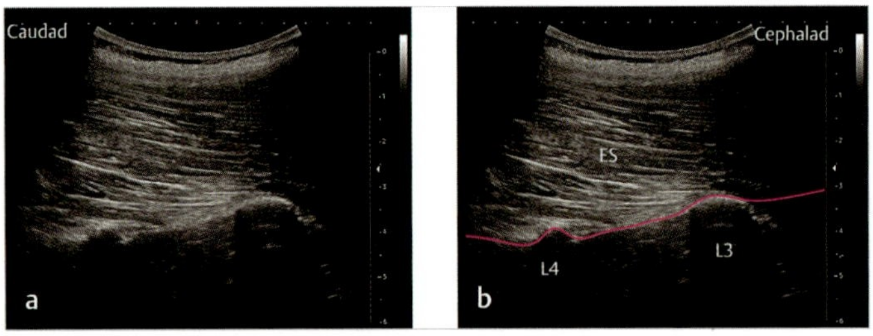

Fig. 4.1 **(a)** Ultrasound image of lumbar spine area using a curvilinear transducer. **(b)** Outline of the anterior border of the erector spinae muscles over the L3 and L4 transverse processes. ES, erector spinae muscle. Depth is in centimeters.

fascia to vertebra, ligaments, and facet joints. The dorsal rami of the spinal nerves innervate all of the aforementioned posterior tissues and bony structures.[5]

- The ESP blocks anesthetize the dorsal rami of the spinal nerves by depositing local anesthetic in the interfascial plane between the erector spinae muscles and the vertebral transverse process.
- While there remains controversy surrounding the definite mechanism of the ESP block in both cadaveric and radiologic studies, block efficacy is thought to be related to the spread of local anesthetic to the paravertebral or epidural space at the corresponding vertebral levels.[2,6]
- This block is safe and ideal for practitioners who do not frequently utilize regional anesthesia. Ultrasound image acquisition is simple, and the endpoint of the transverse process provides a "bony backstop."

4.2.3 Block Performance

- The anesthesia team typically performs the ESP block in the preoperative area with the patient under light sedation, allowing time for the block to onset while the patient is transferred to the operating room (OR) and appropriately positioned for the procedure.[7] However, these blocks can also be performed in the OR.
- After having the patient either in a sitting position (preop) or prone (after induction of anesthesia in the OR), the low-frequency curvilinear ultrasound probe is placed in a parasagittal orientation 1 to 3 cm off midline. The sacrum is identified, and laminar levels are counted in a cephalad direction to the approximate midpoint of the surgical spinal area. After determining the desired location, lateral translation of the probe is necessary to visualize the transverse processes. The optimal image for block performance clearly demonstrates multiple levels of transverse processes with overlying erector spinae muscles.

Expert Tip

The ESP block can be performed with the patient in a sitting position, lateral, or prone based on the operator's preference, patient comfort, or timing of the block.

Expert Tip

While the ideal level for the ESP block is the surgical area's midpoint level, the block performance level is dictated mainly by the clarity of the image and patient anatomy. Suppose conditions do not allow for transverse process contact directly at the midpoint level. In that case, a dilute local anesthetic of approximately 30 mL will spread approximately four lumbar levels, providing some flexibility for block location.

- A chlorhexidine-based prep is used to clean the skin over the area of the needle insertion site; however, other appropriate antiseptics may be used.
- The block needle is then advanced under ultrasound guidance from cranial to caudal via an in-plane approach, passing through the erector spinae muscles until reaching the transverse process.
- The endpoint is needle-to-bone contact on the dorsal surface of the transverse process such that, after negative aspiration, a test injection of saline demonstrates spread along the submuscular plane between the erector spinae and the transverse process in both a cephalad and a caudad direction.

Expert Tip

Intramuscular spread is more common when the needle contacts the top of the transverse process. Aiming for the upper corners of the transverse process increases the chances for successful interfascial plane injection. This will facilitate lifting the muscle and the fascia from the bone when injecting the local anesthetic.

Expert Tip

If the operator is in the correct plane, the local anesthetic injection should expand the interfascial plane area. Once the injection is stopped, the muscle slowly sinks back toward the transverse process, pushing the injectate throughout the interfascial plane. This is called the "breathing sign" and indicates a successful block.

- After location confirmation, the anesthesiologist's local anesthetic of choice will be delivered incrementally in the same plane.
- The same procedure is then performed on the contralateral side.
- These can be performed as single-shot blocks or fascial plane catheters. If implemented as single-shot blocks, they can be prolonged with additive medications such as epinephrine, dexamethasone, dexmedetomidine, or liposomal bupivacaine.
- The addition of liposomal bupivacaine (Exparel, Pacira Biosciences, Tampa, FL) to extend the benefits of the ESP block have been studied for a variety of surgical indications, and may decrease length of hospital stay, time to ambulation, postoperative pain, and narcotic use (▶ Fig. 4.2).[8,9,10]

Expert Tip

In our practice, 20 mL of liposomal bupivacaine (Exparel, Pacira Biosciences) admixed with 30 mL of 0.5% bupivacaine HCl (for a total of 50–25 mL per side) is the local anesthetic of choice for both intraoperative and postoperative analgesia.[11]

4.3 Erector Spinae Plane Data

4.3.1 Data for General Anesthesia in Spine Surgeries

- A growing body of literature surrounds the benefits of adding ESP blocks for postoperative pain control for spine surgeries performed under a general aesthetic.[12]
- Current evidence demonstrates the ESP's ability to reduce opioid utilization significantly, decrease postoperative pain scores, prolong time to first rescue analgesic, lessen the number of patients requiring rescue analgesia, and lower the incidence of postop nausea and vomiting. One notable study of 700 patients revealed a significant decrease in morphine utilization in patients who underwent ESP in the first 24 hours following surgery compared to a control group.[13,14] Additional studies revealed better patient satisfaction and earlier time to ambulation in patients who underwent lumbar spine surgery under general anesthesia supplemented with ESP.[15]
- Randomized controlled trials in patients requiring lumbar spine surgeries exhibit reduced pain scores and decreased opioid consumption compared to control groups.[16] This difference was limited in studies incorporating Enhanced Recovery After Surgery (ERAS) protocols.[17]

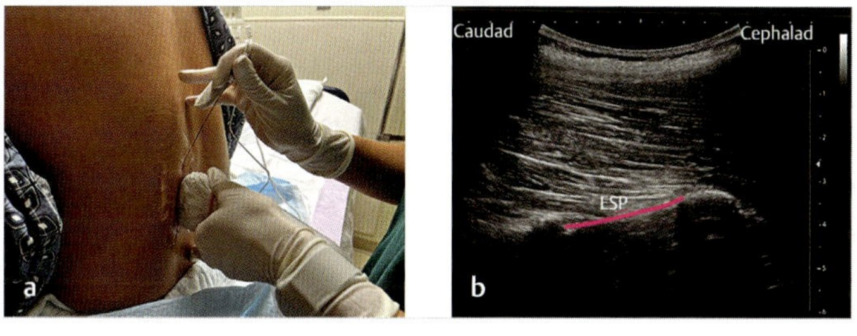

Fig. 4.2 **(a)** The patient is shown positioned sitting for ESP block. **(b)** Block area for ESP block. ESP, erector spinae plane (*pink*). Depth is in centimeters.

4.3.2 Data for Awake Spine Surgery

- Very little research has been published on the niche topic of ESP blocks for awake spine surgery, and current literature searches are limited mainly to case reports.
- One case report demonstrated the successful utility of the ESP block's analgesic properties for minimally invasive endoscopic diskectomy in the awake state.[18]
- Another case report employed ESP block catheters to allow for continuous infusion of local anesthetic to improve the management of acute postoperative pain following minimally invasive transforaminal lumbar interbody fusion.[19]
- The only current prospective randomized controlled trial tested the hypothesis that ESP block plus sedation was as effective as local infiltration anesthesia with fentanyl and propofol plus sedation. In this study, the primary endpoint was the volume of fentanyl and propofol administered during surgery. The authors found that patients who underwent ESP block plus sedation required lower doses of fentanyl and propofol during surgery than those who had local infiltration. The group that received local infiltration anesthesia resulted in the need for deeper sedation and had a higher complication rate, but pain management and patient satisfaction were the same between groups.[20]
- Based on the limited data available on this topic, further research regarding the role of ESP blocks is required to carve out the benefits and ideal population for this anesthetic technique.

4.4 Clinical Example

An 84-year-old woman with right leg radiculopathy presents for L3 laminectomy. Her medical comorbidities include severe chronic obstructive pulmonary disease (on 2 L of O_2 at baseline), coronary artery disease with left ventricular ejection fraction of 35%, hypertension, and type 2 diabetes mellitus. She was offered an awake spine surgery to minimize complications from surgery and anesthesia secondary to her medical issues (possible prolonged intubation and opioid-related side effects). She was given a 10-mg isobaric bupivacaine spinal in the OR, aids in positioning herself on the OR table, and then given bilateral ESP blocks at L3. She was given headphones to listen to a podcast. Surgery proceeds without incident, and she is taken to the postanesthesia recovery area (PACU). She does not ask for or receive any opioid medications in recovery and is monitored overnight, given her comorbidities. She was discharged the following morning.

4.5 Conclusion

The ESP block is a fascial plane block that anesthetizes the dorsal rami of the spinal nerves. Depending on the patient's needs, this regional anesthesia technique can be performed as a single-shot block or with catheter placement. As it has proven beneficial in spine surgery under general anesthesia, integrating ESP blocks for awake spine surgery holds significant promise for patient-centered outcomes. Because of the ease and efficiency of this block, it can be easily integrated into the workflow of the anesthetic and operative teams.

References

[1] Sachdev D, Mamikunian G, Kia C, Zhou H. Narrative review: erector spinae block in spine surgery. J Spine Surg. 2023; 9 (4):454–462

[2] Forero M, Adhikary SD, Lopez H, Tsui C, Chin KJ. The erector spinae plane block: a novel analgesic technique in thoracic neuropathic pain. Reg Anesth Pain Med. 2016; 41(5):621–627

[3] Chin KJ, McDonnell JG, Carvalho B, Sharkey A, Pawa A, Gadsden J. Essentials of our current understanding: abdominal wall blocks. Reg Anesth Pain Med. 2017; 42(2):133–183

[4] Saito T, Steinke H, Miyaki T, et al. Analysis of the posterior ramus of the lumbar spinal nerve: the structure of the posterior ramus of the spinal nerve. Anesthesiology. 2013; 118 (1):88–94

[5] Bajwa SJ, Haldar R. Pain management following spinal surgeries: an appraisal of the available options. J Craniovertebr Junction Spine. 2015; 6(3):105–110

[6] Vidal E, Giménez H, Forero M, Fajardo M. Erector spinae plane block: a cadaver study to determine its mechanism of action. Rev Esp Anestesiol Reanim (Engl Ed). 2018; 65(9): 514–519

[7] Waguia R, Touko EK, Sykes DAW, et al. How to start an awake spine program: protocol and illustrative cases. IBRO Neurosci Rep. 2022; 13:69–77

[8] Dincer A, Wang A, Kanter MJ, et al. Clinical outcomes of liposomal bupivacaine erector spinae block in minimally invasive transforaminal lumbar interbody fusion surgery. Neurosurgery. 2023; 92(3):590–598

[9] Song K, Xu Q, Knott VH, et al. Liposomal bupivacaine-based erector spinae block for cardiac surgery. J Cardiothorac Vasc Anesth. 2021; 35(5):1555–1559

[10] Kumar A, Hulsey A, Martinez-Wilson H, Kim J, Gadsden J. The use of liposomal bupivacaine in erector spinae plane

block to minimize opioid consumption for breast surgery: a case report. A Pract. 2018; 10(9):239–241

[11] Sykes DAW, Tabarestani TQ, Chaudhry NS, et al. Awake spinal fusion is associated with reduced length of stay, opioid use, and time to ambulation compared to general anesthesia: a matched cohort study. World Neurosurg. 2023; 176:e91–e100

[12] Sun Q, Zhang C, Liu S, et al. Efficacy of erector spinae plane block for postoperative analgesia lumbar surgery: a systematic review and meta-analysis. BMC Anesthesiol. 2023; 23 (1):54

[13] Kendall MC, Alves L, Traill LL, De Oliveira GS. The effect of ultrasound-guided erector spinae plane block on postsurgical pain: a meta-analysis of randomized controlled trials. BMC Anesthesiol. 2020; 20(1):99

[14] Liang X, Zhou W, Fan Y. Erector spinae plane block for spinal surgery: a systematic review and meta-analysis. Korean J Pain. 2021; 34(4):487–500

[15] Ueshima H, Inagaki M, Toyone T, Otake H. Efficacy of the erector spinae plane block for lumbar spinal surgery: a retrospective study. Asian Spine J. 2019; 13(2):254–257

[16] Yayik AM, Cesur S, Ozturk F, et al. Postoperative analgesic efficacy of the ultrasound-guided erector spinae plane block in patients undergoing lumbar spinal decompression surgery: a randomized controlled study. World Neurosurg. 2019; 126:e779–e785

[17] Avis G, Gricourt Y, Vialatte PB, et al. Analgesic efficacy of erector spinae plane blocks for lumbar spine surgery: a randomized double-blind controlled clinical trial. Reg Anesth Pain Med. 2022; 47(10):610–616

[18] Reddy A, Barik AK, Bhatia N, Jain K. Ultrasound-guided erector spinae plane block for awake spine surgery: a case report and review of the literature. Saudi J Anaesth. 2024; 18(1): 126–128

[19] Braxton EE, Brena KR, Spears H, Conrad E, Heinze JD. Ultrasound-guided bilateral erector spinae plane nerve blocks: a novel application for the management of acute postoperative pain in awake spine surgery. Illustrative case. J Neurosurg Case Lessons. 2022; 3(18): CASE21633

[20] Barsa M, Filyk O. Erector spinae plane block versus local infiltration anaesthesia for transforaminal percutaneous endoscopic discectomy: a prospective randomised controlled trial. Rev Esp Anestesiol Reanim (Engl Ed). 2023; 70(10): 552–560

5 Anesthesia for Awake Spinal Surgeries—Epidural vs. Spinal Anesthesia

Anjaleekrishna K. and Bikash Ranjan Ray

Abstract

Surgeries of the spine were previously performed almost exclusively under general anesthesia owing to the lack of familiarity in performing neuraxial procedures in spines with pathology or deformity and fear of patients staying awake during the procedures. But awake spinal surgery has gained popularity lately due to evidence of lowering perioperative risks, postoperative opioid consumption, hospital stay after surgery, and cost, especially in lumbar spine surgeries. Detailed studies have shown several advantages in choosing regional anesthesia over general in procedures of the spine affecting limited levels and less durations. This chapter outlines the different advantages and disadvantages of neuraxial procedures (spinal and epidural anesthesia) as well as their safety profile compared to general anesthesia in simple spine surgeries.

Keywords: neuraxial anesthesia, spinal anesthesia, epidural anesthesia, conscious sedation, counseling

Key Points

- Surgeries of the spine are commonly done under general anesthesia.
- Use of regional anesthesia techniques expands the pool of patients getting corrective spinal surgeries by including patients with comorbidities that typically restrict the use of general anesthesia.
- Owing to the difficulty in positioning, duration of surgeries, and ease at expertise, neuraxial techniques are used more common than other nerve blocks.
- Neuraxial techniques can avoid airway manipulation and major hemodynamic changes associated with laryngoscopy, enable patients to position themselves avoiding eye and nerve injuries, and provide better postoperative analgesia with minimal side effects.
- Use of ultrasonography has made performing neuraxial techniques easier in difficult spine deformities.

5.1 Introduction

Surgeries of the spine have been generally performed under general anesthesia (GA).[1] The challenge to the anesthesiologist is to provide optimal surgical conditions at the same time as providing adequate oxygenation to the spinal cord while facilitating the use of intraoperative spinal cord monitoring techniques. The advantages of GA include the facilitation of a rapid securement of airway and loss of consciousness, which ensure less distress to patients and ease of prolongation of anesthesia with extension of surgery. The disadvantages of GA include the risk of aspiration, interference with neuromuscular monitoring, and pulmonary complications. Propofol-based total intravenous anesthesia (TIVA) techniques facilitate easier neuromonitoring, smoother emergence, and rapid awakening along with ease of administration of intraoperative neurological assessment (wake-up test).[2]

Regional anesthesia (RA) provides certain advantages for spinal surgery, when used as either an adjunct or an alternative to GA.[3] RA increases access of patients to safe and opioid-sparing analgesia. Neuraxial anesthesia is not commonly used for spinal surgery but is used only as an analgesic adjunct. RA reduces complications associated with GA due to the airway abnormalities and cardiopulmonary comorbidities and provide better analgesia, but it is associated with a higher incidence of arterial hypotension.[4]

The use of peripheral nerve block techniques for intraoperative and postoperative analgesia is an evolving practice in patients scheduled to undergo spinal interventions.[5] Enhanced Recovery After Surgery (ERAS) protocols have led to the use of different modalities to manage patient pain and improve patient outcomes.[6]

5.2 Mechanism of Action

5.2.1 Spinal Anesthesia

- Spinal anesthesia (SA) (Video 5.1) is the easiest to perform among neuraxial procedures but becomes technically more difficult in patients requiring spine surgery due to difficulty in

positioning, level of deformity, and spinal cord involvement.
- It is commonly performed below the second lumbar vertebra to avoid damage to the spinal cord (▶ Fig. 5.1). Adequate time is given (10–20 minutes) for the intrathecal drug to get fixed at the levels required before the patient is positioned prone to avoid unpredictable ascent of the drug.
- The effect of a single-shot injection usually has onset within 5 minutes and provides SA for about 2 to 4 hours.
- Its use has been described for limited level transforaminal lumbar interbody fusion (TLIF) surgeries and microdiskectomy as the duration of SA cannot be modified after a single injection. As SA wears off in a caudal direction, sacral levels stay anaesthetized longer than thoracic levels.

5.2.2 Epidural Anesthesia

- Epidural anesthesia (EA) is technically more difficult and requires a larger drug dose compared to SA.
- EA can be performed anywhere along the vertebral column including cervical, thoracic, lumbar, and sacral vertebrae. It is usually performed at least two intervertebral levels above the surgical level (e.g., L3–L4 intervertebral space for L5–S1 surgery) as a catheter is inserted to desired levels.[7]
- The onset of analgesia is slower with EA (> 20 minutes) than SA, which provides favorable hemodynamic changes as it causes gradual decrease in blood pressure. For most cases, anesthesia at the level of T6–T10 is adequate for spinal surgery.
- Positioning of the patient can be done immediately after the procedure is performed and anesthesia can be achieved by the time incision is made.
- Two major advantages of using an epidural catheter is that it can be used in case of extended surgeries in terms of levels involved and duration and it can be retained for postoperative analgesia.

Expert Tip

Use of ultrasonography in neuraxial procedures increases the first attempt success rates in patients with deformed spine (▶ Fig. 5.2). Use of epidural catheters can help with cases of unpredictable duration.

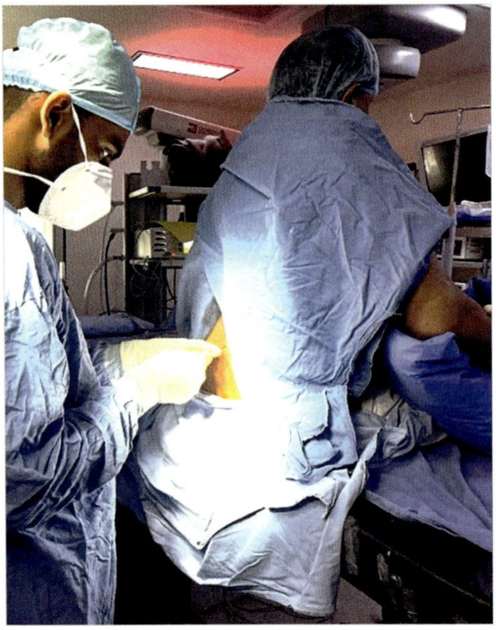

Fig. 5.1 Performing spinal anesthesia in patient posted for L4–L5 transforaminal lumbar interbody fusion (TLIF).

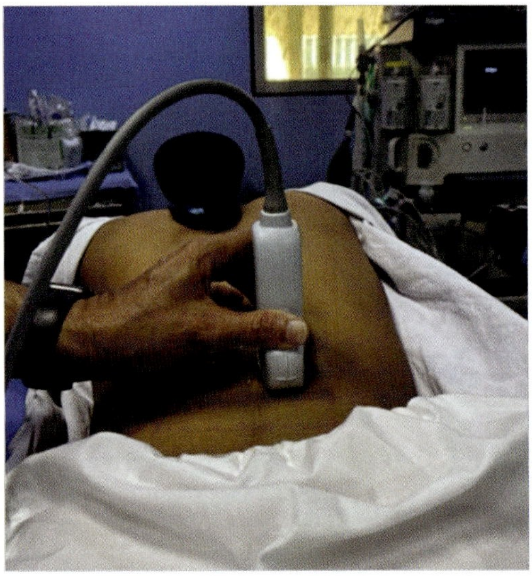

Fig. 5.2 Use of ultrasonography for location of epidural space in awake prone patient.

5.2.3 Patient Selection

- Choosing the right anesthetic technique for the right spine patient can increase the pool of patients recommended against surgery due to the risk associated with GA although duration, complexity, and deformity of the spine pose a major challenge in determining the feasibility and ease of performing regional procedures.
- A list of indications and contraindications that can serve as a guide for appropriate patient selection is given in ▶ Table 5.1. These are suggestive and have to be adapted according to subjects and procedure.

5.3 Managing Awareness during Surgery

- A major concern associated with performing these surgeries under neuraxial or RA is the risk of awareness or rather fear of the patients during the procedures.
- An awake patient positioned in the prone position with SA or EA can position themselves comfortably and remain immobile in the surgical area. The noises in a surgical field can startle a patient during awake surgeries. In addition, the risk of transferred motion due to coughing or the slightest movement of the upper body in a patient can raise major concerns, especially during critical steps of spinal procedures.
- Developing an anesthesia protocol hence starts with ensuring proper patient counseling preoperatively. Often visual aids on the theater setup, how the patient will be positioned, and anticipated communication can alleviate fear and anxiety.

Expert Tip

Patient preparation in advance by the surgeon along with the anesthesiologist is the most important step in successful implementation of an awake spinal surgery protocol. The two major segments of preparation are patient counseling and preemptive analgesia.

- Proper preemptive analgesia is of paramount significance to patient preparation. The most common agents used are gabapentin, pregabalin, paracetamol, dexamethasone and nonsteroidal anti-inflammatory drugs (NSAIDs).[8]
- After routine sign in procedures, the procedure is performed under all aseptic precautions as per the plan and the patient is immediately

Table 5.1 Indications and contraindications for spinal surgery under neuraxial anesthesia

Indications	Contraindications
Patients contraindicated for general anesthesia	Procedures involving more than 2 spinal levels
Procedures requiring intraoperative neuromuscular monitoring	Prolonged/flexible surgical duration
Patients with high risk of delirium, PONV, and opioid tolerance	High BMI patients
Minimally invasive/endoscopic procedures	Patients with OSA
Procedures involving 1–2 spinal levels	Failed back syndrome patients
	Smokers
	Bleeding/coagulation disorders
	Raised ICP/spinal stenosis/arachnoiditis
	Patients with high risk of intraoperative airway or respiratory compromise

Abbreviations: BMI, body mass index; ICP, intracranial pressure; OSA, obstructive sleep apnea; PONV, postoperative nausea and vomiting.

positioned supine. Further monitors, catheters, and equipment can be placed at this time, following which the patient is turned to the prone position.

- Adequate support for headrest and soft face rest should be ensured without strain on the neck. The patient can be allowed to adjust to a comfortable position before site preparation. The patient may be provided with active noise canceling headphone; sedation can be initiated at this time.
- Practice Guidelines for Moderate Procedural Sedation and Analgesia 2018 provides recommendations for patient evaluation and preparation, monitoring of ventilatory function with capnography and pulse oximetry, the need for trained personnel with the knowledge and skills to recognize and treat airway complications, preferential use of sedatives and analgesics such as benzodiazepines and dexmedetomidine, and minimizing or titrating agents for GA (propofol, ketamine, and etomidate) and recovery care.[9]

Expert Tip

The use of agents such as dexmedetomidine and midazolam helps in achieving adequate sedation with arousability for intraoperative monitoring and neurological assessment. These agents carry minimal risk of respiratory depression and lowers the use of postoperative opioids. Use of dexmedetomidine and dexamethasone provides added advantage of analgesia and prolongation of duration of neuraxial blockade.

- ▶ Table 5.2 shows a comparison of the general characteristics of SA and EA.

5.4 Comparison of Efficacy between Epidural and Spinal Anesthesia

Although controlled trials comparing the efficacy of SA and EA are limited, there are systematic reviews and meta-analyses of several case reports and randomized controlled trials (RCTs) that assessed their use in spinal surgeries.

- In 2022, Ní Eochagáin et al published a review on a total of 36 articles about neuraxial anesthesia techniques in spinal surgeries.[10] As per this review, neuraxial techniques were employed most of the times for lumbar diskectomy or laminectomy (36%), spinal fusion surgery (14%), lumbar decompression surgery (11%), and major corrective deformity surgery (8%). The majority of these described neuraxial techniques were the sole anesthetic technique for spinal surgery. SA and thoracolumbar EA were used in almost all the studies. The rest of the studies have used neuraxial techniques for analgesia as an adjunct to GA.
- The most commonly used local anesthetic agent was bupivacaine with or without lidocaine. Lidocaine and ropivacaine are rarely used as sole agents. In all sources describing SA as the technique for anesthesia, bupivacaine was the only agent used, while other agents were used in epidural or combined spinal–epidural techniques.
- The most commonly used adjunct is fentanyl. Other adjuvant medications include morphine, dexmedetomidine, buprenorphine, sufentanil, methyl prednisolone, and even saline.
- Based on this review, the most cited advantages of neuraxial anesthesia were cost efficiency, reduced blood loss, reduced anesthesia-related postoperative complications, better

Table 5.2 Differences between epidural and spinal anesthesia

Differences between epidural and spinal anesthesia		
Features	**Epidural**	**Spinal**
Onset of anesthesia	25–30 min	5 min
Drug dosage	Larger dose	Smaller
Quality of anesthesia	Not dense	Dense blockade
Duration of blockade	Adjustable, prolonged	Brief, 2–4 h depending on adjunct

postoperative analgesia, and its suitability in complex cases where patients are not suitable for GA.

5.5 Comparison of Neuraxial Procedures and General Anesthesia

The literature notes numerous advantages of RA over GA.

- Most notable ones are favorable hemodynamic stability in the perioperative period, lower mortality rates, less intraoperative blood loss, less chance of vascular thrombosis, pulmonary embolism, myocardial infarction, renal dysfunction, and lower incidence of cognitive dysfunction and hypoxic episodes in the postanesthesia care unit (PACU).[11,12,13]
- RA is used alone or in combination with GA or sedation.
- In the case of surgeries of the spine, RA is associated with lower pain scores during PACU stay, shorter anesthesia time, and higher levels of patient satisfaction than GA.[14]
- RA has reduced systemic side effects and less action on the brain; hence, it is seen to be associated with lower incidence of postoperative nausea and vomiting.[15]
- Patients under RA facilitate positioning themselves. This is likely to reduce the chance of injuries associated with positioning such as brachial plexus injury, complications related to head rotation, pressure necrosis of the face, postoperative vision loss, and pressure sores.[16,17,18]
- RA can be employed based on the patient's comorbidities, nature and duration of surgery, ease of positioning, spinal deformity, and relative benefits and risks to the patient.
- Among RA, SA is more time-efficient than GA. Compared to GA, SA for lumbar spine surgery requires 19 minutes of shorter anesthesia time.[19]
- By using EA, postoperative pain and stress response can be better managed. This is due to a combination of sympathetic blockade, vasodilation, and hypotension, along with lower intrathoracic pressure generated by spontaneous breathing in patients.
- Studies show reduced blood loss in patients undergoing spine surgery with RA.[20,21]
- Studies have shown significantly lower incidence of deep venous thrombosis in RA compared to GA. Previous studies have also reported fewer thromboembolic complications in spine surgery patients receiving RA.[22,23] The preventive effect of RA in inhibition of fibrinolysis and faster mobility of the hypercoagulable state that occurs after a major surgery might be the cause of this.
- A Cochrane review by Guay et al in 2014 comparing GA and RA showed a lower mortality rate by approximately 2.5% in surgery with an intermediate to high cardiac risk.[24] Mortality was reduced by a third in patients under RA in a review of multiple RCTs.[11]
- Although there are conflicting results on postoperative pain in RA versus GA, a recent RCT showed a strong association of RA with lower pain scores during PACU stay, lower postoperative nausea and vomiting, and higher levels of patient and surgeon satisfaction.[25,26]
- ▶ Table 5.3 shows a list of advantages and disadvantages of RA over GA.

5.6 Safety Profile

Current literature is limited regarding the safety of RA over GA. In general, RA is considered feasible in patients undergoing surgeries with a duration of less than 3 hours and less anticipated blood loss.[27] As of now, RA is mostly used in decompressive lumbar surgeries. RA is safe for patients with risk of GA-related complications. Currently, patients with American Society of Anesthesiologists (ASA) physical status grade III or IV are not considered safe for spinal surgery under GA. In such cases, RA can be considered a safe and effective choice. In complicated spinal deformities, intraoperative laceration of the dura and loss of cerebrospinal fluid (CSF) does not cause alteration of the SA and effect of SA.

5.7 Complications and Adverse Events

There are certain conflicts to using neuraxial anesthesia in patients with spinal pathology.

- Need for multiple attempts and a risk of failure due to anatomical changes make the procedure

Table 5.3 Advantages and disadvantages of regional anesthesia over GA

Advantages
Lower blood loss
Lower thrombotic events
Lower risk of myocardial infarction
Lower mortality rate
Lower renal failure
Lower pain scores
Lower PONV scores
Fewer hypoxic episodes in PACU
Lower anesthesia time
Better patient satisfaction
Easier positioning
Disadvantages
Higher risk of neurologic complications
Airway not secured
Risk of anesthesia failure
Compromised nerve monitoring
Sympathetic blockade

Abbreviations: GA, general anesthesia; PACU, postanesthesia care unit; PONV, postoperative nausea and vomiting.

technically more complicated. Patients with spine pathology are prone to experience paresthesia during SA. The spinal roots are vulnerable to direct exposure to large doses of anesthetics, leading to irreversible neuron damage. So informed written consent has to be taken for the same if RA is performed.

- GA is preferred in procedures lasting more than 3 hours or involving excessive blood loss.
- There is decreased patient acceptance and a concern regarding securing the airway.[16,17] There is a widespread acceptance of GA in spine patients as secure airway can be achieved in the prone position.
- Intraoperative neuromonitoring may be of limited value with RA since it interferes with neuroaxis transmission.[28,29]
- Although severe neurologic complications are rare, RA has a slight risk of cauda equina syndrome and results in permanent neurologic deficit.[30] SA has been associated with high risk of new deficit.[31] RA can cause features such as radiculopathy or myelopathy in patients with severe spinal stenosis.
- RA can cause blockade of sympathetic fibers originating at thoracic levels T1–T5, leading to severe bradycardia or hypotension.[32]
- As the upper sensory level should be at T10 or higher to provide adequate anesthesia, high levels of motor blockade cause lack of abdominal muscle strength. This causes the inability to breathe deeply in the prone position due to increased abdominal pressure.[16] This makes the use of SA for spine surgery for levels above T10 infeasible.

Expert Tip

The use of neuraxial or regional procedures helps in early detection of complications as the patient remains awake and can complain of any discomfort early on. This is also associated with lower risk of postoperative delirium and better patient satisfaction.

5.8 Current Trends in Anesthesia Choice

- RA is mostly used in lumbar spine surgery, especially in microdiskectomy and lumbar decompression. SA is limited to T10 and lower levels in spine surgery due to the risk of strenuous breathing and the possibility of thoracic sympathetic blockade.
- Literature on the use of RA in lumbar fusion is very limited. Recent evidence suggests the possibility of applying RA in other spinal surgeries. In an article published by Öğrenci et al, SA was used in spinal tumor surgery in elderly patients for tumorectomy and fusion of the spinal columns.[33]
- Cheng and Chen demonstrated the use of RA in thoracic spinal stenosis cases.[34]
- RA was used to perform minimally invasive transforaminal interbody fusion in some RCTs.[35]

- A case report described the use of RA in revision surgery for lumbar pseudoarthrosis in a patient with high risk for GA.[36]

5.9 Future of Regional Anesthesia in Spine Surgeries

Most studies point to the suggestion that RA can be widely used in elderly patients for spine surgeries. With the average life expectancy increasing, elderly patients with comorbidities and high risk of complications with GA may require surgical treatment for spinal surgeries. Therefore, the need for an anesthetic method with low anesthetic risk will be appealing to the geriatric population.

- Deyo et al evaluated the risks of GA in patients aged ≥ 66 years undergoing spinal surgery and reported major medical complications, like cardiorespiratory arrest, acute myocardial infarction, respiratory failure, pulmonary embolism, pneumonia, and stroke.[37]
- A similar report by Lessing et al reported major complications in patients ≥ 70 years undergoing spinal surgery with RA.[28] Older patients are more susceptible to hypoxemic episodes during recovery. Patients who receive RA are associated with a lower risk of hypoxemia than GA.[13]
- A more recent article by Öğrenci et al suggested that it is feasible to use SA in elderly patients with lumbar spinal tumors classified as ASA grade III or IV who are at high risk for GA.[33] All these advantages and studies substantiate the possibility of broadening the spectrum of using RA in lumbar spine surgery.
- A decline in cognition in geriatric patients is associated with postoperative delirium (POD).[38] RCTs show that low depth of anesthesia is associated with POD.[39] The use of RA can combat this incidence of POD in geriatric patients.
- Certain concerns to be taken care of in advanced age is the increased block height due to the low volume and high specific gravity of CSF. CSF volume is negatively correlated to spread of block.[40] As nerve roots are more sensitive to local anesthetics in older patients, a lower drug dose is required.
- RA can be applied in various fields of spinal surgery, especially in minimally invasive surgeries. Research suggests the possibility of using RA in revision spinal fusion, robotic minimally invasive fusion, and spinal tumors.[33,35,36] Studies have also depicted the successful use of continuous EA in lumbar endoscopic surgery, which can be used without time limit, unlike other methods of RA, and as a postoperative epidural analgesia.[41]
- A recent large-scale study using a national registry showed that the type of anesthesia does not affect the outcomes of lumbar decompressions or lumbar fusion.[42]

References

[1] Meng Y, Jiang H, Zhang C, et al. A comparison of the postoperative analgesic efficacy between epidural and intravenous analgesia in major spine surgery: a meta-analysis. J Pain Res. 2017; 10:405–415

[2] Lin WL, Lee MS, Wong CS, et al. Effects of intraoperative propofol-based total intravenous anesthesia on postoperative pain in spine surgery: comparison with desflurane anesthesia—a randomised trial. Medicine (Baltimore). 2019; 98(13):e15074

[3] Finnerty D, Ní Eochagáin A, Ahmed M, Poynton A, Butler JS, Buggy DJ. A randomised trial of bilateral erector spinae plane block vs. no block for thoracolumbar decompressive spinal surgery. Anaesthesia. 2021; 76(11):1499–1503

[4] Ng K, Parsons J, Cyna AM, Middleton P. Spinal versus epidural anaesthesia for caesarean section. Cochrane Database Syst Rev. 2004; 2004(2):CD003765

[5] Christopher S, Gopal TVS, Vardhan V. Thoracolumbar interfascial plane block, way forward for awake endoscopic laminectomies. Indian J Anaesth. 2020; 64(5):436–437

[6] Dietz N, Sharma M, Adams S, et al. Enhanced Recovery after Surgery (ERAS) for spine surgery: a systematic review. World Neurosurg. 2019; 130:415–426

[7] Demirel CB, Kalayci M, Ozkocak I, Altunkaya H, Ozer Y, Acikgoz B. A prospective randomized study comparing perioperative outcome variables after epidural or general anesthesia for lumbar disc surgery. J Neurosurg Anesthesiol. 2003; 15(3):185–192

[8] Rivkin A, Rivkin MA. Perioperative nonopioid agents for pain control in spinal surgery. Am J Health Syst Pharm. 2014; 71 (21):1845–1857

[9] Practice Guidelines for Moderate Procedural Sedation and Analgesia. Practice Guidelines for Moderate Procedural Sedation and Analgesia 2018: A Report by the American Society of Anesthesiologists Task Force on Moderate Procedural Sedation and Analgesia, the American Association of Oral and Maxillofacial Surgeons, American College of Radiology, American Dental Association, American Society of Dentist Anesthesiologists, and Society of Interventional Radiology. Anesthesiology. 2018; 128(3):437–479

[10] Ní Eochagáin A, Singleton BN, Moorthy A, Buggy DJ. Regional and neuraxial anaesthesia techniques for spinal surgery: a scoping review. Br J Anaesth. 2022; 129(4):598–611

[11] Modig J, Karlström G. Intra- and post-operative blood loss and haemodynamics in total hip replacement when performed under lumbar epidural versus general anaesthesia. Eur J Anaesthesiol. 1987; 4(5):345–355

[12] Rodgers A, Walker N, Schug S, et al. Reduction of postoperative mortality and morbidity with epidural or spinal

anaesthesia: results from overview of randomised trials. BMJ. 2000; 321(7275):1493
[13] Moller JT, Wittrup M, Johansen SH. Hypoxemia in the postanesthesia care unit: an observer study. Anesthesiology. 1990; 73(5):890–895
[14] Baenziger B, Nadi N, Doerig R, et al. Regional versus general anesthesia: effect of anesthetic techniques on clinical outcome in lumbar spine surgery: a prospective randomized controlled trial. J Neurosurg Anesthesiol. 2020; 32(1):29–35
[15] Zorrilla-Vaca A, Healy RJ, Mirski MA. A comparison of regional versus general anesthesia for lumbar spine surgery: a meta-analysis of randomized studies. J Neurosurg Anesthesiol. 2017; 29(4):415–425
[16] Mergeay M, Verster A, Van Aken D, Vercauteren M. Regional versus general anesthesia for spine surgery. A comprehensive review. Acta Anaesthesiol Belg. 2015; 66(1):1–9
[17] McLain RF, Bell GR, Kalfas I, Tetzlaff JE, Yoon HJ. Complications associated with lumbar laminectomy: a comparison of spinal versus general anesthesia. Spine. 2004; 29(22):2542–2547
[18] McLain RF, Kalfas I, Bell GR, Tetzlaff JE, Yoon HJ, Rana M. Comparison of spinal and general anesthesia in lumbar laminectomy surgery: a case-controlled analysis of 400 patients. J Neurosurg Spine. 2005; 2(1):17–22
[19] Singeisen H, Hodel D, Schindler C, Frey K, Eichenberger U, Hausmann ON. Signifikant kürzere anästhesiezeit bei lumbaler wirbelsäulenchirurgie: prozess analytischer vergleich von spinalanästhesie und intubation snarkose [Significantly shorter anesthesia time for surgery of the lumbar spine: process analytical comparison of spinal anesthesia and intubation narcosis]. Anaesthesist. 2013; 62(8):632–638
[20] Greenbarg PE, Brown MD, Pallares VS, Tompkins JS, Mann NH. Epidural anesthesia for lumbar spine surgery. J Spinal Disord. 1988; 1(2):139–143
[21] Khajavi MR, Asadian MA, Imani F, Etezadi F, Moharari RS, Amirjamshidi A. General anesthesia versus combined epidural/general anesthesia for elective lumbar spine disc surgery: A randomized clinical trial comparing the impact of the two methods upon the outcome variables. Surg Neurol Int. 2013; 4:105
[22] Tetzlaff JE, Dilger JA, Kodsy M, al-Bataineh J, Yoon HJ, Bell GR. Spinal anesthesia for elective lumbar spine surgery. J Clin Anesth. 1998; 10(8):666–669
[23] Rosenfeld BA, Beattie C, Christopherson R, et al. The effects of different anesthetic regimens on fibrinolysis and the development of postoperative arterial thrombosis. Perioperative Ischemia Randomized Anesthesia Trial Study Group. Anesthesiology. 1993; 79(3):435–443
[24] Guay J, Choi P, Suresh S, Albert N, Kopp S, Pace NL. Neuraxial blockade for the prevention of postoperative mortality and major morbidity: an overview of Cochrane systematic reviews. Cochrane Database Syst Rev. 2014; 2014(1): CD010108
[25] Jellish WS, Thalji Z, Stevenson K, Shea J. A prospective randomized study comparing short- and intermediate-term perioperative outcome variables after spinal or general anesthesia for lumbar disk and laminectomy surgery. Anesth Analg. 1996; 83(3):559–564
[26] Sadrolsadat SH, Mahdavi AR, Moharari RS, et al. A prospective randomized trial comparing the technique of spinal and general anesthesia for lumbar disk surgery: a study of 100 cases. Surg Neurol. 2009; 71(1):60–65, discussion 65
[27] Benyahia NM, Verster A, Saldien V, Breebaart M, Sermeus L, Vercauteren M. Regional anaesthesia and postoperative analgesia techniques for spine surgery: a review. Rom J Anaesth Intensive Care. 2015; 22(1):25–33
[28] Lessing NL, Edwards CC , II, Brown CH , IV, et al. Spinal anesthesia in elderly patients undergoing lumbar spine surgery. Orthopedics. 2017; 40(2):e317–e322
[29] Wehab Z, Tabarestani TQ, Abd-El-Barr MM, Husain AM. Intraoperative electromyography in awake minimally invasive transforaminal lumbar interbody fusion: a case study on nerve activation under the effects of local anesthesia. J Clin Neurophysiol. 2022; 39(7):e26–e29
[30] Hong DK, Lawrence HM. Anterior spinal artery syndrome following total hip arthroplasty under epidural anaesthesia. Anaesth Intensive Care. 2001; 29(1):62–66
[31] Yuen EC, Layzer RB, Weitz SR, Olney RK. Neurologic complications of lumbar epidural anesthesia and analgesia. Neurology. 1995; 45(10):1795–1801
[32] Wetstone DL, Wong KC. Sinus bradycardia and asystole during spinal anesthesia. Anesthesiology. 1974; 41(1):87–89
[33] Öğrenci A, Akar E, Koban O, et al. Spinal anesthesia in surgical treatment of lumbar spine tumors. Clin Neurol Neurosurg. 2020; 196:106023
[34] Cheng XK, Chen B. Percutaneous endoscopic thoracic decompression for thoracic spinal stenosis under local anesthesia. World Neurosurg. 2020; 139:488–494
[35] De Biase G, Chen S, Akinduro O, Quinones-Hinojosa A, Abode-Iyamah K. Awake robotic minimally invasive L4–5 transforaminal lumbar interbody fusion. World Neurosurg. 2021; 148:93
[36] Telfeian AE, Moldovan K, Shaaya E, et al. Awake, endoscopic revision surgery for lumbar pseudarthrosis after transforaminal lumbar interbody fusion: technical notes. World Neurosurg. 2020; 136:117–121
[37] Deyo RA, Mirza SK, Martin BI, Kreuter W, Goodman DC, Jarvik JG. Trends, major medical complications, and charges associated with surgery for lumbar spinal stenosis in older adults. JAMA. 2010; 303(13):1259–1265
[38] Saczynski JS, Marcantonio ER, Quach L, et al. Cognitive trajectories after postoperative delirium. N Engl J Med. 2012; 367(1):30–39
[39] Sieber FE. Postoperative delirium in the elderly surgical patient. Anesthesiol Clin. 2009; 27(3):451–464
[40] Carpenter RL, Hogan QH, Liu SS, Crane B, Moore J. Lumbosacral cerebrospinal fluid volume is the primary determinant of sensory block extent and duration during spinal anesthesia. Anesthesiology. 1998; 89(1):24–29
[41] Xu T, Tian R, Qiao P, Han Z, Shen Q, Jia Y. Application of continuous epidural anesthesia in transforaminal lumbar endoscopic surgery: a prospective randomized controlled trial. J Int Med Res. 2019; 47(3):1146–1153
[42] Wahood W, Yolcu Y, Alvi MA, Goyal A, Long TR, Bydon M. Assessing the differences in outcomes between general and non-general anesthesia in spine surgery: results from a national registry. Clin Neurol Neurosurg. 2019; 180:79–86

6 Paravertebral Blocks for Lumbar Spine

Armaan R. Patel, Nabil Matmati, and Vijay Yanamadala

Abstract

Paravertebral blocks (PVBs) represent an important advancement in regional anesthesia, being more precise and localized with fewer systemic side effects compared to more traditional techniques like epidural and general anesthesia. The objectives of this review are to describe the various techniques for cervical, thoracic, lumbar, and sacral PVB, including their indications, advantages, and complications, and also to evaluate the role of PVBs in providing unilateral somatic and sympathetic nerve blockade with minimal motor block, thereby facilitating early postoperative mobilization. Prone, lateral decubitus, and sitting are some of the positions in which patients can be placed before undergoing PVBs. Success with the block usually depends on the position used and varies with respect to the surgical site and, therefore, access. A combination of long-acting local anesthetics such as bupivacaine, ropivacaine, and lidocaine with adjuvants like dexamethasone and epinephrine prolongs analgesia. Improved accuracy with needle placement, as a result of advances in ultrasound guidance, ensures that complications such as pleural puncture and local anesthetic systemic toxicity are minimized. Fortunately, complications such as incomplete blocks, nerve injury, and catheter misplacement have been minimized by modern techniques. The importance of ongoing research, provider education, and refinement of techniques in order to optimize outcomes cannot be overemphasized. As new clinical applications emerge and techniques continue to evolve, PVBs will most likely continue to play an increasing role in perioperative pain management within an ever-broadening base of surgical specialties.

Keywords: paravertebral block, regional anesthesia, cervical block, thoracic block, lumbar block, sacral block, ultrasound-guided anesthesia, postoperative analgesia, pain management, patient preparation

Key Points

- Paravertebral blocks (PVBs) provide selective anesthesia for spinal nerve roots, enabling effective pain control while preserving motor function and minimizing bilateral side effects like hypotension and urinary retention.
- Lumbar PVBs target the quadratus lumborum and psoas major muscles, making them especially valuable in lumbar spine and hip surgeries that demand precise, segmental analgesia.
- Ultrasound guidance improves procedural safety by clearly visualizing anatomical landmarks, reducing risks such as dural puncture, vascular injury, and inaccurate anesthetic spread.
- Continuous infusion catheters placed in the paravertebral space allow extended postoperative pain management, reducing opioid use and supporting early mobilization.
- Appropriate patient education—including expected benefits, positioning, and procedural risks—is critical to ensure patient cooperation and enhance outcomes in PVB administration.

6.1 Introduction

Paravertebral blocks (PVBs) have solidified their role as a cornerstone technique in regional anesthesia, especially in surgeries that demand precise and effective pain management with minimal systemic impact. These blocks have evolved significantly over the years, providing a targeted approach that anesthetizes specific spinal nerve roots and adjacent tissues, thus enabling effective pain control without the widespread motor or sympathetic block associated with more traditional methods.[1,2]

The rationale behind PVBs lies in their ability to offer localized anesthesia by injecting local anesthetics near the spinal nerves as they emerge from the intervertebral foramina. This process allows the anesthetic to cover a series of dermatomes on one side of the body, creating both somatic and sympathetic nerve blocks. Such focused anesthesia is particularly advantageous for surgeries that require unilateral analgesia, allowing for better pain management and reducing the risk of bilateral side effects like hypotension, motor weakness, and urinary retention that are often seen with epidural anesthesia.[3,4,5]

Historically, epidural anesthesia has been the mainstay for providing extensive analgesia, particularly in thoracic and abdominal surgeries. However, the broad and sometimes unpredictable nature of epidural anesthesia can result in significant bilateral motor block, increased risk of hypotension, and urinary retention. These drawbacks, along with the potential for more serious complications like epidural hematoma and infection, have contributed to the growing preference for PVBs in certain surgical populations. PVBs offer several distinct advantages, including a reduced risk of systemic side effects, decreased incidence of postoperative nausea and vomiting, and the preservation of motor function, which is crucial for early postoperative mobilization and overall recovery.[5,6]

PVBs are incredibly versatile and applicable across a wide range of surgical specialties, including thoracic, abdominal, breast, and spine surgeries. Their efficacy in providing targeted pain relief with minimal systemic impact has made them particularly beneficial in lumbar spine surgery, where precise pain control is essential for optimizing patient recovery. Compared to general anesthesia, which often requires higher doses of anesthetics and analgesics, PVBs provide effective pain relief with lower dosages of local anesthetics such as bupivacaine and ropivacaine, as well as reduced reliance on systemic opioids like morphine or fentanyl, thereby reducing the risk of anesthesia-related complications, particularly in patients with multiple comorbidities or those who are sensitive to systemic opioids.[7,8]

In lumbar spine surgeries, where postoperative pain can significantly hinder recovery, PVBs have been shown to effectively reduce pain scores, minimize opioid consumption, and decrease the incidence of chronic postoperative pain syndromes. Moreover, the advent of ultrasound-guided techniques has significantly enhanced the precision and safety of PVBs, minimizing the risks associated with blind or landmark-based techniques and ensuring that the anesthetic is delivered accurately to the targeted nerves. This precision is particularly important in complex surgeries where pain management plays a critical role in patient outcomes and overall recovery.[9,10]

The following sections will explore the various types of PVBs—cervical, thoracic, lumbar, and sacral—providing an in-depth discussion of their respective techniques, muscle targets, applications, benefits, drawbacks, and specific considerations for their use in different surgical contexts.

6.2 Paravertebral Blocks

6.2.1 Cervical Blocks

Technique and Muscle Targets

Cervical PVBs are employed in surgeries involving the neck, upper thoracic regions, and occasionally the upper limbs.

- These blocks target the cervical nerve roots (C1–C8), which are situated deep to the anterior and middle scalene muscles.
- The procedure typically involves the use of ultrasound guidance to ensure accurate needle placement between these muscles, thereby minimizing the risk of complications such as inadvertent vascular puncture or nerve injury.
- The patient is generally positioned in a supine position with the head turned slightly away from the side being blocked, allowing for optimal exposure of the neck.
- Ultrasound is used to visualize the cervical nerve roots as they emerge from the intervertebral foramina, as well as the surrounding vasculature, which must be carefully avoided during needle insertion.[6,11]

Expert Tip

For cervical PVBs, accurate ultrasound visualization of the cervical nerve roots is crucial. Rotate the patient's head slightly away from the block side for optimal exposure, and use in-plane needle guidance to prevent inadvertent puncture of nearby vascular structures.

- In terms of muscle targets, the cervical PVB focuses on the anterior and middle scalene muscles, which play a crucial role in the blockade of the cervical nerve roots.
- The needle is inserted in-plane with the ultrasound probe, typically using a posterior approach, to deposit the local anesthetic adjacent to the cervical nerve roots.
- This technique not only provides effective analgesia but also preserves respiratory function by avoiding the phrenic nerve, which is responsible for diaphragmatic movement (▶ Fig. 6.1).[12,13]
- Advanced techniques in cervical PVBs may involve the use of nerve stimulation to confirm correct needle placement before anesthetic injection.
- This method is particularly useful in patients with complex cervical anatomy or in situations where ultrasound guidance alone may not provide sufficient visualization of the nerve roots.
- The use of nerve stimulation can help ensure that the anesthetic is delivered precisely where it is needed, thereby enhancing the effectiveness of the block and reducing the risk of complications.

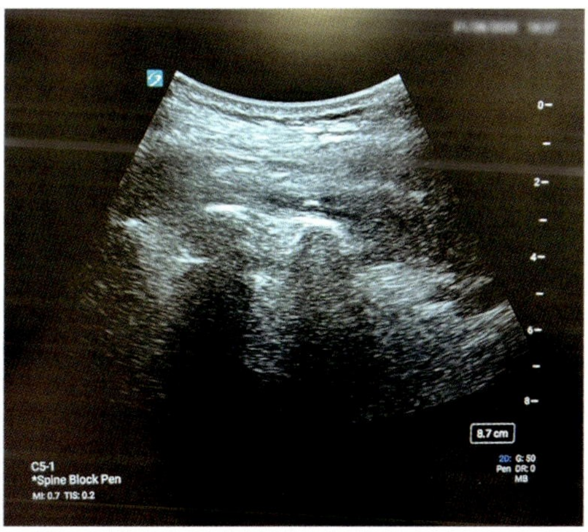

Fig. 6.1 Cervical erector spinae plane block administration with the needle inserted and anesthetic expansion. Ultrasound image demonstrating needle placement (hyperechoic linear structure) in the cervical region for an erector spinae plane block. Anesthetic expansion is visible as a hypoechoic spread within the fascial plane. Depth markers in centimeters are shown on the right.

Summary of Procedure

- The cervical PVB is performed with the patient in a supine position, with the neck slightly extended and rotated away from the side of the block.
- After aseptic preparation of the area, a high-frequency linear ultrasound probe is placed transversely over the lateral neck to identify the relevant cervical vertebrae and nerve roots.
- The needle is inserted using an in-plane approach, with the ultrasound providing real-time guidance to ensure accurate placement adjacent to the nerve roots (▶ Fig. 6.2).
- The local anesthetic is then injected in incremental doses to achieve the desired level of blockade.
- In some cases, a continuous catheter may be placed for prolonged analgesia, particularly in patients undergoing extensive neck or upper thoracic surgery.
- The catheter allows for continuous infusion of local anesthetic, providing sustained pain relief for up to several days postoperatively.
- This technique is especially beneficial in reducing the need for systemic opioids, which can have significant side effects in this patient population.[6,11]

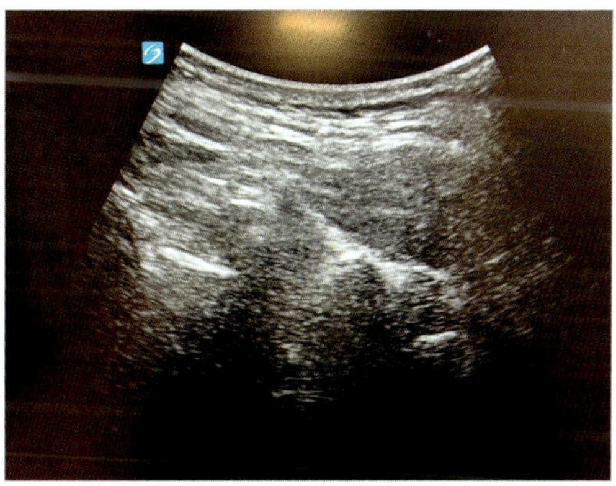

Fig. 6.2 Cervical erector spinae plane block administration with the needle inserted. Ultrasound image showing needle placement (hyperechoic linear structure) within the cervical region for an erector spinae plane block. The needle is positioned in the fascial plane near the target structures, with surrounding tissue visualization.

Patient Preparation

- Patient preparation is crucial for the success of a cervical PVB.
- The patient is usually positioned supine with the neck turned away from the side to be blocked, but the procedure can also be performed in the prone position if necessary to accommodate specific surgical requirements.[14]
- The neck area is thoroughly cleansed with an antiseptic solution and draped in a sterile manner.
- The patient is instructed to remain still during the procedure, as any movement could compromise the accuracy of the needle placement. Sedation may be administered to enhance patient comfort and cooperation, particularly in the cases where anxiety or discomfort is anticipated.
- In addition to physical preparation, patients should be educated about the procedure, including its benefits, risks, and what to expect during and after the block. This education helps alleviate anxiety and ensures patient cooperation during the procedure.
- Informed consent should be obtained after a thorough discussion of the potential risks, including nerve injury, hematoma formation, and the rare but serious risk of phrenic nerve palsy.[15,16]

Type of Medication Used and Duration

- Local anesthetics commonly used for cervical PVBs include bupivacaine (0.25–0.5% solution, 50–150 mg), ropivacaine (0.2–0.5% solution, 40–200 mg), and lidocaine (1–2% solution, < 300 mg). Bupivacaine is favored for its long duration of action, typically lasting between 12 and 24 hours, which is beneficial for extended postoperative pain relief.
- Ropivacaine, another long-acting anesthetic, is often chosen for its lower cardiotoxicity compared to bupivacaine. Adjuvants such as dexamethasone are frequently added to prolong the duration of the block and enhance analgesic efficacy.
- The effects of the block can be extended up to 24 hours with the appropriate use of these adjuvants.[12,13]
- In the cases where prolonged analgesia is required, a continuous infusion of local anesthetic via a catheter can be used. This approach allows for ongoing pain control without the need for repeated injections, making it ideal for complex or extended surgical procedures.
- The choice of anesthetic and adjuvants can be tailored to the specific needs of the patient, taking into account factors such as comorbidities, potential drug interactions, and the expected duration of surgery.[6,11]

Benefits and Drawbacks

- Cervical PVBs offer significant analgesia for neck and upper thoracic surgeries with minimal impact on respiratory function, making them ideal for patients with preexisting respiratory conditions.
- The technique allows for selective blockade, which is particularly advantageous in surgeries that require preserved diaphragmatic function. However, potential complications include phrenic nerve palsy, which can result in diaphragmatic paralysis, and inadvertent vascular puncture, which may lead to hematoma formation or other vascular complications.
- The use of ultrasound guidance has significantly reduced these risks by providing real-time visualization of the relevant anatomy.[4,10]
- Additional considerations include the potential for incomplete block, particularly in patients with complex or variant cervical anatomy. In such cases, the use of adjunctive techniques, such as nerve stimulation or the placement of a continuous catheter, may be necessary to achieve effective analgesia.
- Despite these challenges, the benefits of cervical PVBs in appropriate patients and procedures often outweigh the potential risks, particularly when performed by experienced practitioners.[6,11]

6.2.2 Thoracic Blocks

Technique and Muscle Targets

- Thoracic PVBs are frequently used in thoracic surgeries such as mastectomies, thoracotomies, and rib fracture management.

- These blocks involve the injection of local anesthetic near the thoracic spinal nerves (T1–T12), which are located deep to the intercostal muscles and the paravertebral muscles of the thoracic spine.
- The technique can be performed with the patient in a sitting or lateral decubitus position, depending on the surgeon's preference and the patient's anatomy.
- Ultrasound guidance is often employed to enhance the precision of the needle placement, although landmark-based techniques can also be used effectively.[1,5]
- In performing the thoracic PVB, the ultrasound probe is placed transversely to identify the transverse process of the thoracic vertebra and the associated pleura.
- The needle is then advanced in-plane with the ultrasound probe to reach the paravertebral space, just lateral to the vertebral body.
- The intercostal muscles, which are critical in respiratory function, are also targeted to ensure adequate analgesia across the thoracic dermatomes.
- The precise placement of the needle is crucial to avoid complications such as pleural puncture and pneumothorax, both of which are significant risks associated with this block.[9,10]

Expert Tip

To avoid pleural puncture during thoracic PVB, maintain a shallow needle angle when advancing toward the paravertebral space. Confirm the needle position with ultrasound before injecting to ensure safe delivery of the anesthetic and avoid complications.

- For more complex thoracic surgeries, such as those involving extensive thoracotomy or multiple rib fractures, a continuous infusion technique may be employed. This involves the placement of a catheter in the paravertebral space, allowing for continuous administration of local anesthetic over several days. This approach provides sustained analgesia, reduces the need for systemic opioids, and enhances patient comfort, particularly during the critical early postoperative period.[6,8]

Summary of Procedure

- The thoracic PVB is typically performed with the patient in a sitting or lateral decubitus position.
- The area is prepped and draped in a sterile fashion, and a high-frequency ultrasound probe is used to locate the transverse process of the thoracic vertebra.
- The needle is inserted in-plane with the ultrasound probe, just lateral to the vertebral body, and local anesthetic is injected to block the intercostal nerves at the desired levels.
- This technique provides unilateral analgesia across several thoracic dermatomes, which is particularly beneficial in thoracic surgeries where extensive pain management is required (▶ Fig. 6.3).
- In some cases, the thoracic PVB may be combined with other regional anesthesia techniques, such as epidural anesthesia, to provide more comprehensive pain control.
- This combined approach is particularly useful in patients undergoing extensive thoracic or upper abdominal surgeries, where multimodal analgesia is essential for optimal pain management and recovery.[5,6]

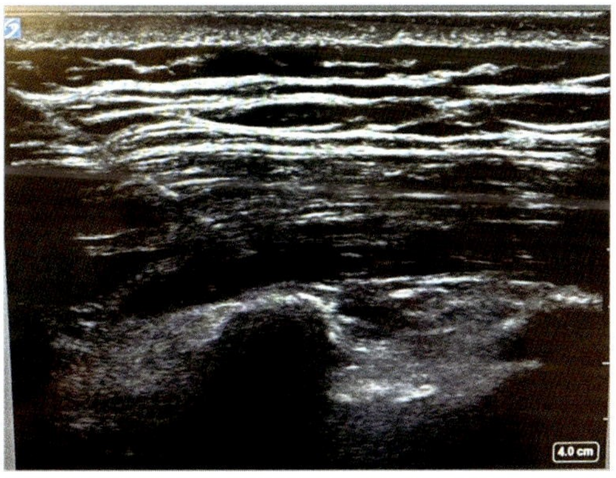

Fig. 6.3 Thoracic erector spinae plane block administration with the needle inserted. Ultrasound image depicting needle placement (hyperechoic linear structure) in the thoracic region for an erector spinae plane block. The needle is positioned within the fascial plane adjacent to the target structures, with surrounding musculature and bony landmarks visible. Depth scale is shown on the right.

Patient Preparation

- The patient is typically positioned in the lateral decubitus or sitting position, though the prone position is also a viable option depending on the surgical setup and access requirements.[14]
- The back is thoroughly cleansed with an antiseptic solution and draped in a sterile manner.
- The patient is instructed to remain still during the procedure to facilitate accurate needle placement. Sedation may be provided to ensure patient comfort and reduce anxiety, especially in the cases where prolonged positioning is required.
- Preprocedural education is also important to ensure patient cooperation and understanding of the procedure. Patients should be informed about the benefits and risks of the thoracic PVB, as well as what to expect during and after the procedure. This includes discussing potential complications, such as pleural puncture, pneumothorax, and systemic toxicity, as well as the steps that will be taken to minimize these risks.[6,11]

Type of Medication Used and Duration

- For thoracic PVBs, long-acting local anesthetics such as ropivacaine (0.2–0.5% solution, 40–200 mg) and bupivacaine (0.25–0.5% solution, 50–150 mg) are commonly used. These anesthetics provide prolonged analgesia, with effects lasting between 12 and 18 hours. In some cases, adjuvants such as clonidine or dexamethasone are added to the anesthetic solution to enhance the duration and quality of the block.
- The use of continuous infusion techniques, such as with a catheter, can further extend the duration of analgesia, making it particularly useful in managing postoperative pain in thoracic surgeries.[6,11]
- In addition to local anesthetics, adjunctive medications such as opioids or nonsteroidal anti-inflammatory drugs (NSAIDs) may be administered to enhance analgesia.
- This multimodal approach to pain management is particularly beneficial in patients undergoing extensive thoracic surgery, where effective pain control is critical to reducing postoperative complications and facilitating recovery.[8,10]

Benefits and Drawbacks

- Thoracic PVBs offer significant pain relief for thoracic surgeries, reducing the need for systemic opioids and enhancing postoperative recovery by allowing for better respiratory function.
- The block is particularly beneficial in patients undergoing thoracotomy, one of the most painful surgical procedures, as it reduces the stress response to surgery and minimizes the risk of pulmonary complications such as atelectasis and pneumonia. However, the main risks associated with thoracic PVBs include the potential for pleural puncture, which can lead to pneumothorax, and the possibility of systemic toxicity if the local anesthetic is absorbed rapidly into the bloodstream.
- The use of ultrasound guidance and careful technique is essential in minimizing these risks.[9,10]
- Additional considerations include the potential for incomplete block, particularly in patients with complex thoracic anatomy or in the cases where the block is performed at multiple levels. In such situations, the use of adjunctive techniques, such as continuous catheter infusion or the combination of PVB with epidural anesthesia, may be necessary to achieve effective pain relief. Despite these challenges, thoracic PVBs remain a valuable tool in the anesthesiologist's arsenal, particularly when performed by experienced practitioners.[5,6]

6.2.3 Lumbar Blocks

Technique and Muscle Targets

- Lumbar PVBs are widely used in lumbar spine surgeries, lower abdominal surgeries, and hip surgeries.
- These blocks target the lumbar nerve roots (L1–L5), providing analgesia to the lower back, abdomen, and lower limbs.
- The quadratus lumborum muscle and the psoas major muscle are key targets in this block, as they play a crucial role in the lumbar plexus.
- The procedure is typically performed with the patient in a lateral decubitus or prone position,

with ultrasound guidance employed to enhance the accuracy of needle placement.
- The ultrasound probe is used to visualize the transverse processes, the quadratus lumborum, and the psoas major muscle, allowing for precise needle placement in the lumbar paravertebral space.[7,9]

Expert Tip

When performing lumbar PVB, positioning the patient in the lateral decubitus or prone position can stabilize the lumbar region, enhancing access to the transverse processes and ensuring optimal ultrasound visualization for precise anesthetic delivery.

- The lumbar PVB can be performed using either a single-shot technique or a continuous infusion technique with the placement of a catheter. The latter is particularly useful in surgeries where prolonged postoperative pain management is required.
- The needle is inserted in-plane with the ultrasound probe, advancing through the muscle layers until it reaches the lumbar paravertebral space.
- The anesthetic is then deposited around the lumbar nerve roots, providing effective pain relief while preserving motor function, which is crucial for early mobilization and rehabilitation.[5,13]
- Advanced techniques in lumbar PVBs may involve the use of fluoroscopic guidance, particularly in patients with complex lumbar anatomy or previous spinal surgeries. This imaging modality provides an additional layer of precision, allowing for accurate needle placement and reducing the risk of complications such as nerve injury or dural puncture.
- Fluoroscopy can also be used to confirm the spread of the anesthetic within the paravertebral space, ensuring effective analgesia across the targeted dermatomes.[6,8]

Summary of Procedure

- The lumbar PVB is performed with the patient in a lateral or prone position, depending on the surgical approach (Video 6.1).
- The back is prepped and draped in a sterile manner, and an ultrasound probe is used to identify the transverse processes and the paravertebral space.
- The needle is inserted under ultrasound guidance, with real-time visualization ensuring accurate placement near the lumbar nerve roots. Local anesthetic is then injected to achieve the desired level of blockade, providing unilateral analgesia to the lower back, abdomen, and lower extremities.
- In some cases, the lumbar PVB may be combined with other regional anesthesia techniques, such as transversus abdominis plane (TAP) block and femoral nerve block, to provide more comprehensive pain control.
- This combined approach is particularly useful in patients undergoing extensive lower abdominal or pelvic surgeries, where multimodal analgesia is essential for optimal pain management and recovery.[5,13]

Patient Preparation

- Patients are most often positioned in the lateral decubitus or prone position for better access to the lumbar region, but the prone position may be preferred for certain surgeries.[14]
- The area is draped in a sterile fashion, and the patient is instructed to remain still during the procedure. Sedation may be administered to ensure patient comfort and to minimize movement during needle insertion.
- In addition to physical preparation, patients should be educated about the procedure, including its benefits, risks, and what to expect during and after the block. This education helps alleviate anxiety and ensures patient cooperation during the procedure. Informed consent should be obtained after a thorough discussion of the potential risks, including nerve injury, dural puncture, and the rare but serious risk of epidural hematoma.[6,11]

Type of Medication Used and Duration

- Commonly used anesthetics for lumbar PVBs include bupivacaine (0.25–0.5% solution, 50–150 mg), ropivacaine (0.2–0.5% solution, 40–200 mg), and occasionally lidocaine (1–2% solution, < 300 mg), depending on the required duration of anesthesia.

- Bupivacaine is favored for its prolonged duration of action, typically lasting between 12 and 24 hours. Ropivacaine is another popular choice due to its lower risk of cardiotoxicity. In some cases, epinephrine (~5 µg/mL) is added to prolong the duration of the block and reduce systemic absorption.
- Adjuvants such as dexamethasone (4–10 mg/mL) are also commonly used to extend the duration of the block and enhance analgesic efficacy.[4,5]
- In patients requiring prolonged postoperative pain management, a continuous infusion of local anesthetic via a catheter may be used. This approach allows for ongoing pain control without the need for repeated injections, making it ideal for complex or extended surgical procedures.
- The choice of anesthetic and adjuvants can be tailored to the specific needs of the patient, taking into account factors such as comorbidities, potential drug interactions, and the expected duration of surgery.[6,9]

Benefits and Drawbacks

- Lumbar PVBs are particularly beneficial in lumbar spine and lower abdominal surgeries, offering significant pain relief while preserving motor function, which is crucial for early mobilization. This allows for faster recovery and reduced hospital stays.
- The block is also effective in managing postoperative pain in hip surgeries, where early mobilization is essential for ensuring the block adequately covers the pelvic region, particularly in surgeries like proctectomies and lower limb procedures.
- The sacral block is typically performed with ultrasound guidance, which helps identify the sacral hiatus—a key landmark for this injection.
- Given the complexity of the pelvic anatomy, accurate placement of the needle in the sacral canal is crucial to avoid nerve damage and ensure effective anesthesia.

6.2.4 Sacral Blocks

Summary of Procedure

- The sacral PVB is performed with the patient in the prone position.
- The lower back is disinfected and draped in a sterile manner. An ultrasound probe is positioned over the sacrum to locate the sacral cornua and the sacral hiatus, through which the needle will be introduced.
- The needle is carefully guided to the target area where the local anesthetic is deposited.
- This block is often used for analgesia in surgeries involving the pelvic floor, lower limbs, and perineal area, providing significant pain relief without extensive motor block, which is crucial for early postoperative mobilization.

Patient Preparation

- Thorough patient preparation is vital for a successful sacral block.
- The prone position is commonly used, allowing for optimal access to the sacral hiatus, although other positions may be employed depending on the surgical context.[14]
- The sacral area is cleaned and draped to maintain sterility. Patients are typically given mild sedation to ensure comfort and minimize movement during the procedure.
- It is important to educate patients about the procedure to help reduce anxiety and ensure cooperation. They should be informed of the potential sensations they might experience during the injection, such as pressure or a brief sting, and reassured about the measures taken to minimize discomfort.

Type of Medication Used and Duration

- For sacral blocks, long-acting local anesthetics such as bupivacaine and ropivacaine are preferred due to their duration and effectiveness.
- The addition of adjuvants like epinephrine or dexamethasone can prolong the effects of the block, typically ensuring analgesia for 12 to 24 hours postprocedure.
- In procedures requiring prolonged pain management, a continuous infusion catheter may be placed, allowing for extended delivery of the anesthetic.

Benefits and Drawbacks

- The sacral PVB is highly effective for managing perioperative pain in lower extremity, pelvic, and perineal surgeries. It offers the advantage of

targeted pain relief without significant impacts on motor function, facilitating early postoperative rehabilitation.
- However, the technique requires precise needle placement to avoid complications such as nerve damage and inadequate block coverage.
- The anatomical variability of the sacral region can pose challenges, making ultrasound guidance a critical component of the procedure.

6.3 Safety Issues

The administration of PVBs, while highly effective, carries potential risks that must be carefully managed to ensure patient safety. The most common concerns involve the risk of local anesthetic systemic toxicity (LAST), nerve injury, and inadvertent puncture of adjacent structures.

6.3.1 Local Anesthetic Systemic Toxicity

LAST is a serious complication associated with the accidental intravascular injection of local anesthetic. Symptoms can range from mild, such as metallic taste and tinnitus, to severe, including seizures, cardiac arrhythmias, and cardiac arrest. The risk of LAST can be minimized through the use of ultrasound guidance to avoid vascular structures, careful monitoring of anesthetic dosage, and readiness to manage complications should they arise.

Expert Tip

To minimize the risk of LAST, administer incremental doses of anesthetic, observing patient reactions after each injection. Ensure lipid emulsion is on hand to address any rapid-onset symptoms such as seizures or cardiac irregularities, which are critical to manage immediately.

6.3.2 Nerve Injury

While rare, nerve damage can occur if the needle directly injures a nerve or if the local anesthetic is injected directly into the nerve sheath. This risk is mitigated by the use of ultrasound guidance, which allows for real-time visualization of the needle's path and the surrounding nerves.

Expert Tip

Using ultrasound guidance and slow needle advancement significantly reduces the risk of nerve injury during PVB. Real-time imaging allows you to avoid direct nerve contact and monitor the spread of the anesthetic, ensuring safer, more effective blocks.

6.3.3 Inadvertent Puncture

The risk of puncturing adjacent structures such as the pleura in thoracic blocks and the dura mater in lumbar and sacral blocks remains a concern. These risks can lead to complications like pneumothorax or dural puncture, which may result in prolonged recovery or additional interventions. Using ultrasound and adhering to precise anatomical guidelines can significantly reduce these risks.

6.4 Conclusion

PVBs offer numerous advantages over traditional methods such as epidural anesthesia and general anesthesia, which tend to have broader systemic effects like hypotension, urinary retention, and significant motor block. In contrast, PVBs provide localized pain relief, reducing the need for opioids and allowing faster mobilization with fewer side effects.

Cervical PVBs enable precise pain control in neck and upper thoracic surgeries without compromising respiratory function, using an elective targeting of the cervical nerve roots, making them particularly useful in patients with respiratory comorbidities. The ability to block specific dermatomes while preserving diaphragmatic function is a major advantage.

Thoracic PVBs are frequently employed in thoracic surgeries, such as mastectomies and rib fractures, providing effective analgesia while avoiding the complications of thoracic epidurals, like bilateral motor block or hypotension. By limiting the block to the necessary dermatomes, patients experience improved respiratory function, reduced risk of pneumonia, and lower rates of chronic postsurgical pain.

In **lumbar PVBs**, the targeted analgesia for lumbar spine or hip surgeries allows for excellent pain relief with preserved motor function. This enables early mobilization and reduces the length of hospital stays. By decreasing reliance on systemic opioids, lumbar PVBs also help mitigate opioid-related complications such as nausea, constipation, and addiction.

As techniques evolve, especially with advancements in ultrasound guidance, the precision, safety, and efficacy of PVBs will continue to improve. Ongoing education for anesthesia providers on these evolving techniques and safety protocols, combined with research into optimal anesthetic combinations and adjuvant therapies, ensures that PVBs remain a cornerstone of perioperative pain management across various patient populations.

References

[1] D'Ercole F, Arora H, Kumar PA. Paravertebral block for thoracic surgery. Curr Anesthesiol Rep. 2018; 8(3):299–306

[2] Thavaneswaren J, Rudkin GE, Graham SE, et al. Systematic review of paravertebral blocks for anesthesia. Anaesth Intensive Care. 2010; 38(4):654–660

[3] Chelly JE. Paravertebral blocks. Curr Opin Anaesthesiol. 2012; 25(5):501–507

[4] Ardon AE, Mellender SJ, Blasi R, et al. Paravertebral block: anatomy and relevant safety issues. Reg Anesth Pain Med. 2020; 45(4):292–299

[5] Boezaart AP, Koorn R, Rosenquist RW, et al. Paravertebral block: cervical, thoracic, lumbar, and sacral. Pain Med. 2009; 10(7):1189–1194

[6] Qiu Y, Zhang TJ, Hua Z. Erector spinae plane block for lumbar spinal surgery: a systematic review. J Pain Res. 2020; 13: 1611–1619

[7] Nair A, Sharma S, Prabhakar H, et al. Paravertebral blocks and novel alternatives. Curr Opin Anaesthesiol. 2020; 33(5): 621–627

[8] Brandão MP, Oliveira JN, Filho C, et al. Lumbar erector spinae plane block: successful control of acute pain after lumbar spine surgery: a clinical report. Braz J Anesthesiol. 2019; 69 (6):622–625

[9] Scarfe AJ, Schuhmann-Hingel S, Duncan JK, et al. Continuous paravertebral block for post-cardiothoracic surgery analgesia: a systematic review and meta-analysis. Eur J Anesthesiol. 2016; 33(12):867–871

[10] Pawa A, Weller R, Awad IT, et al. Paravertebral blocks: anatomical, practical, and future concepts. Anaesthesia. 2016; 71(5):478–488

[11] Pratheep K, Gupta R, Kushwah P, et al. Transient paraplegia in lumbar spine surgery: a potential complication following erector spinae plane block. Indian J Anaesth. 2022; 66(2): 169–171

[12] Weltz CR, Klein SM, Arbo JE, et al. Paravertebral block anesthesia for inguinal hernia repair. Anesth Analg. 2003; 96(2): 601–602

[13] Greengrass RA, Klein SM, D'Ercole F, et al. Paravertebral anaesthesia/analgesia for ambulatory surgery. Anesth Analg. 2002; 95(2):487–491

[14] Mandal MC, Das S, Gupta S, Ghosh TR, Basu SR. Paravertebral block can be an alternative to unilateral spinal anaesthesia for inguinal hernia repair. Indian J Anaesth. 2011; 55(6): 584–589

[15] Tighe PJ, Greene MD, Rajesh MS. Paravertebral block. Anesthesiol Clin. 2010; 28(4):677–704

[16] Singh S, Choudhary NK, Lalin D, et al. Bilateral ultrasound-guided erector spinae plane block for postoperative analgesia in lumbar spine surgery: a randomized control trial. Indian J Anaesth. 2020; 64(8):716–717

[17] Media of Cervical, Thoracic, and Lumbar Erector Spinae Plane Blocks. IAA Regional. 2025

7 Paravertebral Blocks for Cervical Spine

Debesh Bhoi, Ashwin M., and Sukriti Jha

Abstract

Cervical spine surgeries have become more common in recent times owing to an aging population, rising prevalence of degenerative cervical spine pathologies, and advances in imaging. General anesthesia is a necessity for these surgeries to take place. However, regional anesthesia techniques enhance quality and rate of recovery by offering effective pain relief and reducing the need for systemic opioids. Prominent techniques include fascial plane blocks and plexus blocks. Cervical erector spinae plane blocks and paraspinal interfascial plane blocks (including *multifidus cervicis plane block, inter-semispinal plane block*, and *retrolaminar blocks*) have been utilized to reduce opioid requirement without compromising neuromuscular monitoring. Cervical plexus blocks and paravertebral blocks have been used in other surgeries involving the neck like carotid endarterectomy and thyroid and parathyroid surgeries, as well as to alleviate chronic pain conditions. They have been successfully applied to spine surgeries at the cervical level. A combination of above-mentioned blocks may be adapted in spine programs to enhance recovery after surgery. This chapter explores the anatomy, techniques, clinical applications, and outcomes of these blocks in cervical spine surgeries, emphasizing their role in enhancing surgical outcomes and patient comfort.

Keywords: cervical spine surgery, cervical erector spinae plane block, cervical plexus block, paraspinal interfascial plane block, cervical paravertebral block

Key Points

- Paraspinal interfascial plane blocks (PIPBs) target the dorsal rami of the spinal nerves in the posterior neck by injecting local anesthetic into the interfascial plane.
- Three variants have been described: multifidus cervicis plane block, inter-semispinal plane block, and retrolaminar block.
- Major vessels (vertebral and carotid arteries) and spinal cord are remote from the site of injection, making it safer to perform these blocks.
- These block provide targeted pain relief without affecting intraoperative neuromonitoring.
- Cervical erector spinae plane (ESP) block involves depositing a local anesthetic deposited in the fascial plane between the erector spinae muscle and the transverse processes of the cervical vertebrae.
- The spread is extensive from the occiput to the upper thoracic region and the analgesic coverage is substantial due to injectate advancing to the paravertebral region and cervical nerve roots.
- Similar to PIPBs, the ESP block is preferred for analgesia due to its distance from vascular and neural structures.
- *Superficial cervical plexus block (CPB):* Subcutaneous injection at the posterior border of the sternocleidomastoid (SCM) muscle to block the superficial branches of the cervical plexus.
- *Intermediate CPB:* The needle is placed between the SCM muscle and the prevertebral fascia at the C4 level, which targets superficial branches as well as branches to the SCM muscle.
- *Deep CPB:* The needle is placed between the prevertebral fascia and cervical nerve roots at C2–C4 to target both superficial and deep branches of the cervical plexus simultaneously.
- Ultrasound guidance is recommended for intermediate and deep CPBs.
- It may provide complete anesthesia of the neck when combined with the fascial plane block.

7.1 Introduction

Cervical spine surgeries are becoming prevalent due to rising incidence of cervical spine pathologies. The pathologies treated include radiculopathy, myelopathy, instability caused by degeneration or trauma, infection, and tumors. Surgical strategies include decompression of neural elements and stabilization when necessary, through an anterior, posterior, or combined approach. These surgeries address conditions such as degenerative disk diseases and traumatic injuries, which are crucial for pain relief, restoring function, and preventing neurological deterioration. The incidence is rising due to an aging population, increased prevalence of degenerative spinal conditions, and advancements in diagnostic imaging.

Regional anesthetic techniques have significantly advanced the management of cervical spine surgeries by providing effective pain relief and minimizing the need for systemic opioids. Among these techniques, cervical erector spinae plane (ESP) blocks, paraspinal interfascial plane blocks (PIPBs), cervical plexus blocks (CPBs), and paravertebral blocks (PVBs) are prominent. This chapter delves into the anatomy, techniques, clinical applications, and outcomes of these blocks in cervical spine surgeries, highlighting their role in improving surgical outcomes and patient comfort.

7.2 Cervical Paraspinal Interfascial Plane Blocks

7.2.1 Introduction

Cervical PIPBs are a regional anesthetic technique that targets the dorsal rami of the spinal nerves. This method involves the injection of a local anesthetic (LA) into the interfascial plane between the muscles in the posterior neck.

Initially, the concept of interfascial plane blocks was applied to the thoracic and lumbar spine.[1,2] Following the success in these regions, the technique was adapted for the cervical spine. The first cervical interfascial plane block was reported in 2017, although the original article was later retracted. Subsequently, the multifidus cervicis plane (MCP) block was introduced, offering a new method for providing analgesia during cervical spine surgeries. Since then, two additional cervical blocks—the inter-semispinal plane (ISP) block in 2018 and the retrolaminar block in 2021—have been developed and described in the literature. These blocks have shown promise as alternatives to neuraxial blockade for various procedures.[3,4,5]

These blocks provide effective analgesia by targeting the interfascial planes between muscles in the posterior neck, ensuring motor function preservation. The significant advancements in ultrasound technology have facilitated the precise administration of these blocks, enhancing their efficacy and safety. Unlike traditional PVBs, where the injection site is close to the neuraxis, PIPBs are performed relatively farther from the spinal cord, making them simpler and safer to administer. This section will discuss three specific variants: the MCP block, the ISP block, and the retrolaminar block.

7.2.2 Relevant Anatomy

The cervical paraspinal region is composed of several critical muscles and nerves (▶ Fig. 7.1).

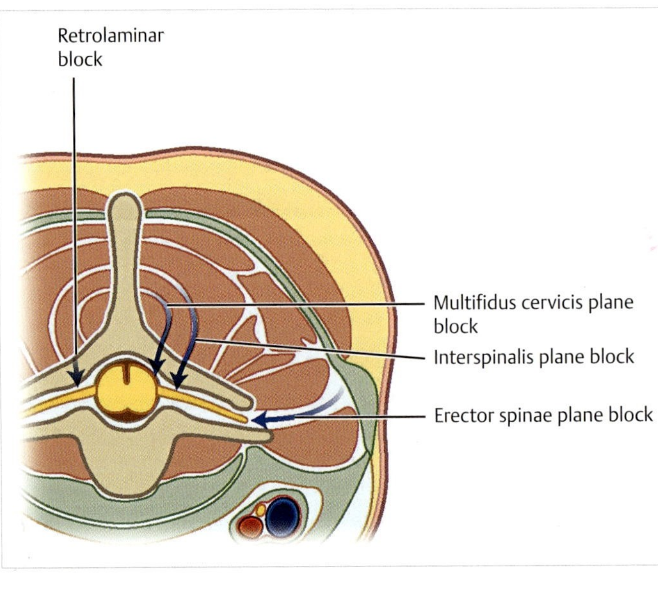

Fig. 7.1 Axial cross-section at the C6 vertebral level showing paraspinal muscles and interfascial planes. The *arrows* mark the fascial plane targets for drug deposition for multifidus cervicis plane block, inter-semispinal plane block, retrolaminar block, and erector spinae plane block. (Illustration created by Brenda L. Bunch, MA, MS/©Thieme.)

Key anatomical structures include the following:

- **Multifidus cervicis muscle:** It is situated deep within the posterior neck, adjacent to the cervical vertebrae, providing stability.
- **Semispinalis cervicis and semispinalis capitis:** It is positioned more superficially, running longitudinally along the spine and assisting in head and neck movement.
- **Dorsal rami of cervical spinal nerves:** These nerves exit the intervertebral foramina and traverse through the interfascial planes, innervating the muscles involved.

7.2.3 Technique

Expert Tip

Before proceeding for the block, place the patient prone in a comfortable position and do a prescan, identify relevant anatomical structures, and then prepare the required volume and concentration of the drug. Positioning the patient in a comfortable position will decrease the patient's anxiety and tolerance to undergo the block.

Multifidus Cervicis Plane Block

- **Patient positioning:** The patient is placed in the prone position. [3,4,5,6,7]
- **Ultrasound guidance:** Using a high-frequency linear transducer, the ultrasound probe is placed transversely over the cervical spine to identify the relevant anatomical landmarks, including the transverse processes (TPs) and multifidus cervicis muscle.
- **Needle insertion:** A 22-gauge needle is inserted in-plane with the ultrasound beam and advanced between the multifidus cervicis and semispinalis cervicis muscles.
- **Drug and dosage:** 0.25% ropivacaine is used, with a typical dosage of 10 mL each injected into the interfascial plane bilaterally (total volume of 20 mL).
- **Injection site:** The LA is delivered into the plane between the multifidus cervicis and semispinalis cervicis muscles, ensuring effective spread and analgesia.

Inter-Semi Spinal Plane Block/ Cervical Semispinalis Cervicis Plane Block

- This block involves injecting LA between the semispinalis cervicis and semispinalis capitis muscles. The patient is positioned in the same manner as for the MCP block.
- The ultrasound probe is placed transversely to visualize the semispinalis muscles.
- The needle is inserted in-plane and advanced into the ISP and LA is injected after confirming the needle's position.

Retrolaminar Block

- The retrolaminar block targets the space posterior to the lamina of the cervical vertebrae with the patient positioned prone as described previously.
- The needle is inserted in-plane and advanced until it contacts the lamina and LA is then injected posterior to the laminae (▸ Fig. 7.2).

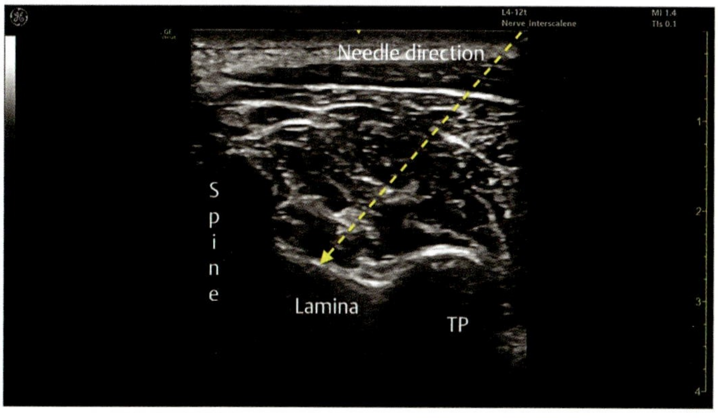

Fig. 7.2 Sonoanatomy of the cervical retrolaminar plane block. TP, transverse process.

7.2.4 Clinical Applications

Cervical Spine Surgeries Utilizing PIP Blocks

- Posterior cervical laminectomy.[7]
- Cervical laminoplasty.[4]

Additional Advantages

- *Intraoperative neuromonitoring:* Tseng et al[7] reported no adverse effects on somatosensory evoked potentials and motor evoked potentials with the use of PIP blocks, ensuring safe and effective pain management without compromising neurophysiologic monitoring.
- Reduced opioid consumption.
- Enhanced patient recovery and satisfaction.[3,7] due to better pain control and fewer complications.

7.2.5 Summary

PIP blocks, including the MCP block, ISP block, and retrolaminar block, provide targeted pain relief without affecting intraoperative neuromonitoring. These blocks enhance patient outcomes by reducing opioid consumption and facilitating faster recovery, making them a valuable addition to multimodal analgesia in cervical spine surgeries.

7.3 Cervical Erector Spinae Plane Block

Expert Tip

- *At the cervical level, the practitioner must identify the C6 posterior tubercle, C7 posterior tubercle, and the T1 tubercle during prescan. Understanding the relevant anatomy and sonographic appearance is critical for success.*
- *Before proceeding for the block, any vascular bridge must be excluded through the needle path as the neck area is highly vascular. Using the Doppler feature on ultrasound is helpful for identifying vascular anatomy.*

7.3.1 Introduction

The cervical ESP block involves the administration of LA into the fascial plane between the erector spinae muscle and the TPs of the cervical vertebrae. Initially described by Forero et al in 2016 for thoracic neuropathic pain, the ESP block was later adapted for the cervical region.[8] The first documented case of the cervical ESP block was reported by Chin et al in 2017, who demonstrated effective postoperative analgesia for surgery in the neck.[9]

Clinical studies and cadaveric investigations have validated the efficacy and safety of the cervical ESP block, demonstrating its advantages in reducing opioid consumption, enhancing recovery, and providing effective analgesia for a range of cervical spine procedures. This chapter will explore the detailed anatomy relevant to the cervical ESP block, the precise techniques for its administration, and its clinical applications, supported by key studies and clinical evidence.

7.3.2 Relevant Anatomy

The cervical ESP block involves the injection of LA into the fascial plane between the erector spinae muscle and the TPs of the cervical vertebrae (▸ Fig. 7.1).

Key anatomical structures relevant to this block include the following:

- **Erector spinae muscle:** It is a group of muscles located bilaterally along the spine, including the spinalis, longissimus, and iliocostalis muscles. In the cervical region, the relevant muscles are the spinalis cervicis, longissimus cervicis, and iliocostalis cervicis.
- **TPs:** These are bony projections from the sides of the cervical vertebrae, serving as landmarks for needle insertion and spread of LA.
- **Fascial plane:** The target plane for LA injection lies between the erector spinae muscle and the TPs.

The spread of LA in the cervical ESP block extends craniocaudally from the occiput to the upper thoracic levels. According to Diwan et al,[10] the injectate spreads along the dorsal rami, paravertebral space, and dorsal to the ventral cervical roots, providing extensive analgesic coverage. This spread can be visualized using ultrasound, ensuring precise placement and effective analgesia without compromising motor function or intraoperative neuromonitoring.

Elsharkawy et al[11] conducted a dye spread test on five cadavers to assess the craniocaudal and mediolateral extent of spread when a cervical ESP block is administered at the C6 and C7 levels under ultrasound guidance. The dye consistently stained the C5, C6, and C7 roots deeply in all cadavers. Cranial spread was limited, with faint staining of C4 in only one cadaver (5%), while caudal spread showed 75% staining of C8 and 30% staining of T1 roots. The phrenic nerve was deeply stained in one sample and faintly in two others, highlighting the safety of the cervical ESP block. The dorsal rami area from C4 to T1 was stained in all samples, confirming widespread dye spread. Critical nerves associated with shoulder and cervical spine procedures, such as the long thoracic, dorsal scapular, and suprascapular nerves, were deeply stained, suggesting the potential of the ESP block for comprehensive analgesia. The study did not examine the epidural space or verify potential paravertebral and epidural spread. They concluded that ultrasound-guided cervical ESP injections at the C6 and C7 levels consistently stain the roots of the brachial plexus and dorsal rami. This study suggests that the cervical ESP block could effectively provide analgesia for patients undergoing shoulder and cervical spine surgeries.

7.4 Technique

The cervical ESP block is performed under ultrasound guidance to ensure precise needle placement and effective spread of LA. [9,12,13] The detailed steps of the technique are the following:

- **Patient positioning:** The patient is placed in the prone or lateral decubitus position with the head turned slightly away from the side to be blocked.
- **Preparation:** The area is cleaned and prepped using standard aseptic techniques.
- **Ultrasound guidance:** A high-frequency linear transducer (5–13 MHz) is placed transversely or longitudinally over the cervical spine to identify the TPs of the cervical vertebrae. The relevant structures such as the erector spinae muscle and the TPs are visualized (▶ Fig. 7.3, ▶ Fig. 7.4).
- **Needle insertion:** A 22-gauge, 80- to 100-mm needle is typically used. The needle is inserted

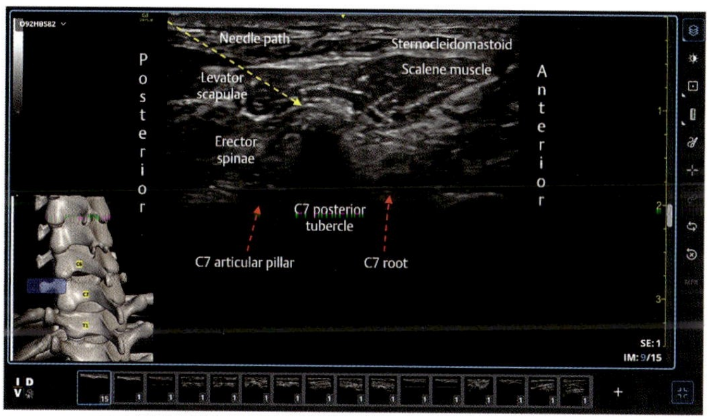

Fig. 7.3 Sonoanatomy of the cervical erector spinae block: transversely placed probe.

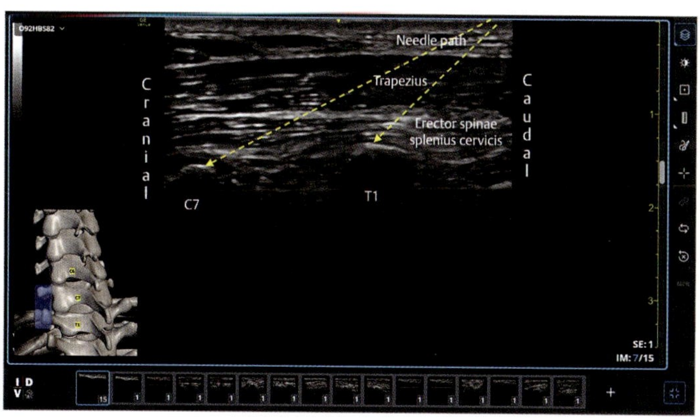

Fig. 7.4 Sonoanatomy of the cervical erector spinae plane block: longitudinally placed probe.

in-plane with the ultrasound beam and advanced until the tip is located in the fascial plane between the erector spinae muscle and the TPs. The needle position is confirmed by injecting a small amount of saline to ensure proper placement within the fascial plane.

- **Injection of LA:**
  - *Drug and dosage:* Typically, 15 to 20 mL of 0.25% bupivacaine or ropivacaine is used.
  - *Injection:* The LA is injected slowly with intermittent aspiration to avoid intravascular injection. The spread of the anesthetic is monitored in real time using ultrasound, ensuring it extends craniocaudally along the fascial plane.

Expert Tip

During final LA deposition, intermittent aspiration is of paramount importance to exclude intravascular injection and must ensure safe deposition after hydrodissection.

7.5 Clinical Applications of the Cervical ESP Block

The cervical ESP block is used for perioperative analgesia in both posterior and anterior cervical spine surgeries.

Cervical spine surgeries utilizing the cervical ESP block include the following:

- *Anterior cervical diskectomy and fusion (ACDF) surgeries.*[12,13] : These surgeries provide significant pain relief and reduce opioid consumption.
- *Posterior cervical decompression and fusion surgery:* In the study by Diwan et al,[14] four patients undergoing posterior cervical decompression and fusion surgery received bilateral continuous cervical ESP blocks at T1–T2.
- The ESP block provided intense analgesia, significantly reducing the need for perioperative anesthetic drugs and ensuring opioid-free postoperative pain management.
- Computed tomography (CT) contrast imaging shows extensive paravertebral spread of the LA, with no encroachment into the surgical field, allowing effective pain relief and stable hemodynamic conditions throughout the perioperative period.
- The block facilitated rapid recovery and tolerance of the endotracheal tube, with minimal need for additional analgesics postoperatively. These applications highlight the block's versatility and efficacy in managing postoperative pain across various cervical spine surgeries.

7.6 Potential Complications of the Cervical ESP Block

The cervical ESP block is generally considered safe, but it can be associated with some complications. The study by Kamel et al reported the following complication rates for patients who underwent cervical ESP blocks[12]:

- Nausea: 17.2%.
- Vomiting: 6.9%.
- Bradycardia: 10.3%.
- Hypotension: 10.3%.
- Phrenic paresis.
- Horner's syndrome.
- Unintended motor blockade.
- Local anesthetic systemic toxicity (LAST).

7.7 Cervical Paravertebral Block

7.7.1 Introduction

The cervical paravertebral block (CPVB) involves the injection of an LA into the paravertebral space, where spinal nerves exit the intervertebral foramen. Unlike thoracic and lumbar nerve roots, cervical nerves emerge above the vertebral bodies. This block has its history dating back to 1905, with significant advancements over the decades, including a notable modern approach described by Boezaart et al in 2003 for continuous paravertebral infusion.[15] Cervical paravertebral space also serves a window to posterior approach to brachial plexus.

7.7.2 Relevant Anatomy

Key anatomical structures for this block include the following:

- Cervical paravertebral space:
  - Located in the posterior triangle of the neck.
  - The floor of this triangle is formed by the deep cervical fascia, paravertebral muscles, and cervical vertebra.

- This space also contains various vascular structures, lymph nodes, and elements of the cervical and brachial plexus.[16]
- The proximity to the carotid sheath and neuraxis poses technical challenges and requires expertise. Clinicians should also be aware of the proximity of radicular arteries, which originate from the vertebral, ascending cervical, and deep cervical arteries, to the spinal nerves in this area.
- Since dural sleeves extend with the nerve roots into the paravertebral region, a risk of dural puncture and inadvertent intrathecal injection remains.
- The injectate is deposited close to the emergence of the spinal nerves, achieving a unilateral blockade of somatic and sympathetic nerves.

Expert Tip

When an LA injection is administered deep to the prevertebral fascia between C2 and C4 for a deep CPB, it is considered a PVB.

Similarly, a deep injection to the prevertebral fascia between C5 and C7 for the posterior approach to the interscalene brachial plexus also qualifies as a PVB.

7.7.3 Technique

The cervical paravertebral space can be accessed via the posterior triangle of the neck or posteriorly at the back of the neck. Landmark techniques may lead to disastrous complications; hence, ultrasound guidance is preferred.

- Approach from the back of the neck:
  Patient positioning: The patient is placed in a lateral decubitus or sitting position, with the nape of the neck exposed.
  Preparation: The area is cleaned and prepped using standard aseptic techniques.
  Ultrasound guidance:
  A high-frequency linear probe (5–13 MHz) is placed transversely on the nape of the neck.
  The spinous process, spinal canal, and lamina of the cervical vertebrae are identified.
  The probe is then moved laterally from the midline, identifying posterior elements such as muscle layers, lamina, interlaminar space, facet joint, and TPs at the same level.
  The carotid and vertebral arteries are identified with Doppler.
  Needle insertion: Under ultrasound guidance, an echogenic needle is inserted in-plane to the transducer, targeting the paravertebral space adjacent to the TP.
  Injection of LA: After confirming negative aspiration, 10 to 20 mL of LA is injected just lateral to the TP.
  Drug and dosage: 0.25% of bupivacaine or 0.2 to 0.375% ropivacaine is used.

Expert Tip

Drug deposition varies across studies, with some targeting the area between the prevertebral fascia and TP, while others deposit the drug after contacting the bony TP.[17,18,19,20]

This technique is relatively safe because the cervical foramen remains away from the needle path, and the vertebral artery can be easily identified using ultrasonography. The analgesic solution spreads to adjacent levels within the cervical region due to the open communication of the paravertebral space, allowing a single-level injection to produce the desired effect.

- Approach to cervical paravertebral space in the posterior triangle of the neck:
  - The technique is like the deep CPB, which is described later.

7.7.4 Clinical Use for Cervical Spine Surgery

Ultrasound-guided CPVB has primarily been used for pain management in cervicogenic headache, proving to be as effective as the fluoroscopic-guided technique.[19] It also offers the added benefit of identifying important vascular structures.

Chronic cervical pain conditions like radiculopathy and disk displacement also utilize CPVB.

> **Expert Tip**
>
> *It has not been used for postoperative pain management or as an anesthetic technique yet, probably due to familiarity with CPBs.*
>
> *Continuous LA infusion even in the paravertebral soft tissue in posterior cervical fusion procedures achieved lower pain scores and opioid use with improvement in multiple postoperative outcomes.*[23] *However, there are limited clinical studies to analyze the safety and efficacy of the procedure.*

7.7.5 Limitations and Complications

- Vertebral artery or carotid artery puncture.
- Hematoma and airway obstruction.
- Intravascular LA administration.
- Hypotension.
- Epidural/intrathecal injection.
- Spinal cord injection/injury.
- Phrenic nerve paresis.
- Ultrasound usage lowers the incidence of these complications.

7.8 Cervical Plexus Block

7.8.1 Introduction

The CPB targets the cervical plexus formed by the C1–C4 spinal nerves. It can be performed at three depths and is named as such: deep, intermediate, and superficial, each offering different levels of anesthesia and analgesia for various surgical procedures.

7.8.2 Relevant Anatomy

Cervical Plexus

The cervical plexus is located deep to the sternocleidomastoid (SCM) muscle between the longus capitis and middle scalene muscles, beneath the prevertebral fascia but not in the interscalene groove.

It comprises two nerve loops formed by the anterior spinal nerves from C2 to C4, giving off four superficial sensory branches:

- Lesser occipital (C2, C3).
- Great auricular (C2, C3).
- Transverse cervical (C2, C3).
- Supraclavicular nerves (C3, C4).

Course

- These branches run posteriorly, pierce the prevertebral fascia, and travel through the interfascial space between the SCM and prevertebral muscles to reach the skin and superficial neck structures.
- The ansa cervicalis, formed by fibers from C1–C3, supplies motor branches to the infrahyoid and SCM muscles. The anterior rami of C3 and C4 join C5 to form the phrenic nerve.
- The cervical plexus also connects with several cranial nerves and the sympathetic trunk.

7.8.3 Technique

Administering an LA injection deep to the prevertebral fascia between C2 and C4 for a deep CPB is classified as a PVB.

For the deep CPB performed at the C2–C4 levels, the needle is directed toward the TPs. Intermediate and superficial blocks are performed at shallower depths, targeting the deep cervical fascia layer. Ultrasound guidance enhances precision, with the LA injected after confirming needle placement (▶ Fig. 7.5, ▶ Fig. 7.6).

Intermediate and Deep Cervical Plexus Block

Patient position: The patient lies supine with the neck turned to define the SCM muscle.[18]

Preparation: The area is cleaned and prepped using standard aseptic techniques.

Ultrasound guidance:

A high-frequency linear probe (5–13 MHz) is placed transversely at the level of cricoid cartilage.

The posterior triangle of the neck is scanned.

The levator scapulae muscle (LSM) is visualized beneath the SCM muscle. The fascial band between these muscles and cervical TPs is identified.

Color Doppler can be used to locate the vertebral vessels.

Needle insertion:

Under ultrasound guidance (out-of-plane technique), a needle is advanced into the fascial band between the SCM and LSM muscles and drug is injected. This is the intermediate CPB.

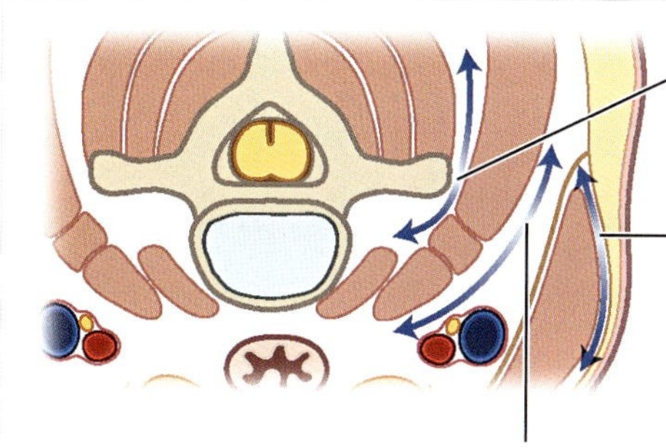

Fig. 7.5 Cross-section of the neck at the C4 vertebral level showing drug deposition in superficial, intermediate, and deep cervical plexus block. (Illustration created by Brenda L. Bunch, MA, MS/©Thieme.)

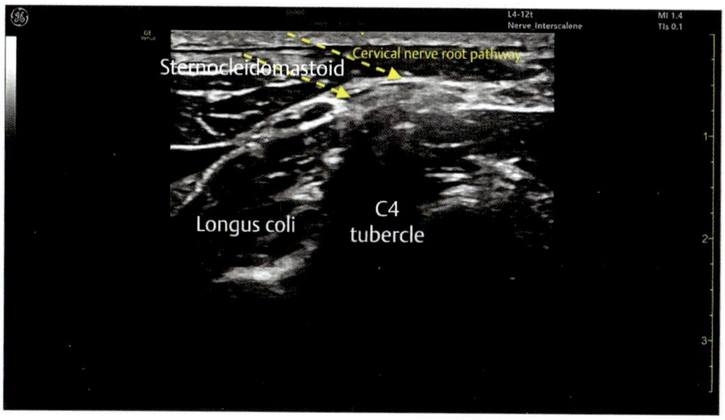

Fig. 7.6 Ultrasound-guided intermediate cervical plexus block.

The needle is then advanced between the levator scapulae and the hyperechoic contour of the cervical TP, and the same volume can be injected at this point, resulting in a deep CPB.

Injection of LA: After confirming negative aspiration, 10 to 20 mL of LA is injected just lateral to the TP.

Drug and dosage: 0.25% of bupivacaine or 0.2 to 0.375% of ropivacaine solution is used.

Superficial Cervical Plexus Block

Patient position: The patient lies supine with the neck turned to define the SCM muscle.

Preparation: The area is cleaned and prepped using standard aseptic techniques.

Ultrasound guidance:

A high-frequency linear transducer is placed transversely at the level of cricoid cartilage.

The SCM muscle is identified, and the transducer moved laterally until the tapered posterior edge of the SCM is centered on the screen.

At this point, the interscalene groove between the anterior and middle scalene muscles can be seen.

The cervical plexus appears as hypoechoic nodules beneath the SCM and resting on the deep cervical fascia.

Needle insertion

A 5-cm echogenic needle passes through the skin, platysma, and investing layer of the deep cervical fascia to place the tip adjacent to the plexus.

Given the shallow position of the target, both in-plane (from the medial or lateral sides) and out-of-plane approaches can be used.

Injection of LA: About 5 to 15 mL of drug is deposited to envelop the plexus.

Drug and dosage: 0.25% of bupivacaine or 0.2 to 0.375% ropivacaine is used.

The literature suggests that performing a deep CPB at a single level can also anesthetize adjacent levels. Boezaart et al demonstrated that injecting LA with contrast into the C4 paravertebral space extends the anesthetic from the base of the skull to the fifth cervical vertebra.[22] The technique of performing deep CPB with either one or multiple injection points is well-documented, showing comparable efficacy, with the primary difference being the time required to achieve an effective blockade with a single injection.

7.8.4 Clinical Use for Cervical Spine Surgery

- CPB has been used in ACDF and cervical arthroplasty, providing excellent pain control and allowing for intraoperative neurological monitoring. It is also utilized in carotid endarterectomy and thyroid surgeries.
- Superficial CPB has been used to provide analgesia in ACDF surgeries and thyroid and/or parathyroid surgeries.[23]
- Kamel et al conducted a randomized controlled trial comparing intermediate CPB and cervical ESP blocks in 58 patients undergoing anterior cervical spine surgery. Both groups received 15 mL of 0.25% bupivacaine at the designated site. Patients in the intermediate CPB group requested rescue analgesia significantly earlier than those in the ESP group. However, the intermediate CPB had shorter times for block performance and onset of effect, which were secondary outcomes. The authors concluded that intermediate and superficial CPBs affect the terminal sensory branches of the ventral rami of the C2–C4 spinal nerves and the C2–C4 dermatomes, without blocking the motor branches of the ventral rami C1–C4 or the dorsal rami supplying the posterior neck muscles. The cervical erector spinae muscles, which attach to the TPs of C2–C6, allow drug spread from the occiput to the upper thoracic levels.[12]
- Wang et al used a combination of superficial and deep CPB to facilitate awake single-level ACDF in 176 patients ($N = 356$). Although patients reported lesser satisfaction in the deep CPB group, pain control was significantly better when compared to the general anesthesia (GA) group. No case was converted to GA. The authors attributed lesser patient satisfaction to anxiety related to pressure on the trachea and esophagus during surgical manipulation. Intraoperative hemodynamics were better regulated in GA. Surgeon satisfaction did not differ significantly between groups.[24]

Expert Tip

Using CPB as the sole anesthetic technique offers benefits such as reduced anesthetic exposure, decreased opioid requirements, faster recovery, and less postoperative nausea and vomiting. However, there is an important caveat that conversion to GA may be necessary. Patients who incur high risk of morbidity or mortality if operated under GA can undergo surgery with CPB.

7.8.5 Limitations and Complications

Deep CPB has the potential to cause extreme complications, by the virtue of being in the vicinity of important structures. It should be regarded as a peridural block.

- Carotid and vertebral artery puncture.
- Hematoma and airway obstruction.
- Epidural injection.
- Dural puncture and intrathecal injection (may lead to cardiopulmonary arrest).
- Horner's syndrome.
- Phrenic nerve paresis.

7.9 Conclusion

Current evidence suggests that fascial plane blocks and plexus blocks could play crucial roles in multimodal analgesia and enhanced recovery after surgery. Fascial plane blocks, while limited to providing analgesia, are considered safer than plexus blocks. Plexus blocks may offer effective anesthesia for the neck but have been associated with patient discomfort in initial studies. To ensure safety and accuracy, ultrasound guidance is recommended for CPBs due to the proximity of vital structures. Proper patient and procedure selection is essential for achieving effective anesthesia when using these blocks or their combinations.

References

[1] Hand WR, Taylor JM, Harvey NR, et al. Thoracolumbar interfascial plane (TLIP) block: a pilot study in volunteers. Can J Anaesth. 2015; 62(11):1196–1200

[2] Ueshima H, Sakai R, Otake H. Clinical experiences of ultrasound-guided thoracolumbar interfascial plane block: a clinical experience. J Clin Anesth. 2016; 33:499

[3] Ohgoshi Y, Izawa H, Kori S, Matsukawa M. Multifidus cervicis plane block is effective for cervical spine surgery. Can J Anaesth. 2017; 64(3):329–330

[4] Ohgoshi Y, Nishizakura R, Takahashi Y, et al. Novel ultrasound-guided inter-semispinal plane block: a comparative pilot study in healthy volunteers. J Anesth. 2018; 32(1):143–146

[5] Hochberg U, de Santiago Moraga J. Ultrasound-guided retrolaminar cervical block. Reg Anesth Pain Med. 2022; 47(1): 73–74

[6] Mohamed ZE, Zarad CA, Flifel ME, Abou Elmaaty AA. The efficacy of ultrasound-guided multifidus cervicis plane block versus greater occipital nerve block for cervicogenic headache. Egypt J Neurol Psychiatr Neurosurg. 2021; 57:11

[7] Tseng V, Cole C, Schmidt MH, Abramowicz AE, Xu JL. Analgesic efficacy of paraspinal interfascial plane blocks performed with the use of neurophysiology monitoring for posterior cervical laminectomy surgery: a case series. J Spine Surg. 2021; 7(1):109–113

[8] Forero M, Adhikary SD, Lopez H, Tsui C, Chin KJ. The erector spinae plane block: a novel analgesic technique in thoracic neuropathic pain. Reg Anesth Pain Med. 2016; 41(5):621–627

[9] Chin KJ, Adhikary SD, Sarwani N, Forero M. The analgesic efficacy of pre-operative bilateral erector spinae plane (ESP) blocks in patients having ventral hernia repair. Anaesthesia. 2017; 72(4):452–460

[10] Diwan S, Blanch XS, Nair A, Shah D. Anatomic and radiological correlation of injectate spread from first thoracic costotransverse junction in cervical erector spinae plane. Autops Case Rep. 2021; 11:e2021275

[11] Elsharkawy H, Ince I, Hamadnalla H, Drake RL, Tsui BCH. Cervical erector spinae plane block: a cadaver study. Reg Anesth Pain Med. 2020; 45(7):552–556

[12] Kamel AAF, Fahmy AM, Fathi HM, Elmesallamy WAEA, Khalifa OYA. Regional analgesia using ultrasound-guided intermediate cervical plexus block versus cervical erector spinae block for anterior cervical spine surgery: a randomized trial. BMC Anesthesiol. 2024; 24(1):153

[13] Goyal A, Kamath S, Kalgudi P, Krishnakumar M. Perioperative analgesia with erector spinae plane block for cervical spine instrumentation surgery. Saudi J Anaesth. 2020; 14(2): 263–264

[14] Diwan S, Koh WU, Chin KJ, Nair A. Bilateral high thoracic continuous erector spinae plane blocks for postoperative analgesia in a posterior cervical fusion. Saudi J Anaesth. 2020; 14(4):535–537

[15] Boezaart AP, Koorn R, Rosenquist RW. Paravertebral approach to the brachial plexus: an anatomic improvement in technique. Reg Anesth Pain Med. 2003 May-Jun; 28(3): 241–244

[16] Sinnatamby CS. Head and neck and spine. In: Sinnatamby CS, ed. Last's Anatomy: Regional and Applied. 11th ed. London: Churchill Livingstone; 2006:341–372

[17] Perisanidis C, Saranteas T, Kostopanagiotou G. Ultrasound-guided combined intermediate and deep cervical plexus nerve block for regional anaesthesia in oral and maxillofacial surgery. Dentomaxillofac Radiol. 2013; 42(2):29945724

[18] Saranteas T, Kostopanagiotou GG, Anagnostopoulou S, Mourouzis K, Sidiropoulou T. A simple method for blocking the deep cervical nerve plexus using an ultrasound-guided technique. Anaesth Intensive Care. 2011; 39(5):971–972

[19] Wan Q, Yang H, Li X, et al. Ultrasound-guided versus fluoroscopy-guided deep cervical plexus block for the treatment of cervicogenic headache. BioMed Res Int. 2017; 2017: 4654803

[20] Sandeman DJ, Griffiths MJ, Lennox AF. Ultrasound guided deep cervical plexus block. Anaesth Intensive Care. 2006; 34 (2):240–244

[21] Elder JB, Hoh DJ, Liu CY, Wang MY. Postoperative continuous paravertebral anesthetic infusion for pain control in posterior cervical spine surgery: a case-control study. Neurosurgery. 2010; 66(3) Suppl Operative:99–106, discussion 106–107

[22] Boezaart AP, Nosovitch MA. Carotid endarterectomy using single injection posterior cervical paravertebral block. Anesth Analg. 2005 Dec; 101(6):1885–1886

[23] Mariappan R, Mehta J, Massicotte E, Nagappa M, Manninen P, Venkatraghavan L. Effect of superficial cervical plexus block on postoperative quality of recovery after anterior cervical discectomy and fusion: a randomized controlled trial. Can J Anaesth. 2015; 62:883–890

[24] Wang H, Ma L, Yang D, et al. Cervical plexus anesthesia versus general anesthesia for anterior cervical discectomy and fusion surgery: a randomized clinical trial. Medicine (Baltimore). 2017; 96(7):e6119

8 Abdominal Wall Blocks

Stephen Davies and W. Michael Bullock

Abstract

Multimodal pain control for surgical interventions is the gold standard for patient care and has shown a myriad of benefits. As a component of multimodal analgesia, regional anesthesia has become a more consistent modality in various surgeries. Truncal blocks, in particular, have become a cornerstone of multimodal pain control for procedures involving the anterior abdominal wall. They are an excellent adjunct for postoperative analgesia and demonstrate a significant reduction in postoperative opiate consumption, which has been shown to have many other benefits, such as reduced rates of ileus, hospital length of stay, and new chronic opiate dependence. The two most utilized truncal blocks for spine surgery are the transversus abdominis plane (TAP) blocks and quadratus lumborum (QL) blocks. While the QL block can cover anterior or posterior approaches, TAP blocks only cover anterior surgical approaches. The relevant anatomy and physiology, utility, and evidence for each of these techniques will be outlined in this chapter.

Keywords: truncal, transversus abdominis plane, quadratus lumborum, regional anesthesia, ERAS, abdominal wall block, spine surgery

Key Points

- Multimodal pain control has proven effective for multiple patient cohorts, including spine surgery; both TAP and QL blocks can significantly reduce postoperative pain and opiate consumption in appropriately selected patients and procedures.
- QL blocks provide more visceral analgesia and broader dermatomal coverage than TAP blocks can achieve; they have also been successfully employed for combined anterior and posterior approach lumbar surgeries.
- Given their ease of performance and safety profile, TAP blocks have been successfully integrated into many ERAS protocols. They have repeatedly demonstrated benefits to patients and are an effective addition to anterior approach procedures.
- Truncal blocks have a long history of safety; given their distance from the surgical site, they can be a preferred location for neural blockade with a very low risk of motor weakness.

8.1 Introduction

The term "truncal block" refers to a technique where local anesthetic is deposited in an interfascial plane in the thoracoabdominal region, providing analgesia to various locations within the chest, back, abdomen, and groin, depending on the location of injection. They have been a part of multimodal analgesia protocols for multiple procedures for over 40 years.[1] Given they are a fascial plane block, many of these methods cannot provide singular surgical anesthesia (apart from paravertebral blocks); however, they have proven their utility in providing benefit to patients with reliable decreases in postoperative pain, opiate consumption, and nausea/vomiting.[2] This, coupled with their safety profile, has led to the integration of truncal blocks into many Enhanced Recovery After Surgery (ERAS) protocols with proven success.[3] In the realm of spine surgery, the most applicable and utilized truncal blocks are the quadratus lumborum (QL) and transversus abdominis plane (TAP) blocks.

Expert Tip

Consultation with a qualified anesthesiologist is crucial in determining the indication of truncal block for a particular surgery. While erector spinae plane (ESP) blocks (Chapter 4) can be used for analgesia after cervical, thoracic, and lumbar surgeries, other truncal blocks are further localized and may not be advantageous for a particular surgery.

Expert Tip

The vast majority of truncal blocks are best utilized for postoperative analgesia, after either awake spine surgery (ESP blocks indicated) or spine surgery with general anesthesia (e.g., QL and TAP).

8.2 Quadratus Lumborum Block

8.2.1 Background

- The QL block originated as a variant of the TAP block and was first described in 2007.[4]
- The use of this technique continued to be relatively sparse until 2016 when new prospective studies demonstrated a reliably significant reduction in pain scores and opiate consumption after abdominal surgery when QL blocks were performed.[5]
- Since then, indications for QL blocks have rapidly increased, ranging from gynecologic, colorectal, and general abdominal surgery to, more recently, spine surgery.

8.2.2 Anatomy

- The QL muscle (QLM) creates a lateral border for the lumbar spine (▶ Fig. 8.1, ▶ Fig. 8.2).
- It spans from the iliac crest to the 12th rib and inserts onto the transverse processes of the lumbar vertebrae.
- Identifying the erector spinae muscle group posteriorly and the psoas major (PM) anteriorly is imperative. These muscles are enveloped by the thoracolumbar fascia, creating a conduit for spreading local anesthetic to the paravertebral space.[4]
- The thoracolumbar fascia also allows for the spread of local anesthetic around the sympathetic trunk and celiac plexus, which confers visceral abdominal analgesia.[6]

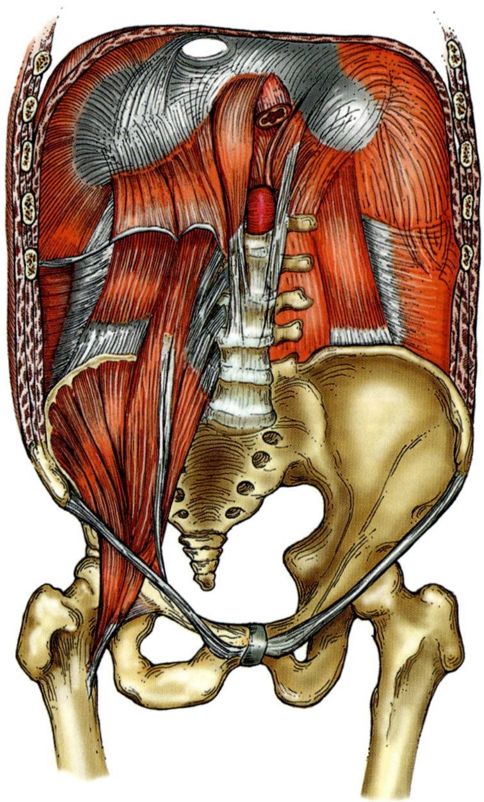

Fig. 8.1 The diaphragm attaches to the lumbar spine at the transverse process. The lumbocostal arches then traverse the quadratus lumborum and psoas muscles and attach to the ventral spine. Mobilization of the diaphragmatic crus is frequently required in thoracolumbar approaches. (Reproduced from Perez-Cruet M, Fessler R, Wang M, ed. An Anatomic Approach to Minimally Invasive Spine Surgery. 2nd ed. New York, NY: Thieme; 2018.)

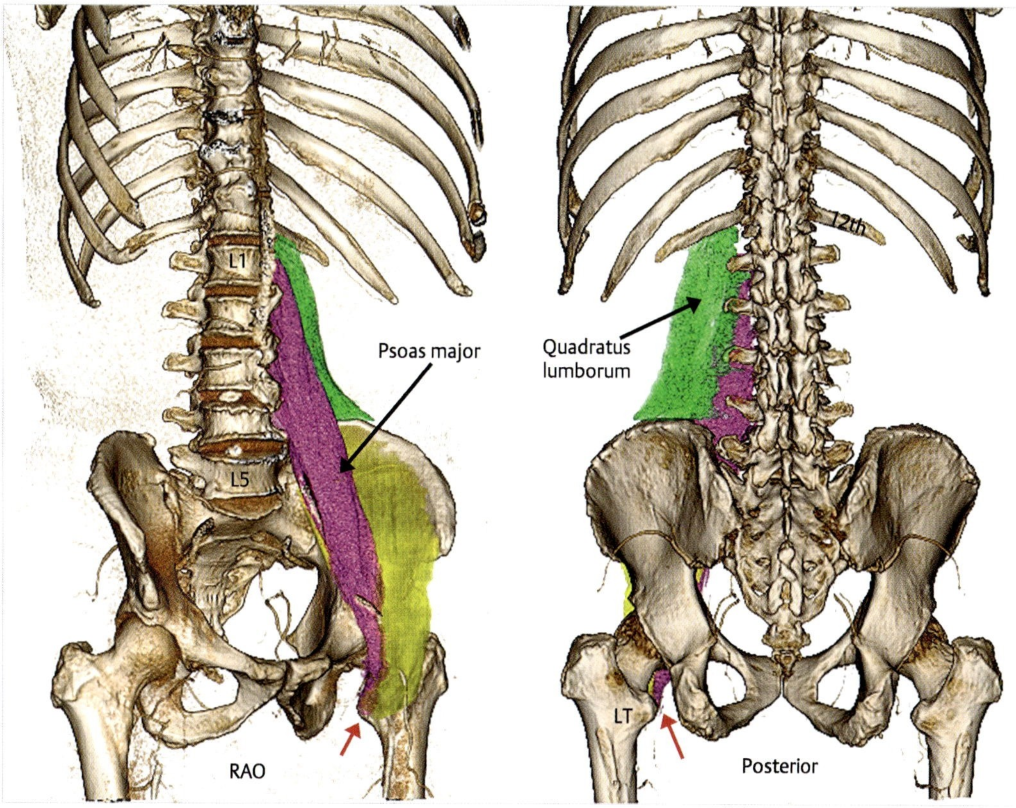

Fig. 8.2 Color-coded right anterior oblique (RAO) and posterior abdominal views showing the anatomical relationship of the psoas major (*purple*), iliacus (*yellow*), and quadratus lumborum (*green*) muscles to the adjacent bones. The psoas has fibrous attachments to the anterior aspects of L1 to L5 transverse processes and to the anteromedial aspect of all lumbar disks and adjoining bodies with the exception of the L5 body. The iliacus muscle originates at the superior two-thirds of the iliac fossa. The quadratus lumborum muscle lies lateral to the lumbar spine and connects the ilium to the 12th rib and to the lumbar vertebrae. The iliopsoas tendon is usually a conjoint tendon (*red arrows*) of the psoas major and iliacus muscles that connects to the lesser trochanter (LT). (Reproduced from Saremi F, ed. Imaging Anatomy: Text and Atlas. Vol. 3: Bones, Joints, Muscles, Vessels, and Nerves. 1st ed. New York, NY: Thieme; 2023.)

8.2.3 Variations

- The QL block, as originally described, entailed the deposition of local anesthetic on the lateral aspect of the QLM, where it joins with the transversalis fascia as the transversus abdominis aponeurosis spreads laterally and posteriorly.
- Since this description, four additional techniques have been described, all with the common goal of depositing local anesthetic around the QLM such that there is spread in the thoracolumbar fascia (▶ Fig. 8.3).[7,8]

Lateral QL Block (Formerly QL1)

- Local anesthetic is deposited at the lateral border of the QLM, deep to the transversus abdominis aponeurosis.
- This allows for spread between the anterior and middle layers of the thoracolumbar fascia.[1]

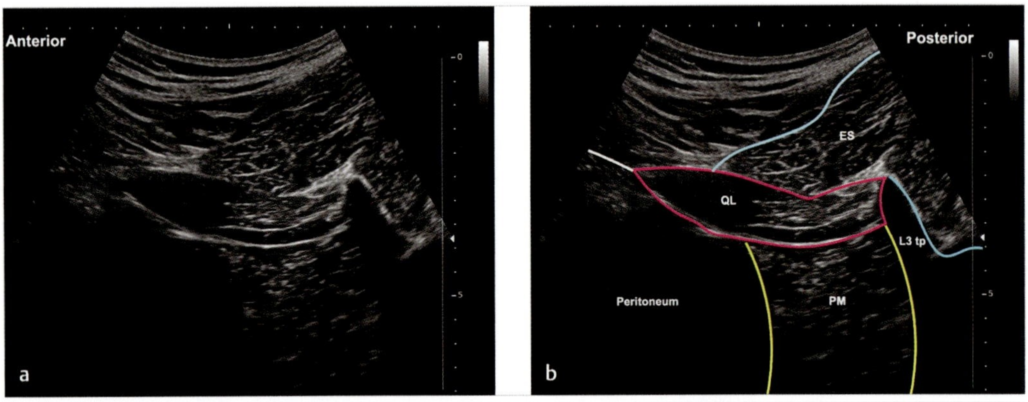

Fig. 8.3 (a) Ultrasound image of "shamrock" using a curvilinear transducer. **(b)** Outlines of muscles in "shamrock." ES, erector spinae (*blue*); L3 tp, L3 transverse process; PM, psoas major (*yellow*); QL, quadratus lumborum (*pink*). Depth in centimeters.

Expert Tip

Only the lateral QL block can be performed in the supine position. The other techniques require the patient to be in the sitting, lateral, or prone.

Posterior QL Block (Formerly QL2)

- Local anesthetic is deposited posterior to the QLM.
- Spread occurs between the posterior and middle layers of the thoracolumbar fascia.
- More recently, it has been suggested that the lumbar interfascial triangle is the target for local anesthetic deposition in this block. This region is where the lumbar fascia joins the retinacular sheath on the lateral edge of the erector spinae muscle group.[1]

Anterior or Transmuscular QL Block (Formerly QL3)

- Local anesthetic is deposited on the anterior aspect of the QLM.
- This block utilizes the classic "shamrock sign" on ultrasound guidance, which denotes the PM anteriorly, erector spinae posteriorly, and QL laterally.[7]
- Injection occurs between the QLM and PM muscles.

Expert Tip

The anterior QL block, in particular, is considered a deep block and caution should be employed in patients taking anticoagulants or presenting with a coagulopathy to decrease risk of bleeding with inadvertent vascular disruption.

Intramuscular QL Block

- Local anesthetic is deposited within the QL.
- The crux of this block involves spread of local anesthetic to the anterior aspect of the QL where many of the targeted divisions of spinal nerves lie.
- Unfortunately, no dye spread studies currently confirm the mechanism of this variation of the QL block (▶ Fig. 8.4).[9]

8.2.4 Block Coverage

- The QL block typically provides analgesia in the T7–L1 dermatomes.
- As noted previously, spread into the thoracolumbar fascia allows blockade of sympathetic fibers as well as hypothesized paravertebral spread.
- This spread aids in providing visceral analgesia, which is unique to QL blocks in relation to TAP blocks.[7]

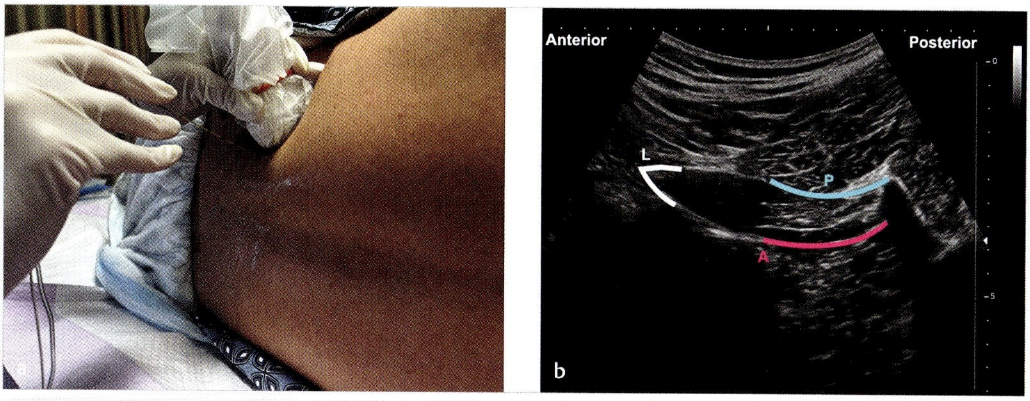

Fig. 8.4 **(a)** The patient is positioned in the lateral decubitus position for the quadratus lumborum (QL) block. **(b)** Block areas for QL block variations. A, anterior or transmuscular QL (*pink*); L, lateral QL (*white*); P, posterior QL (*light blue*). Depth in centimeters.

8.2.5 Block Technique

- At our institution, we most commonly perform the transmuscular or anterior QL block (QL3).
- Patients can be positioned in a sitting, lateral, or prone position.
- There are two approaches, both using the curvilinear probe, to achieve proper imaging.
  - Medial-to-lateral approach:
    - Beginning midline, the probe is placed in a transverse orientation to visualize the spinous process of (typically) L3.
    - The probe translated laterally to visualize the lamina and then the transverse process.
    - The QLM is attached to the transverse process.
  - Lateral-to-medial approach:
    - Beginning at the midaxillary line, the probe is placed in a transverse orientation between the costal margin and the iliac crest.
    - Oblique abdominal wall muscles are identified.
    - The probe is translated medial and posterior to identify the L3 transverse process.
    - Structures identified at the L3 transverse process: erector spinae anteriorly, QL laterally, and PM posteriorly.[5]
    - The interfascial plane is identified deep or anterior to the QLM.
- The skin is prepared with chlorhexidine, and subcutaneous local anesthetic is injected to aid with block tolerance.
- The block needle is then advanced in-plane through the QL to its anterior fascial plane.
- Saline is injected to hydrolocate the appropriate interfascial plane between the PM and the QL.
- At this time, 20 mL of local anesthetic is deposited into the space, and the PM should be slightly depressed by the local anesthetic.
- The block is repeated on the contralateral side for full effect.

Expert Tip

A nerve stimulation device typically used for regional anesthesia can help identify the interfascial plane between the QLM and the PM. Increasing the stimulator current to 1.5 to 2 V causes direct local muscle stimulation of the QLM. As the needle is advanced into the interfascial plane, the stimulation stops. Test the location with saline, and if determined to be in the correct location, inject local anesthetic.

Expert Tip

Ensure local anesthetic is injected between the QLM and the PM, as any injection into the PM may cause anterior lower extremity muscle weakness due to nerve blockade of the lumbar plexus, which is contained within the PM.

8.2.6 Application in Spine Surgery

- The most common indication for QL blocks currently is posterior approach lumbar surgery.
- Indeed, a recent randomized controlled trial (RCT) of 60 patients undergoing single-level lumbar microdiskectomy/hemilaminectomy demonstrated that QL blocks were more effective than local infiltration by the surgical team. The QL group showed improved pain scores up to 16 hours and required significantly less rescue analgesia. Postoperative nausea and vomiting (PONV) was also decreased in the QL block cohort.[10]
- Another retrospective cohort study demonstrated that continuous analgesia via QL catheters led to a significant reduction in postoperative opioid consumption in patients undergoing lumbar fusion surgeries. This study found the standard postoperative regimen group to require, on average, more than two times the amount of morphine milliequivalents (MME) than the group that had QL catheters placed.[11]
- Internationally, a retrospective cohort study from Turkey with 45 patients undergoing single-level lumbar diskectomy again demonstrated that the application of bilateral QL blocks significantly reduced postoperative opiate consumption and postoperative pain scores.[12] These results were congruent with a separate RCT showing efficacy of posterior QL blocks as part of the analgesic regimen for single-level lumbosacral spine surgery.[13]
- Given that QL blocks have been successfully employed in ERAS protocols for many types of abdominal surgery, QL blocks are used for anterior lumbar interbody fusion (ALIF) and lateral lumbar interbody fusion (LLIF) in our institution.[14]

Expert Tip

For awake spine surgery, it is technically easier and just as efficacious to perform ESP blocks for postoperative analgesia.

8.3 Transversus Abdominis Plane Block

8.3.1 Background

- As advocated by Hebbard in 2007, the ultrasound-guided technique has gained popularity given its enhanced reliability and efficacy compared to the landmark-based technique.[15]
- Indications for TAP blocks have increased and have been incorporated into many different types of ERAS protocols.
- Many small, single-center studies showed benefit, and more recently, a meta-analysis of various abdominal surgeries and patient cohorts demonstrated a significant reduction in postoperative MME consumption and a concurrent significant decrease in PONV rates.[16]

8.3.2 Anatomy

- The anterior abdominal wall comprises four muscles: the rectus abdominis, external oblique, internal oblique, and the transversus abdominis.
- The rectus abdominis muscle is the most anterior and midline abdominal wall muscle.
- The three oblique muscles converge medially to form the aponeurosis that invests the rectus abdominis muscle at the linea semilunaris.
- The TAP exists between the internal oblique and transversus abdominis muscles.
- This interfascial plane is where the anterior divisions of the thoracolumbar spinal nerves T6–L1 traverse and subsequently provide somatosensory innervation to the lateral and anterior abdominal wall (▶ Fig. 8.5).[3]

8.3.3 Variations

Classical (Lateral)

- This is the most common approach for the TAP block.
- The TAP is visualized between the internal oblique and the transverse abdominis at the space superior to the iliac crest and inferior to the subcostal margin, roughly at the midaxillary line.
- This reliably anesthetizes T10–12 dermatomes.[17]

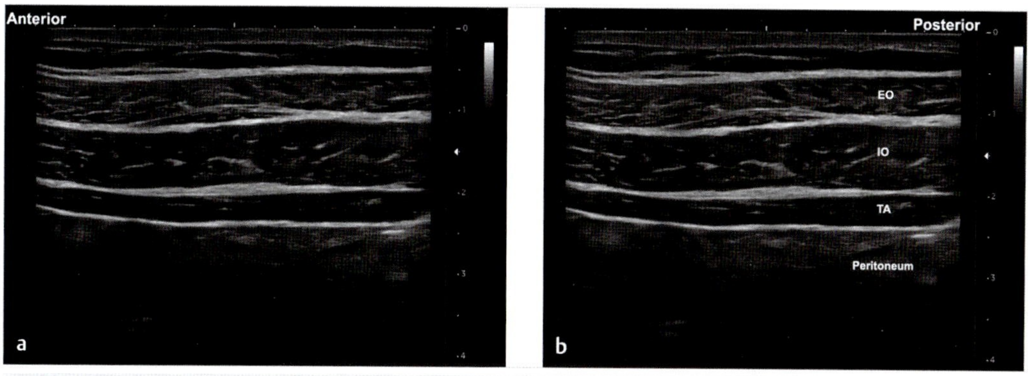

Fig. 8.5 **(a)** Ultrasound image of classical TAP block using a linear transducer. **(b)** Outlines of muscles in the classical TAP block. EO, external oblique; IO, internal oblique; TA, transversus abdominis. Depth in centimeters.

- These blocks are volume dependent and typically require 30 mL of dilute local anesthetic to be injected per side.

Expert Tip

The TAP blocks are typically performed once the patient is under general anesthesia, increasing patient satisfaction and acceptance of this regional anesthetic technique.

Subcostal

- This is a more recent variation of the TAP block that aims to maximize analgesia of the abdominal wall.
- This is performed more anteriorly, at the level of the anterior axillary line, just inferior to the costal margin.
- The goal is to deposit local anesthetic between the transversus abdominis and the posterior rectus sheath.
- This will provide analgesia to the T6–T9 dermatomes.[17]
- These blocks are less volume dependent than classical TAP blocks and typically require 10 to 15 mL of dilute local anesthetic to be injected per side.

Expert Tip

If subcostal TAP blocks are added, the volume injected to each classical TAP block may need to be decreased. Reducing the classical TAP volume to 20 mL per side is appropriate in this case.

8.3.4 Block Coverage

- As noted previously, the anterior and lateral cutaneous branches of the thoracolumbar spinal nerves of T6–L1 traverse the TAP and are anesthetized by this field block.
- Additionally, the ilioinguinal and iliohypogastric nerves, which arise from the lumbar plexus, travel within the TAP and are also anesthetized.[3]
- This results in reliable somatic analgesia from roughly the umbilicus to the pubic symphysis.
- Some have proposed adding the subcostal TAP to the traditional method to maximize block coverage. This has demonstrated coverage from L1 up to T6.[17]

8.3.5 Block Technique

- Classical TAP block (▶ Fig. 8.6).
  - Position the patient supine.
  - Either a linear or curvilinear probe is placed onto the abdominal wall between the iliac crest and the costal margin at about the anterior axillary line.
  - The oblique muscles are identified.

Expert Tip

Linear probes are generally higher in frequency than curvilinear probes and provide greater resolution but sacrifice depth. For deeper blocks or patients with large BMI, consider using the curvilinear probe as it may provide a better ultrasonographic image.

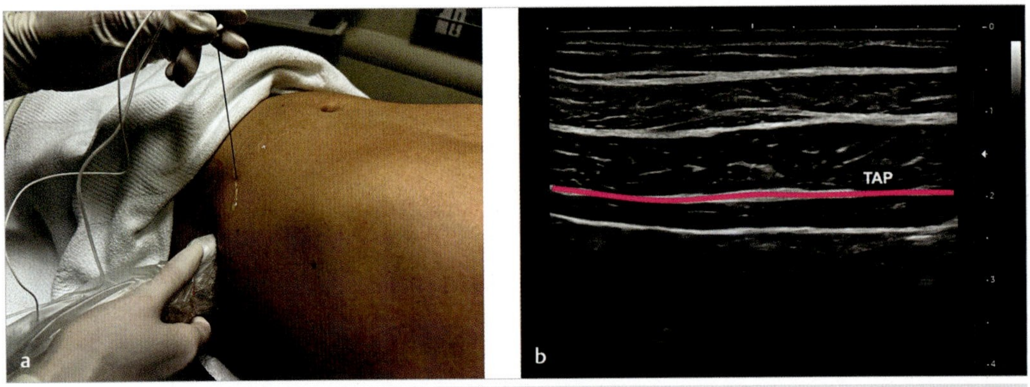

Fig. 8.6 **(a)** The patient is positioned supine for the classical TAP block. **(b)** Block plane for TAP block (*pink*). TAP, transversus abdominis plane. Depth in centimeters.

Expert Tip

Translating the probe or tilting the probe back and forth craniocaudally shows the muscle fibers of the external and internal oblique muscles moving in opposite directions. This is useful if the provider is unsure of the location and needs confirmation of appropriate structures.

Expert Tip

The inferior epigastric artery or its branches may be visualized, and care is taken to ensure the intended needle path does not intersect any of these structures.

- The skin is sterilized with chlorhexidine or an appropriate antiseptic solution.
- An echogenic needle is advanced through the skin into the TAP.
- Hydrolocation is used by injecting saline to confirm the correct placement.
- If the needle is placed in the correct location, the fascia "zippers apart" as it expands to accommodate the injectate.
- Once the correct location is confirmed, 20 to 30 mL of dilute local anesthetic is injected into the space.
- The procedure is then repeated on the contralateral side.

Expert Tip

Depending on provider preference, catheters or adjunctive additives may be used to prolong the analgesic effect of the block. Additives include dexamethasone, dexmedetomidine, and liposomal bupivacaine.

8.3.6 Application in Spine Surgery

- TAP blocks are now widely integrated into the practice of spine ERAS protocols.
- Multiple studies have proven their efficacy in immediate postoperative MME consumption.
  - A retrospective review of nearly 100 patients undergoing ALIF procedures, of which 47 received preoperative TAP blocks. Those who received TAP blocks consumed significantly less opiates on postop days 1 to 5. Pain scores were reduced in the TAP block group on post-op days 3 to 4; otherwise, they were not significantly different.[18] These results are congruent with a multitude of studies demonstrating the ability of TAP blocks to reduce postoperative opiate consumption and pain scores for many different types of abdominal surgeries.[19]
  - A separate analysis for those undergoing staged anterior and posterior procedures, for which a subset received TAP blocks, demonstrated no significant difference in postoperative pain scores, MME consumption,

nor length of stay (LOS)—demonstrating the limitations of TAP coverage to anterior abdominal dermatomes.[19]
- Retrospective review of 250 patients undergoing ALIF or LLIF, 129 of whom underwent pre-incisional TAP block. Those who received a TAP block as part of a standard multimodal analgesic approach had significantly reduced opiate consumption, LOS, and PONV.[16]
- Retrospective review of 109 patients, 68 of whom received a multimodal regimen during their single-level ALIF. Postoperative opiate consumption was decreased by 62%. While no differences in LOS or hospital cost were identified, it is postulated that the decreased postoperative opiate consumption would reduce rates of ileus, a known factor for increased LOS.[20]

8.4 Case Example

A 62-year-old man presents for L4/L5 ALIF due to radiculopathy that has been unresponsive to conservative measures. He has a history of obesity, obstructive sleep apnea (OSA) on continuous positive airway pressure, and chronic pain on oxycodone 10 mg three times daily at home. In the preoperative holding area, 30 mL of 0.5% bupivacaine was admixed with 20 mL of liposomal bupivacaine (Exparel, Pacira BioSciences, Tampa, FL), and bilateral transmuscular (anterior) QL blocks were performed with a total of 25 mL injected per side to optimize anterior and posterior coverage given the patient's history of OSA and chronic opiate use. The patient is then brought to the operating room, where general endotracheal anesthesia is induced. The patient is given ketamine, 0.5 mg/kg of ideal body weight, before incision and maintained on total intravenous anesthesia for neuromonitoring purposes. Surgery proceeds without incident, and the patient is extubated and brought to the postanesthesia care unit. He is provided with oxycodone 15 mg every 4 hours as needed in addition to scheduled acetaminophen and ketorolac. He has a return of bowel function on postoperative day 2 and is discharged home on postoperative day 3.

References

[1] Akerman M, Pejčić N, Veličković I. A review of the quadratus lumborum block and ERAS. Front Med (Lausanne). 2018; 5: 44

[2] Chakraborty A, Khemka R, Datta T. Ultrasound-guided truncal blocks: a new frontier in regional anaesthesia. Indian J Anaesth. 2016; 60(10):703–711

[3] Young MJ, Gorlin AW, Modest VE, Quraishi SA. Clinical implications of the transversus abdominis plane block in adults. Anesthesiol Res Pract. 2012; 2012:731645

[4] Blanco R. TAP block under ultrasound guidance: the description of a "non pops technique." Reg Anesth Pain Med. 2007; 32:130

[5] Ueshima H, Otake H, Lin JA. Ultrasound-guided quadratus lumborum block: an updated review of anatomy and techniques. BioMed Res Int. 2017; 2017:2752876

[6] Bordoni B, Varacallo M. Anatomy, Abdomen and Pelvis, Quadratus Lumborum. Treasure Island, FL: StatPearls Publishing; 2024

[7] Elsharkawy H, El-Boghdadly K, Barrington M. Quadratus lumborum block: anatomical concepts, mechanisms, and techniques. Anesthesiology. 2019; 130(2):322–335

[8] Willard FH, Vleeming A, Schuenke MD, Danneels L, Schleip R. The thoracolumbar fascia: anatomy, function and clinical considerations. J Anat. 2012; 221(6):507–536

[9] Yoshida K, Tanaka S, Watanabe K, Obara S, Murakawa M. The effectiveness of the intramuscular quadratus lumborum block in postoperative analgesia after cesarean section with vertical incision: a randomized, double-blinded placebo-controlled study. J Anesth. 2020; 34(6):849–856

[10] Alver S, Bahadir C, Tahta AC, et al. The efficacy of ultrasound-guided anterior quadratus lumborum block for pain management following lumbar spinal surgery: a randomized controlled trial. BMC Anesthesiol. 2022; 22(1):394

[11] Wilton J, Chiu H, Codianne N, Knapp H, Escolar VR, Burns S. Continuous quadratus lumborum block as post-operative strategy for pain control in spinal fusion surgery. Indian J Anaesth. 2020; 64(10):869–873

[12] Sertçakacılar G, Yıldız GÖ. Evaluation of the efficacy of posterior approach quadratus lumborum block for postoperative analgesia after lumbar discectomy surgery; retrospective observational study. Dünya Sağlık Ve Tabiat Bilimleri Dergisi. 2022; 5(1):12–22

[13] Canikli Adıgüzel Ş, Akyurt D, Bahadır Altun H, et al. Posterior quadratus lumborum block or thoracolumbar interfascial plane block and postoperative analgesia after spinal surgery: a randomized controlled trial. J Clin Med. 2023; 12(23):7217

[14] Blanco R, Ansari T, Girgis E. Quadratus lumborum block for postoperative pain after caesarean section: a randomised controlled trial. Eur J Anaesthesiol. 2015; 32(11):812–818

[15] Rafi AN. Abdominal field block: a new approach via the lumbar triangle. Anaesthesia. 2001; 56(10):1024–1026

[16] Reisener MJ, Hughes AP, Okano I, et al. The association of transversus abdominis plane block with length of stay, pain and opioid consumption after anterior or lateral lumbar fusion: a retrospective study. Eur Spine J. 2021; 30(12): 3738–3745

[17] Lee TH, Barrington MJ, Tran TM, Wong D, Hebbard PD. Comparison of extent of sensory block following posterior and subcostal approaches to ultrasound-guided transversus abdominis plane block. Anaesth Intensive Care. 2010; 38(3): 452–460

[18] Brogi E, Kazan R, Cyr S, Giunta F, Hemmerling TM. Transversus abdominal plane block for postoperative analgesia: a systematic review and meta-analysis of randomized-controlled trials. Can J Anaesth. 2016; 63(10):1184–1196

[19] Colón LF, White CC, Miles DT, et al. Transversus abdominis plane block as part of a multimodal analgesic regimen in patients undergoing anterior lumbar interbody fusion: a retrospective cohort study. Int J Spine Surg. 2023; 17(3):426–433

[20] Ogura Y, Gum JL, Steele P, et al. Multi-modal pain control regimen for anterior lumbar fusion drastically reduces in-hospital opioid consumption. J Spine Surg. 2020; 6(4): 681–687

9 Patient Anxiety in Awake Spine Surgery

Arnav Sharma and Basma Mohamed

Abstract

Awake spine surgery aims to reduce postoperative complications, length of hospital stay, and patient discomfort. Over the last two decades, spine surgeons and anesthesiologists have advocated for employing regional anesthesia techniques to expedite recovery, allow for multimodal analgesia, and reduce overall costs. In addition, economic analyses demonstrated that using conscious sedation combined with spinal anesthesia reduced the total cost of lumbar decompression surgery. However, awake spine surgery presents potential challenges, including patient discomfort, patient movement, and challenging sedation techniques while surgery is performed in a prone position. Anxiety has been identified as a contraindication to proceed with awake spine surgery. Anxiety occurs in one-third of spine surgery patients and is an important predictor for perioperative outcomes, including pain, physical impairment, and overall quality of life. Factors contributing to anxiety include inadequate information, clinical environment, and demographic and psychological factors. Nonpharmacological interventions such as music therapy, virtual reality, progressive muscle relaxation, guided imagery, hypnosis, cognitive behavioral therapy, and massage are effective in managing anxiety. Pharmacological interventions such as benzodiazepines, alpha-2-agonists, propofol, ketamine, and gabapentin have also been evaluated in awake surgery. In addition, preoperative education and counseling can be crucial in managing anxiety, improving patient preparedness for surgery, and enhancing perioperative outcomes while achieving the optimal goal for awake spine surgery.

Keywords: awake spine surgery, anxiety during awake surgery, anxiety management, preoperative predictors of anxiety, nonpharmacological management of anxiety, conscious sedation

Key Points

- Awake spine surgery uses regional anesthesia with or without conscious sedation to reduce postoperative complications, hospital stays, and patient discomfort.
- Challenges include intraoperative hypotension, spinal anesthesia masking intraoperative complications, intraoperative movements, and airway protection during conscious sedation techniques.
- Managing patient anxiety is crucial as it can significantly impact patient experience and outcomes.
- Anxiety occurs in one-third of patients undergoing spine surgery and can lead to more significant pain, physical impairment, and lower quality of life.
- Effective nonpharmacological interventions for anxiety include music therapy, virtual reality, progressive muscle relaxation, guided imagery, hypnosis, cognitive behavioral therapy, aromatherapy, and massage.
- Pharmacological options for managing anxiety include benzodiazepines, alpha-2 agonists, propofol, ketamine, and gabapentin.
- Preoperative education and counseling are crucial for reducing anxiety, improving preparedness, and enhancing postoperative outcomes.
- Postoperative anticipation of the impact of anxiety on perioperative outcomes allows for a tailored approach to individual patients to improve their outcomes and patient satisfaction.

9.1 Introduction

- Awake spine surgery, which employs minimally invasive techniques, using regional anesthesia techniques and often conscious sedation, aims to reduce postoperative complications, hospital stays, and patient discomfort.[1] In the past 20 years, spine surgeons and anesthesiologists have advocated for methods requiring only regional anesthesia, potentially offering reduced patient costs, enhanced recovery, and improved outcomes.[2]
- An increasing number of studies have shown the clinical advantages of performing operations under regional anesthesia, including reduced intraoperative blood loss, fewer complications related to general anesthesia, and better postoperative pain management when compared to general anesthesia.[3,4,5] In addition to clinical benefits, recent economic analyses have shown that using conscious sedation with spinal anesthesia instead of general anesthesia reduced the total cost of lumbar diskectomy and laminectomy by 40%. This cost reduction is attributed to factors such as shorter operation times, decreased anesthesia duration, and lower estimated blood loss.[6]
- However, awake spine surgery can be associated with potential challenges, including intraoperative hypotension, spinal anesthesia masking intraoperative complications, intraoperative movements, and a challenging conscious sedation technique.[7] In addition, awake spine surgery presents unique challenges in managing patient anxiety, which can significantly impact patient experience and outcomes.
- As a result, careful patient selection and a multidisciplinary approach are crucial for successfully implementing awake spine surgery.[1,7] In addition, anticipating different challenges and proactive preparation for the best outcome is crucial to achieving the best perioperative outcomes. As a result, a multidisciplinary perioperative care team approach is crucial for planning awake spine surgery.[1,3,8]
- Patients with a history of anxiety face one of the highest challenges in intraoperative care. Current literature focused on excluding patients with a history of anxiety from performing awake spine surgery to minimize perioperative complications; however, excluding patients with preexisting anxiety may not reduce the risk of experiencing anxiety by patients who are undiagnosed or underdiagnosed.
- Anxiety occurs in one-third of patients undergoing spine surgery. Preoperative anxiety is an important predictor of perioperative outcomes, including greater pain, physical impairment, and lower quality of life.[9] It is estimated that at least 7% of spine surgery patients have the underlying diagnosis of anxiety as a preexisting condition.

9.2 Factors Contributing to Anxiety in Awake Spine Surgery

- Being conscious during surgery poses a challenge for the patients and the perioperative care team during awake spine surgery. As a result, identifying factors that contribute to the increased severity of anxiety is crucial for the perioperative care team to mitigate anxiety effectively. Identifying these factors can lead to adopting various techniques that can minimize anxiety and allow for a better perioperative experience while maximizing the benefits of performing surgery while awake without compromising patient care and surgical outcomes.
- In a recent systematic integrative review, Strøm et al found five categories of interacting factors that influenced symptoms of anxiety and depression both before and after spine surgery. These factors include pain, lack of information, disability, return to work, and mental health. Information and perioperative counseling appear to have a regulating effect on anxiety and depression.[9]

9.2.1 Fear of Pain and Being Awake

- Patients undergoing awake spine surgery may fear experiencing pain or discomfort during surgery, which can increase their level of anxiety dramatically.
- The anticipation of being conscious during surgery is what most likely drives the highest level of anxiety. In addition, the potential feeling or sensing the operating room environment might be distressing for many patients, mainly for those undergoing awake surgery for the first time.[10]
- The fear and anticipation of pain have been addressed in studies as one of the most

common contributing factors to anxiety reported by patients before surgery.[11]

- In a survey of surgical patients who underwent surgery under conscious sedation, a patient survey analyzing the causes of intraoperative anxiety revealed multiple aspects of their fear, mainly the fear of requiring more than one injection, being awake, hearing the surgeons, feeling the surgery, seeing the body cut open, and the anticipation that regional anesthesia and local anesthesia will be painful.[10]

9.2.2 Inadequate Information and Communication

- Lack of preparation, adequate information, and a predictable set of expectations about the procedure and anesthesia can exacerbate anxiety. Patients who expect a higher level of detailed information may experience an increased level of anxiety if they do not receive the appropriate details before surgery.[12]
- Effective communication and comprehensive preoperative education and counseling regarding the upcoming surgery and the intraoperative expectation can help alleviate fears by addressing misconceptions and providing reassurance.[12]

9.2.3 Influence of the Clinical Environment

- The operating room that is designed for mainly unconscious patients can be intimidating for awake surgery. Understanding the environment and addressing various aspects that may heighten patient anxiety is crucial for a better experience.
- Nonpharmacological approaches to managing patient anxiety can emphasize certain modifications of the environment, such as light, noise, communication, and attitude of the operating room personnel.

9.2.4 Demographic and Psychological Factors

- Anxiety levels are usually higher in specific populations, such as younger patients, females, and those with a high need for information.[13]
- Preexisting psychological factors such as depression, fear avoidance, and catastrophizing are significant predictors of anxiety in this patient population and can contribute to worse postoperative surgical outcomes.

Expert Tip

Factors Contributing to Patient Anxiety

- Being conscious during surgery, pain, lack of information, disability, return to work, and mental health.
- Fear of experiencing pain, discomfort, sensing the operating room environment, fear of requiring more than one injection, hearing the surgeons, feeling the surgery, seeing the body cut open, and anticipation of painful anesthesia.
- Lack of preparation, inadequate information, unpredictable expectations, need for detailed information, effective communication, and preoperative education and counseling
- Intimidating operating room, nonpharmacological approaches, modification of environment such as light, noise, communication, and attitude of personnel.
- Higher anxiety in younger patients, females, high need for information, and preexisting psychological factors like depression, fear avoidance, and catastrophizing.

9.3 Implications of Anxiety on Perioperative Outcomes

- Patient anxiety is considered a contraindication to proceed with awake spine surgery in the current literature[2,14]; however, experiencing anxiety in the preoperative period and during surgery can be inevitable. The impact of anxiety on perioperative outcomes can be multifaceted, including physiological and psychological consequences.
- Preoperative anxiety has been shown to increase the intensity of postoperative pain, leading to higher doses of anesthesia and analgesia, all of which can lead to a cycle of

dissatisfaction and potential side effects of increased doses of analgesic medications.[15]

- In one study, anxiety was found to provoke a glucocorticoid signaling that impaired the GABAergic system in the spine cord, as a result causing hyperalgesia and increased postoperative pain medications.[16]
- Patients with preoperative anxiety are at increased risk of postoperative complications, including surgical site infection and higher reoperation rates.[17,18] In addition, anxiety has been associated with an increased incidence of postoperative delirium[19]; all these factors can result in prolonged length of hospital stay and increased health care utilization costs, which contradict the primary purpose of adopting awake spine surgery as a method to enhance patient recovery and improve outcome and health care utilization.
- Patient anxiety can negatively impact patient-reported outcomes, such as patient satisfaction and patient-reported physical function and quality of life.[18,20,21] Patients with anxiety usually report lower satisfaction scores and worse functional outcomes compared to those without anxiety. In addition, the presence of anxiety combined with depression can result in suboptimal recovery and increased health care utilization.[22]
- Patient anxiety has been associated with higher rates of delirium, readmission, more extended hospital stay, and higher rates of nonroutine discharges after spine surgery; in addition, its association with increased use of postoperative opioids has an impact on health care resource utilization and health care economics.[23,24]

9.4 Nonpharmacological Interventions for Perioperative Management of Patient Anxiety

- Nonpharmacological interventions to address patient anxiety during awake surgery can be effective, mainly when there are contraindications, lack of anticipated effectiveness, or side effects of pharmacological interventions. Several approaches that have been evaluated in the literature are discussed here.

9.4.1 Music Therapy

- Music therapy is one of the most frequently utilized interventions to mitigate anxiety for patients during awake surgery. It has been demonstrated to reduce anxiety levels during procedures by providing a calming auditory stimulus that diverts patients' attention from the surgical environment.[25,26]
- Research indicates that music therapy can significantly decrease preoperative anxiety, with a demonstrated efficacy rate exceeding 70% across various surgical procedures.[26]
- This approach is efficacious in the preoperative phase of care before the day of surgery and can be implemented during and after surgical interventions.

9.4.2 Virtual Reality

- Another cutting-edge method used to address anxiety in surgical patients is virtual reality (VR). By engaging patients in an immersive digital environment, VR distracts from the surgical procedure, thus helping lower anxiety levels.[25,27]
- The effectiveness of VR has been particularly notable in pediatric settings, where it has been utilized to create soothing and captivating experiences that help alleviate preoperative anxiety.[27]
- VR is another approach applicable in the perioperative setting, before, during, and after awake spine surgery.

9.4.3 Progressive Muscle Relaxation and Guided Imagery

- Two relaxation techniques, progressive muscle relaxation and guided imagery, are employed to alleviate anxiety in patients. The former involves methodically tensing and relaxing different muscle groups, while the latter utilizes mental visualization.
- These approaches help patients shift their focus from the impending surgical procedure to their physical sensations and mental images, thereby reducing anxiety levels.[25,28]
- These methods are frequently combined with other therapeutic interventions, such as music therapy, to enhance their efficacy.[28]

- Lack of knowledge or expertise regarding these techniques may limit their utility during and after surgery. However, consulting with experienced personnel may be an innovative approach to add to the value of awake spine surgery.

9.4.4 Hypnosis and Cognitive Behavioral Therapy

- Anxiety in surgical patients has been addressed utilizing two psychological interventions: hypnosis and cognitive behavioral therapy (CBT). Hypnosis aims to induce a state analogous to trance, facilitating relaxation and anxiety reduction. Conversely, CBT targets the negative thought patterns that contribute to anxiety.[26,28]
- Research has demonstrated the efficacy of both approaches in alleviating anxiety, with hypnosis exhibiting particular promise for highly suggestible individuals.[26]

9.4.5 Aromatherapy and Massage

- Nonpharmacological approaches such as aromatherapy, which utilizes essential oils to induce relaxation and massage therapy, have been employed to alleviate anxiety in patients undergoing surgery. These techniques function by offering sensory input that can divert patients' attention from the surgical setting and foster a sense of tranquility.[28,29]
- Research has demonstrated that these interventions can effectively decrease anxiety levels, with aromatherapy showing a significant effect size in reducing preoperative anxiety.[29]

9.5 Pharmacological Interventions for Perioperative Management of Patient Anxiety

- Sedation techniques that focus on one or a combination of sedating medications have been described in the setting of monitored anesthesia care (MAC) procedures and short-acting anesthetics that would allow immediate recovery in case of oversedation.
- Medications that have been in current use include benzodiazepines, alpha-2-agonists, propofol, gabapentin, ketamine, and short-acting opioids.

9.5.1 Benzodiazepines

- Benzodiazepines play an important role in managing patient anxiety during awake spine

Expert Tip

Nonpharmacological Interventions for Patient Anxiety

Intervention	Description	Effectiveness	Additional notes
Music therapy	Calming auditory stimulus during surgery	Reduces anxiety levels, efficacy rate > 70%	Applicable preoperative, during, and after surgery
VR	Immersive digital environment as a distraction	Notable in pediatric settings	Applicable before, during, and after surgery
Progressive muscle relaxation and guided imagery	Relaxation techniques involving muscle tensing and mental visualization	Reduces anxiety levels	Can be combined with music therapy
Hypnosis and CBT	Psychological interventions for relaxation and targeting negative thought patterns	Effective in alleviating anxiety	Hypnosis beneficial for highly suggestible individuals
Aromatherapy and massage	Use of essential oils and massage to induce relaxation	Effectively decreases anxiety levels	Aromatherapy shows significant effect but may not be practical in the operating room

surgery, mainly through their anxiolytic and sedation properties.
- Midazolam is the most commonly used anxiolytic of this group among surgical patients; however, it may lead to adverse outcomes if not managed effectively.
- Suppose the decision was made to proceed with awake spine surgery to avoid the impact of general anesthesia on the incidence of delirium in the geriatric population or those at high risk of delirium. In that case, benzodiazepines may not be the best choice due to their association with a higher incidence of postoperative delirium and potential postoperative cognitive dysfunction.
- Benefits of benzodiazepines:
  - *Anxiolysis and sedative effects:* Benzodiazepines are effective in decreasing anxiety through their action of GABA-A receptors, which facilitate inhibitory neurotransmission. Remimazolam, an ultrashort-acting GABA-A receptor agonist, may be a useful new benzodiazepine in future anesthetic practice.[30]
  - *Amnestic properties:* Midazolam produces anterograde amnesia that can prevent memories of intraoperative events, hence reducing the risk of anesthesia awareness and the associated psychological stress.
  - Midazolam has a rapid onset and short duration of action, which makes it suitable for awake spine surgery, given the prone positioning and the potential impact of positioning on the respiratory status.
- Risks and considerations:
  - *Respiratory depression and oversedation:* This side effect of benzodiazepines can defeat the purpose of performing awake spine surgery, which might lead to the need to convert to general anesthesia to secure the patient's airway and respiratory status. Flumazenil can be used to reverse the sedative effects. However, flumazenil is short acting and can result in seizures in a select group of patients.
  - *Postoperative delirium:* Benzodiazepines have been linked to a higher incidence of postoperative delirium, mainly in the geriatric patient population. This might complicate recovery and contradict the goals of performing awake spine surgery, which are expedited recovery, decreased complication rates, and decreased length of hospital stay.[13]
  - *Variability in practice:* Variability among institutions in the use of benzodiazepines can result in variability in outcomes. Some practices opt to focus on using benzodiazepines as an adjunct and not as the sole sedative during awake surgery. The adoption of this practice will allow for minimizing the risks and adverse events associated with benzodiazepines.
- Remimazolam, a novel benzodiazepine that exerts sedative, anxiolytic, and amnestic properties similar to midazolam, has a short half-life of 5 to 10 minutes, faster onset, and faster recovery.[31] Remimazolam is effective in procedures requiring short-acting sedation, such as endoscopies, and has been effective without the need for rescue therapy. In a case series of three patients undergoing awake craniotomy in adolescents, Remimazolam infusion was used in combination with dexmedetomidine and remifentanil, and Remimazolam was discontinued 30 minutes before the planned awake assessments. Patients emerged calmly without side effects. Also, Remimazolam was predictable and provided adequate sedation, maintenance of spontaneous respiration, and rapid awakening without compromising the patient's assessments.[32]

Expert Tip

Benzodiazepines Use for Patient Anxiety

Drug	Properties	Benefits	Risks	Considerations
Midazolam	Anxiolytic, sedative, amnestic	Rapid onset, short duration, anterograde amnesia	Respiratory depression, postoperative delirium	May need conversion to general anesthesia, variability in practice
Remimazolam	Ultrashort-acting GABA-A receptor agonist	Short half-life, faster onset, faster recovery	Minimal	Effective for short-acting sedation, predictable, maintains spontaneous respiration

9.5.2 Alpha-2 Agonists

- Alpha-2 agonists, particularly dexmedetomidine and clonidine, have been increasingly recognized for their efficacy in managing anxiety during awake surgical procedures. These agents exhibit anxiolytic, sedative, and analgesic properties without causing significant respiratory depression, rendering them suitable for awake interventions.
- The utilization of these agents in awake surgery is substantiated by their capacity to maintain stable hemodynamics and mitigate the requirement for opioids, potentially resulting in a reduction of adverse effects and complications.
- **Anxiolytic and sedative properties:**
  - Dexmedetomidine and clonidine provide sedation, hypnosis, anxiolysis, amnesia, and analgesia in a dose-dependent effect through their effects on the noradrenergic neurons in the locus ceruleus of the brainstem, which is the primary site that modulates wakefulness.[33]
  - Dexmedetomidine has amnestic effects less than that of benzodiazepines and does not cause retrograde amnesia.
- **Hemodynamic stability:**
  - Dexmedetomidine has a biphasic effect on hemodynamics, including initial hypertension followed by dose-dependent hypotension and bradycardia.[30] When the loading dose is given a 20-minute infusion period, this minimizes the transient initial hypertension. Bradycardia can be easily managed using anticholinergic medications.
  - Clonidine and dexmedetomidine have been shown to reduce perioperative oxygen consumption and blunt the sympathetic response to surgery.[30,34]
- **Respiratory effects:**
  - Dexmedetomidine has a limited impact on the respiratory drive, which allows for a wide safety margin, mainly in awake spine surgeries performed in the prone position. When using dexmedetomidine, the hypercapnic arousal is maintained, and the apnea threshold is decreased.[33]
  - Given the respiratory effects of dexmedetomidine, it can be safely used in prone awake spine surgery; the only disadvantage is when combined with other sedatives that compromise the respiratory status, such as when combined with opioids and benzodiazepines.
- **Reduction in opioid use:**
  - The alpha-2 agonists exert their analgesic effects through the activation of alpha-2C and alpha-2A receptors in the dorsal horn, which directly inhibits pain signals by decreasing the release of pain-promoting neurotransmitters and substance P and glutamate.
  - When administered systemically, dexmedetomidine reduces the need for opioids during and after surgery. This benefit is particularly valuable for patients at risk of perioperative respiratory depression, such as awake spine surgery in a prone position.[30]
  - Alpha-2 agonists can diminish the requisite dosage of opioids, which are frequently associated with adverse effects such as respiratory depression, nausea, and pruritus.

This reduction is advantageous in awake surgeries where maintaining patient alertness and minimizing side effects are crucial.[35]
  - Studies have demonstrated that combining alpha-2 agonists with local anesthetics can prolong the duration of sensory block, thereby reducing the need for additional analgesics.[35]
- **Safety and efficacy**:
  - The safety profile of alpha-2 agonists is generally favorable, with most studies indicating minimal adverse effects when used appropriately. However, there are concerns about potential hypotension and bradycardia, particularly in elderly patients or those with preexisting cardiovascular conditions.[30]
  - Dexmedetomidine has been associated with a reduced risk of postoperative cognitive dysfunction, mainly in the elderly population.[36]
  - Despite the safety profile of the alpha-2 agonists, no reversal agents are available. When combined with other sedative agents, such as benzodiazepines, low-dose propofol, or opioids, disinhibition and lack of patient cooperation might fail awake surgery.
- While alpha-2 agonists offer several advantages in the management of anxiety during awake spine surgeries, their use is not without challenges. The variability in hemodynamic responses and the potential for adverse effects such as hypotension and bradycardia necessitate careful patient selection and monitoring.
- Further research is needed to optimize dosing regimens and better understand these agents' long-term effects in various surgical settings. Nonetheless, their role as adjuncts in awake spine surgery continues to be promising, offering a balance between effective sedation and patient safety.

Expert Tip

Role of Alpha-2 Agonists in Patient Anxiety	
Alpha-2 agonists in use	Dexmedetomidine and clonidine
Anxiolytic and sedative properties	Provide sedation, hypnosis, anxiolysis, amnesia, and analgesia
Hemodynamic stability	Biphasic effect on hemodynamics, including initial hypertension followed by dose-dependent hypotension and bradycardia
Respiratory effects	Limited impact on respiratory drive, maintains hypercapnic arousal, and decreases apnea threshold
Reduction in opioid use	Reduces need for opioids, diminishes dosage, and prolongs sensory block duration
Safety and efficacy	Generally favorable safety profile, minimal adverse effects, and concerns about hypotension and bradycardia
Challenges	Variability in hemodynamic responses, potential for adverse effects, and careful patient selection and monitoring needed

9.5.3 Propofol

- Propofol is a commonly used anesthetic during awake procedures, and when used at the appropriate dosing for sedation, it can minimize discomfort and manage anxiety during awake spine surgery.
- Its rapid onset and short duration of action make it an appropriate choice for achieving patient comfort when combined with regional or neuraxial anesthesia without compromising airway management.
- The short plasma half-life allows for its use in fast titration, and rapid recovery is required intraoperatively and postoperatively.[37] When compared to midazolam, propofol was found to have the advantage of providing faster onset and rapid recovery with a quick return to baseline

mental status and less postoperative impairment of cognitive function.[38]

- Potential side effects of propofol include apnea and respiratory depression, mainly if used in higher doses (which can be derived from patient discomfort and inadequate regional analgesia).
- Given the effectiveness of propofol, it is an excellent choice for alleviating patient anxiety while maintaining the expected fast recovery and increased patient satisfaction; all promote the goals of awake spine surgery. However, there should be caution in titrating the dose to effects and to consider patient factors and the surgical context when being used as the only sedative versus in combination with other sedatives.

9.5.4 Ketamine

- Ketamine has been described as a versatile agent in the management of sedation and anxiety in various awake surgical procedures.
- Ketamine, as an N-methyl-D-aspartate (NMDA) receptor antagonist, provides analgesic and anxiolytic effects without compromising respiratory status commonly associated with other sedatives. This makes ketamine a unique choice for a select group of patients who have multiple risk factors for anxiety, discomfort, and risk of respiratory compromise while having awake spine surgery in the prone position (such as obese patients).
- Ketamine might have a bad reputation related to its role in increasing intracranial pressure, the pro-epileptic effects, and the potential for hallucination and psychiatric side effects. However, recent studies showed the impact of low-dose ketamine on alleviating anxiety, reducing inflammation, and improving perioperative analgesia without compromising the respiratory or hemodynamic status.[39]
- The anxiolytic effects of low-dose ketamine have led to its use as a treatment for a few psychiatric illnesses, such as anxiety and depression.[39]
- The analgesic effects of ketamine can mask any discomfort experienced by patients when the duration of the regional or neuraxial techniques starts to dissipate.
- Potential side effects of ketamine use during awake spine surgery include hallucination, disinhibition, and postoperative delirium. Those are not experienced when combined with other sedatives such as propofol and benzodiazepine. However, caution should be applied when combined with other sedation medications so as not to compromise the respiratory benefits of ketamine.

9.5.5 Gabapentin

Gabapentin, an anticonvulsant medication, shows potential in managing anxiety and sedation during awake spine surgery.

- Gabapentin has been found to reduce preoperative anxiety in various surgical settings, with studies showing significant decreases in anxiety scores without causing sedation or memory impairment, making it useful for awake procedures where patient cooperation is essential.[40]
- Gabapentin's sedative effects are generally mild, making it suitable for procedures requiring patient alertness. It has been associated with fewer side effects like dizziness and drowsiness than other medications.[41,42]
- Gabapentin has been effective in reducing postoperative pain and analgesic requirements, which can indirectly reduce anxiety and improve patient satisfaction during awake spine surgery.

Expert Tip

Role of Low-Dose Anesthetics and Gabapentin

Medication	Uses	Advantages	Potential side effects
Propofol	Anesthetic during awake procedures	Rapid onset, short duration, fast recovery, minimizes discomfort, manages anxiety	Apnea, respiratory depression
Ketamine	Management of sedation and anxiety	Analgesic, anxiolytic, does not compromise respiratory status	Hallucination, postoperative delirium
Gabapentin	Managing anxiety and sedation	Reduces preoperative anxiety, mild sedative effects, fewer side effects	Dizziness, drowsiness

9.6 Preoperative Evaluation and Consideration for Patients with Anxiety before Awake Spine Surgery

- Patient anxiety is a challenging factor in the perioperative management of patients undergoing awake spine surgery. Despite the lack of formal diagnosis of anxiety, patients undergoing spine surgery experience a heightened level of anxiety given the stress of surgery, the fear of experiencing the unpredictable intraoperative events, and the lack of knowledge of what to expect.
- Perioperative management of patient anxiety should focus on a multifactorial and multidisciplinary approach based on preoperative predictors of anxiety, the presence of anxiety as a comorbid condition, the severity of patient anxiety, and associated risk factors such as pain, mental health, and employment status.

9.6.1 The Role of Preoperative Patient Education and Counseling

- **Reduction in anxiety levels:** Preoperative education has been shown to reduce anxiety levels in patients significantly. For instance, a study found that a hospital-based education class led to a statistically significant reduction in anxiety among surgical spine patients.[43] Similarly, video education was effective in reducing preoperative anxiety by providing interactive and engaging information.[44]
- **Normalization of expectations:** Interventions such as the Preoperative Spinal Education (POSE) program contribute to reducing patient anxiety and aligning their expectations by acquainting them with surgical procedures and possible outcomes.[43]
- **Improved preparedness:** Individuals who undergo organized educational programs prior to surgery report feeling more prepared, which is associated with decreased anxiety levels and enhanced postsurgery outcomes.[45,46]
- Structured educational programs should focus on essential information regarding surgery, recovery, hospitalization expectations, and potential expectations. Focusing on these elements will prevent information overload and enhance the patients' preparedness for surgery while alleviating anxiety.
- Comprehensive knowledge of preoperative, intraoperative, and postoperative processes reduces patient anxiety, promoting a more favorable psychological state that benefits both patients and medical personnel.
- Increased preparedness and reduced anxiety contribute to improved postoperative outcomes, such as enhanced recovery, pain perception, complication rates, compliance with postoperative instructions, and engagement in rehabilitation.
- Approaching patient education as a comprehensive multidisciplinary structural program ensures inclusion of all necessary and important information for the patients.
- Potential components of educational programs:
  - Detailed surgical procedure explanations.
  - Information on anesthesia and pain management.

- Expected recovery timeline.
- Potential risks and complications.
- Postoperative care instructions.
- Rehabilitation exercises and activities

9.6.2 Methods of Delivering Education

- **In-person and literature-based education:** The POSE program, which includes a 60-minute in-person session with accompanying literature, has been effective in reducing anxiety and hospital length of stay for spinal fusion patients.[43]
- **Video education:** Utilizing video as a medium for delivering educational content has proven effective in reducing anxiety, as it allows for a more engaging and comprehensive delivery of information.[44]
- **Peer education:** Peer education, where patients learn from others who have undergone similar procedures, has been shown to significantly reduce anxiety by improving morale and providing relatable experiences.[47]

9.6.3 Counseling and Psychological Support

- **Counseling interventions:** Counseling that involves explaining the surgical procedure, diagnosis, and anesthesia can significantly reduce preoperative anxiety. A study demonstrated that counseling reduced anxiety scores from 44.1 to 29.8% in the counseled group.[48]
- **Addressing psychological concerns:** Anxiety can lead to adverse physiological responses, such as hypertension, which can affect surgical outcomes. Therefore, addressing psychological concerns through education and counseling is crucial.[46,49]
- While patient education and counseling are effective in reducing anxiety, it is important to consider individual patient differences and preferences. Some studies have shown that not all educational interventions lead to statistically significant reductions in anxiety, suggesting that factors such as personal beliefs and previous experiences may also play a role.[46,48]
- Additionally, the uptake of educational programs like POSE can be low, indicating potential barriers that need to be addressed to maximize their effectiveness.[43]
- Overall, a tailored approach that considers the unique needs and preferences of each patient may be necessary to optimize the benefits of education and counseling in minimizing anxiety in awake spine surgery.

Expert Tip

Patient Education and Counseling Approaches Reduction in Anxiety Levels
Preoperative education significantly reduces anxiety in patients. Hospital-based education and video education are effective methods.

Normalization of Expectations
Programs like POSE help reduce anxiety and align patient expectations by familiarizing them with procedures and outcomes.

Improved Preparedness
Organized educational programs make patients feel more prepared, reducing anxiety and improving postsurgery outcomes.

Educational Focus
Programs should cover surgery, recovery, hospitalization expectations, and potential outcomes to prevent information overload.

Comprehensive Knowledge
Understanding preoperative, intraoperative, and postoperative processes reduces anxiety and benefits patients and medical personnel.

Improved Postoperative Outcomes
Increased preparedness and reduced anxiety lead to enhanced recovery, pain perception, lower complication rates, and better compliance.

Educational Program Components
Includes surgical procedure explanations, anesthesia and pain management, recovery timeline, risks, postop care, and rehabilitation.

Methods of Delivering Education
In-person sessions with literature (POSE), video education, and peer education are effective in reducing anxiety.

Counseling Interventions
Counseling about procedures, diagnosis, and anesthesia can significantly reduce preoperative anxiety.

Addressing Psychological Concerns
Education and counseling address anxiety-related physiological responses, improving surgical outcomes.

Individual Differences
Not all educational interventions reduce anxiety significantly; personal beliefs and experiences play a role.

Barriers to Uptake
Programs like POSE may have low uptake, indicating barriers that need addressing to maximize effectiveness.

Tailored Approach
Considering unique patient needs and preferences optimizes the benefits of education and counseling in reducing anxiety.

9.7 Patient Anxiety in the Postoperative Phase of Care after Awake Spine Surgery

- Patient anxiety can impact patients' postoperative recovery after awake spine surgery. Patient anxiety can be influenced by multiple factors, such as baseline preoperative anxiety, pain before, during, and after surgery, and unmet information needs. The postoperative phase of care is critical in patient recovery and postoperative outcomes, including the return of physical functions, pain management, and patient satisfaction.[19]
- Preoperative anxiety is a significant predictor of postoperative outcomes. It has been shown to cause increased pain perception, higher analgesic requirements, and postoperative delirium. One-third of patients undergoing spine surgery have experienced preoperative anxiety. Addressing anxiety early in the preoperative phase is crucial in alleviating further consequences in the postoperative phase.[9]
- Postoperative anxiety is usually related to pain and physical disability. Patients with higher level of pains report higher anxiety scores, which can result in poor recovery. Pain management is crucial in alleviating patient anxiety and improving postoperative recovery. Multimodal analgesia and nonpharmacological approaches to pain management have shown promise in managing anxiety in the perioperative period.[25]
- Lack of information or education can be a significant source of anxiety in patients undergoing awake spine surgery. Patients with preoperative high anxiety levels often report greater need for information, and failure to do so can exacerbate anxiety. Providing detailed information to the patients and their families will allow for clear communication between the perioperative care teams and patients, alleviate anxiety, and improve patient satisfaction.[12]
- Anxiety and depression are common among patients undergoing spine surgery. Identifying those comorbidities in the preoperative phase can allow for an improved postoperative care by addressing the anticipated adverse events. Preoperative planning is key in preventing the impact of anxiety on postoperative outcomes.[21,23]
- It is crucial to emphasize the role of sociodemographic status, access to mental health resources, and individual patient characteristics in addressing the severity of their anxiety and in using a precision clinical pathway, rather than a standardized approach, in alleviating anxiety and improving perioperative outcomes. A holistic approach that considers these factors, alongside targeted interventions for anxiety and pain management, can enhance the overall care experience for patients undergoing awake spine surgery.[20,23]

9.8 Clinical Example

A 69-year-old man is presenting with lumbar degenerative spine disease requiring lumbar transforaminal interbody fusion. The patient has a list of comorbidities, including anxiety, depression, chronic obstructive pulmonary disease, and congestive heart failure. His body mass index is 39 kg/m^2. The preoperative assessment shows the elevated risk of postoperative delirium and postoperative cognitive dysfunction, and high anxiety and distress scores related to the expectations of surgery and the patient's baseline anxiety. After consulting with the multidisciplinary team, it was advised to proceed with awake lumbar spine fusion surgery using spinal anesthesia and conscious sedation. The following was the perioperative management plan for this patient's anxiety.

- The preoperative phase of care:
  - Preoperative assessment, including risk stratification and current status of patient comorbidities.
  - Preoperative referral to neuropsychological testing for detailed assessment of neurocognitive conditions and anxiety, including recommendations for further management of anxiety.
  - Preoperative referral to pain management for a holistic approach to perioperative patient's risk of higher levels of anxiety and pain.
  - Recommendations for a nonpharmacological approach to anxiety include music therapy and CBT.
  - Patient education protocol that allows for the appropriate teaching methods for this unique patient and emphasizes spaced repetition and teaching back methods for ensuring a detailed understanding of the procedure-related expectations.
- Intraoperative phase of care:
  - Discussion among surgery, anesthesiology, and nursing teams regarding expectations during surgery.
  - Repeat the preoperative education items that the patient received and reiterate the patient's current understanding, including potential clarification for patient and family questions.
  - Patient and family discussion with the anesthesiologist regarding appropriate choices for sedation medications. Remimazolam was the better benzodiazepine; however, with the risk of postoperative cognitive dysfunction, dexmedetomidine was a better choice for sedation during this procedure in combination with spinal and regional anesthesia to provide intraoperative anesthesia and postoperative pain management, respectively.
- The postoperative phase of care:
  - Inpatient admission versus ambulatory decision will be based on the patient's current status regarding pain, independence, and ability to care for self when home.
  - Postoperative evaluation of the patient's level of anxiety and pain.
  - Postoperative discharge instructions are tailored to explain expectations regarding recovery as a measure to alleviate anticipated anxiety.
  - Postoperative explanation of early signs of any potential surgery-related complications for the patient and family, including contact information for the care team.

9.9 Conclusion and Future Directions

Awake spine surgery, through regional anesthesia and conscious sedation, offers significant clinical and economic benefits, including fewer complications and better perioperative pain management; however, managing patient anxiety remains a critical challenge to the perioperative team. Patient anxiety can significantly impact perioperative outcomes and patient satisfaction. Effective management of anxiety through pharmacological and nonpharmacological approaches is essential in maximizing the benefits of awake spine surgery. Future research should focus on optimizing patient selection criteria and broadening the selection to include those with anxiety while implementing comprehensive anxiety management protocols tailored to this patient population. In addition, exploring innovative nonpharmacological interventions, such as VR and progressive muscle relaxation, can enhance patient experience and overall surgical outcomes. The continued evaluation of pharmacological agents such as Remimazolam and dexmedetomidine in awake spine surgery patients will be crucial in refining the sedation techniques while ensuring patient safety and favorable outcomes. Finally, a multidisciplinary approach involving surgeons, anesthesiologists, and mental health professionals will be key in advocating for optimizing patient anxiety before, during, and after awake spine surgery while striving to improve patient outcomes.

References

[1] Letchuman V, Agarwal N, Mummaneni VP, et al. Awake spinal surgery: simplifying the learning curve with a patient selection algorithm. Neurosurg Focus. 2021; 51(6):E2

[2] Fiani B, Reardon T, Selvage J, et al. Awake spine surgery: an eye-opening movement. Surg Neurol Int. 2021; 12:222

[3] Abode-Iyamah K, Ghaith AK, Bhandarkar AR, et al. Single-level awake transforaminal lumbar interbody fusion: a Mayo Clinic institutional experience and national analysis. Neurosurg Focus. 2021; 51(6):E4

[4] Garg B, Ahuja K, Sharan AD. Awake spinal fusion. J Clin Orthop Trauma. 2020; 11(5):749–752

[5] Garg B, Ahuja K, Sharan AD. Regional anesthesia for spine surgery. J Am Acad Orthop Surg. 2022; 30(17):809–819

[6] Agarwal P, Pierce J, Welch WC. Cost analysis of spinal versus general anesthesia for lumbar diskectomy and laminectomy spine surgery. World Neurosurg. 2016; 89:266–271

[7] Adler JG. Awake Lumbar Fusion: A Case Report on the Use of Spinal Anesthesia During Lumbar Fusions. JBJS Journal of Orthopaedics for Physician Assistants. 2022; 10(2):e21.00035

[8] Kai-Hong Chan A, Choy W, Miller CA, Robinson LC, Mummaneni PV. A novel technique for awake, minimally invasive transforaminal lumbar interbody fusion: technical note. Neurosurg Focus. 2019; 46(4):E16

[9] Strøm J, Bjerrum MB, Nielsen CV, et al. Anxiety and depression in spine surgery: a systematic integrative review. Spine J. 2018; 18(7):1272–1285

[10] Mitchell M. Conscious surgery: influence of the environment on patient anxiety. J Adv Nurs. 2008; 64(3):261–271

[11] Lakra D, Kujur SP. Patient perception regarding preoperative information to anxiety towards surgery. J Evol Med Dent Sci. 2015; 4(51):8839–8845

[12] Fischbeck S, Petrowski K, Renovanz M, Nesbigall R, Haaf J, Ringel F. Anxiety is associated with unfulfilled information needs and pain at the informed consent consultation of spine surgery patients: a longitudinal study. Eur Spine J. 2021; 30(8):2360–2367

[13] Friedrich S, Reis S, Meybohm P, Kranke P. Preoperative anxiety. Curr Opin Anaesthesiol. 2022; 35(6):674–678

[14] Boddeti U, Polavarapu H, Patel S, et al. Current status of awake spine surgery: a bibliometric analysis. World Neurosurg. 2024; 187:194–201.e2

[15] Stamenkovic DM, Rancic NK, Latas MB, et al. Preoperative anxiety and implications on postoperative recovery: what can we do to change our history. Minerva Anestesiol. 2018; 84(11):1307–1317

[16] Wu H, Huang Y, Tian X, et al. Preoperative anxiety-induced glucocorticoid signaling reduces GABAergic markers in spinal cord and promotes postoperative hyperalgesia by affecting neuronal PAS domain protein 4. Mol Pain. 2019; 15:1744806919850383

[17] Katsnelson BM, Rancu AL, Winter AD, Grauer JN. Preoperative anxiety: an important risk factor of postoperative adverse events and increased reoperation rates in patients undergoing single-level anterior cervical diskectomy and fusion. JAAOS Glob Res Rev. 2024; 8(10):e24.00204

[18] Deshpande N, Hadi M, Mansour TR, et al. The impact of anxiety and depression on lumbar spine surgical outcomes: a Michigan Spine Surgery Improvement Collaborative study. J Neurosurg Spine. 2024; 40(6):741–750

[19] Freedman Z, Hudock N, Hallan DR, Kelleher J. Anxiety as a risk factor for postoperative delirium in elective spine deformity surgeries: a national database study. Cureus. 2022; 14(9):e28984

[20] Rahman R, Ibaseta A, Reidler JS, et al. Changes in patients' depression and anxiety associated with changes in patient-reported outcomes after spine surgery. J Neurosurg Spine. 2020; 32(6):871–890

[21] Toll BJ, Yolcu YU, Passer JZ, et al. Impact of depression and anxiety on patient reported outcomes measures after lumbar fusion. World Neurosurg. 2024; 186:e391–e397

[22] Jain N, Sharma M, Wang D, Ugiliweneza B, Drazin D, Boakye M. The phenotypes of anxiety and depression: analysis of combined comorbidity and treatment in patients undergoing spinal fusion. Neurosurgery. 2022; 91(1):103–114

[23] Holbert SE, Wertz S, Turcotte J, Patton C. The impact of depression and anxiety on perioperative outcomes and patient-reported outcomes measurement information system physical function after thoracolumbar surgery. Int J Spine Surg. 2022; 16(6):1095–1102

[24] Jackson KL, Rumley J, Griffith M, Agochukwu UF, DeVine JG. Correlating psychological comorbidities and outcomes after spine surgery. Global Spine J. 2020; 10(7):929–939

[25] Lim K, Jung S, Kim H. Integrative review of non-pharmacological intervention and multidimensional evaluation for intraoperative anxiety under spinal anaesthesia. J Clin Nurs. 2023; 32(9–10):2114–2127

[26] Weisfeld CC, Turner JA, Bowen JI, et al. Dealing with anxious patients: an integrative review of the literature on nonpharmaceutical interventions to reduce anxiety in patients undergoing medical or dental procedures. J Altern Complement Med. 2021; 27(9):727–737

[27] Llerena GE, Krzykwa E, Huzior M, et al. Exploring novel non-pharmacologic approaches to address preoperative anxiety and postoperative pain in pediatric patients undergoing in-patient surgical procedures: a scoping review. Cureus. 2024; 16(1):e52006

[28] Wang R, Huang X, Wang Y, Akbari M. Non-pharmacologic approaches in preoperative anxiety: a comprehensive review. Front Public Health. 2022; 10:854673

[29] Kim HY, Lee MN. Effects of non-pharmacological interventions for preoperative anxiety in surgical patient: a systematic review and meta-analysis. J Korean Acad Fundam Nurs. 2019; 26(4):248–259

[30] Gropper MA, Miller RD, Cohen NH, eds. Miller's Anesthesia. Vol. 1. 9th ed. Philadelphia, PA: Elsevier; 2020

[31] Lee A, Shirley M. Remimazolam: a review in procedural sedation. Drugs. 2021; 81(10):1193–1201

[32] Smith A, Kalsotra S, Tobias JD. The use of Remimazolam during awake craniotomy for seizure foci resection in adolescents: a case series. J Clin Med Res. 2024; 16(6):319–323

[33] Afonso J, Reis F. Dexmedetomidine: current role in anesthesia and intensive care. Rev Bras Anestesiol. 2012; 62(1):118–133

[34] Cormack JR, Orme RM, Costello TG. The role of α2-agonists in neurosurgery. J Clin Neurosci. 2005; 12(4):375–378

[35] LA Via L, Santonocito C, Bartolotta N, et al. α-2 agonists vs. fentanyl as adjuvants for spinal anesthesia in elective cesarean section: a meta-analysis. Minerva Anestesiol. 2023; 89 (5):445–454

[36] Yu H, Kang H, Fan J, Cao G, Liu B. Influence of dexmedetomidine on postoperative cognitive dysfunction in the elderly: a meta-analysis of randomized controlled trials. Brain Behav. 2022; 12(8):e2665

[37] Patel JN, Maliwad JF, Mehta PJ, Damor RD, Shringarpure KS. Sedative effect of propofol and midazolam in surgery under spinal anaesthesia: a comparative study. Indian J Clin Anaesth. 2020; 7(1):187–191

[38] El Kady GAAER, El-Sersi MH, Kassem AA, Hussein AYM. Comparison of propofol versus midazolam infusion for conscious sedation during spinal anaesthesia in patients undergoing inguinal hernia repair. QJM: Int J Med. 2023; 116 Suppl 1:hcad069.017

[39] Erdman HB, Kornilov E, Kahana E, et al. Asleep DBS under ketamine sedation: proof of concept. Neurobiol Dis. 2022; 170:105747

[40] Roushdy ASI, Gadelrub AT, Abdo KA. Gabapentin plus celecoxib as preemptive analgesia in complex spine surgery for improving perioperative patient anxiety and satisfaction: is it effective? Randomized double-blind controlled clinical trial. Minia J Med Res. 2023; 34(1):42–52

[41] Ménigaux C, Adam F, Guignard B, Sessler DI, Chauvin M. Preoperative gabapentin decreases anxiety and improves early functional recovery from knee surgery. Anesth Analg. 2005; 100(5):1394–1399

[42] Adam F, Bordenave L, Sessler DI, Chauvin M. Effects of a single 1200-mg preoperative dose of gabapentin on anxiety

and memory. Ann Fr Anesth Réanim. 2012; 31(10):e223–e227

[43] Edwards R, Gibson J, Mungin-Jenkins E, Pickford R, Lucas JD, Jones GD. A preoperative spinal education intervention for spinal fusion surgery designed using the rehabilitation treatment specification system is safe and could reduce hospital length of stay, normalize expectations, and reduce anxiety : a prospective cohort study. Bone Jt Open. 2022; 3 (2):135–144

[44] Cakmak M, Kose I, Zinzircioglu C, et al. Effect of video-based education on anxiety and satisfaction of patients undergoing spinal anesthesia. Braz J Anesthesiol. 2018; 68(3):274–279

[45] Kalliyath AK, Korula SV, Mathew A, Abraham SP, Isac M. Effect of preoperative education about spinal anesthesia on anxiety and postoperative pain in parturients undergoing elective cesarean section: a randomized controlled trial. J Obstet Anaesth Crit Care. 2019; 9(1):14–17

[46] Bell J, Paul S, Sesti J, Granger B. Improving self-reported preoperative anxiety through a preoperative education program: a quality improvement project. J Dr Nurs Pract. 2019; 12(1):117–124

[47] Raoufian F, Sahbaeiroy F. The effect of peer education on pre- and post-operative anxiety in patients with spinal stenosis referred to selected hospitals of Iran University of Medical Sciences in 2020. Med Sci J Islam Azad Univ. 2022; 32(2):204–214

[48] Shah P, Kezo A, Solanki HD, Dhengle Y. Effect of counseling on preoperative anxiety levels in surgical patients, a randomized controlled trial in a teaching institution. Bharati Vidyapeeth Med J. 2022; 2(2):3–7

[49] Wilson CJ, Mitchelson AJ, Tzeng TH, et al. Caring for the surgically anxious patient: a review of the interventions and a guide to optimizing surgical outcomes. Am J Surg. 2016; 212 (1):151–159

10 General Anesthesia—Not Just Going to Sleep

Maya Blasingame and Amanda H. Kumar

Abstract

General anesthesia has had a vital role in revolutionizing surgery, dating back to the mid-19th century. The first successful demonstration of modern anesthesia began with the use of ether anesthesia by William T.G. Morton, marking the foundation of the development of anesthetic agents in an effective manner. Throughout the years, general anesthesia has evolved significantly and has diversified its incorporation of a variety of substances that are used as anesthetic agents. Despite the vital role of general anesthesia, it is associated with a range of adverse effects. Effects range from common and intermediate symptoms including nausea, vomiting, and sore throat to more severe and rare complications including malignant hyperthermia, cardiovascular instability, and cognitive effects. This chapter outlines a brief history of general anesthesia and its use to optimize surgical operating conditions and the risk profile associated with the use of general anesthesia.

Keywords: general anesthesia, complications, postoperative complications, adverse effects, risk stratification

Key Points

- Through development and innovation in the field of anesthesiology, there have been several iterations of anesthetic agents used to provide safe and efficient operating conditions.
- Common side effects of general anesthesia include nausea, vomiting, sore throat, drowsiness, and confusion.
- General anesthesia can have significant effects on different organ systems including cardiovascular, respiratory, and neurological systems.
- Careful selection of anesthetic technique is essential to provide safe perioperative patient care.

10.1 Introduction

The history of general anesthesia details the innovation within medicine that has transformed both the field of surgery and patient care, enhancing patient comfort. In 1846, Dr. William T. Morton laid the groundwork for the development and refinement of anesthetic agents providing a pivotal moment in surgical operating conditions.[1] Dr. Morton used inhaled ether to show its properties as a safe and effective anesthetic, shaping the role of anesthetics for decades to come.

- 1847: Dr. James Y. Simpson began the use of chloroform for women during childbirth and the use of chloroform as an obstetric anesthetic is popularized by Dr. John Snow in 1853.[2]
- 1932: Dr. John Lundy described the use of sodium thiopental and other barbiturates as intravenous (IV) anesthetics.[3]
- 1942: Drs. Harold Griffith and Enid Johnson establish the use of the first muscle relaxant as an anesthetic.
- 1960s: Drs. Gunter Corssen and Robert Virtue began human trials of the IV anesthetic ketamine and inhaled anesthetic enflurane.
- 1963: Dr. Edmon I. Eger develops the characterization of the minimum alveolar concentration, the concentration of inhaled anesthetic that enacts immobility in 50% of patients.[4]
- 1977: Propofol became a widely used IV medication that provided antiemetic effects in addition to anesthetic effects.[5]
- 1990s: Desflurane and sevoflurane are introduced as inhaled anesthetics.[6]

The primary role of general anesthesia is to render the patient unconscious and decrease the perception of pain during procedures. The innovation of anesthetics provided a pivotal turning point in the focus of patient-centered care, not only providing improved patient safety and comfort but also creating efficient operating environments for surgical teams. Various anesthetic techniques are used for both the induction and maintenance of general anesthesia. Modern anesthetic techniques incorporate monitoring systems that maximize patient safety while minimizing the risk of complications and side effects. Although these innovations have been vital for surgery, general anesthesia is not without risks and adverse effects.

10.2 Cardiovascular Effects of General Anesthesia

- Common anesthetic induction agents, including inhaled anesthetics and IV anesthetics, such as propofol, can have significant impacts on the cardiovascular system. These effects include decreased systemic vascular resistance, decreased myocardial contractility, decreased stroke volume, increased myocardial irritability, and other hemodynamic consequences.[7]
- Inhaled anesthetics cause vasodilation, which can lead to decreased blood pressure and overall decreased systemic vascular resistance.
- General anesthesia diminishes the forcefulness of the heart muscle, leading to decreased cardiac output and a reduction in stroke volume.
- The heart muscle can become more susceptible to arrhythmias with the use of anesthetics.
- Patients with preexisting heart conditions are more susceptible to the cardiovascular effects of anesthesia and are monitored to regulate and avoid any adverse complications that could occur during surgical operations.[8]
- General anesthesia has a role in modifying autonomic reflex control of circulation upon induction of the anesthetic.[9]
- In patients undergoing noncardiac surgery, there is a risk of cardiac complications perioperatively including mortality as a result of cardiac incidents from the physiological stress of surgery (e.g., blood loss, anesthesia effects, and hemodynamic changes).[10]
- Patients with preexisting conditions such as coronary artery disease are at an increased risk of perioperative myocardial infarction several days after surgery as a result of prolonged imbalance between myocardial oxygen supply and demand and inflammatory responses.[10]
- The stress of surgery and/or the effects of anesthesia and other medications can lead to the disruption of normal electrical activity of the heart, triggering the onset of arrhythmias during noncardiac surgery. Anesthesia can affect the autonomic regulation of the heart rate and rhythm, leading to arrhythmias.[11]
- To reduce these perioperative complications, careful patient selection and close hemodynamic monitoring is essential. The anesthetic plan should be carefully crafted, taking into account the patient's preexisting conditions. A frank discussion between the anesthesiology and surgical teams is helpful to ensure open communication about the length of the procedure, expected intraoperative blood loss, and other surgical considerations that may impact the anesthetic plan. A frank discussion with the patient about these risks and benefits is always necessary.
- Should a major cardiac event occur perioperatively, the anesthesiologist would first medically stabilize the patient. Cardiology consultation and/or escalation in postoperative level of care (i.e., admission to intensive care unit) may be necessary in certain situations.

Expert Tip

Perioperative risk stratification is a key part of curating a safe anesthetic plan.

10.3 Respiratory Effects of General Anesthesia

- General anesthesia for a surgical operation involves manipulation of the airway in patients and can lead to several adverse outcomes that include direct injury, challenges with airway management, and physiological responses.[12]
- Difficulty with ventilation or intubation can occur after induction of general anesthesia, resulting in desaturation, pulmonary compromise, and/or aspiration during airway manipulation. As a result, alternative methods may be required in order to secure the airway and continue a safe and effective operation.

Expert Tip

Preoperative examination and evaluation can determine the likelihood of difficult ventilation and difficult intubation. The American Society of Anesthesiologists Task Force on Management of the Difficult Airway has a published difficult airway algorithm.

- Laryngospasm and negative pressure pulmonary edema are other complications from airway manipulation that can result in hypoxemia, hypercarbia, hypotension, and pulmonary edema.
- During airway manipulation, physiological responses may occur such as increased heart rate and blood pressure or bronchospasm.
- Inhaled anesthetics have been indicated in their role as irritants of the airway of asthmatics leading to bronchospasm as a result of exposure to noxious anesthetic agents.[6]
- Anesthesia leads to decreased muscle tone and relaxation of respiratory muscles, including the diaphragm; overall, this can lead to shallower breaths and a decrease in lung volumes during surgery.[13]
- Induction of anesthesia leads to the reduction of the functional residual capacity of the patient; this could lead to hypoxemia as a result of ventilation/perfusion mismatch.[13]
- General anesthesia can result in the collapse of airways, which leads to blocked airway flow during exhalation and alveolar collapse, thus promoting hypoxemia.[14]
- After a procedure, postoperative pulmonary complications can persist including suppressed cough reflex, atelectasis, ventilation/perfusion mismatch, and an increased risk of acute respiratory distress syndrome.
- Patients are at increased risk of infections and inflammatory processes postoperatively, including pneumonia and pleurisy.[15]
- The respiratory complications that can arise with the use of general anesthesia can be mitigated but not eliminated with careful preoperative airway assessment, selection of appropriate airway equipment, and vigilant and continuous monitoring of ventilation and oxygenation intraoperatively.
- Patients with respiratory compromise may require prolonged intubation after surgery until they meet the extubation criteria. Surgeries in the prone position add another layer of complexity as airway edema may compromise the ability to extubate patients at the end of surgery. A cuff leak test is one procedure that may help predict the likelihood of postextubation airway obstruction from laryngeal edema.

10.4 Other Complications of General Anesthesia

10.4.1 Postoperative Nausea and Vomiting

- One of the most common adverse effects of general anesthesia is one that arises from the chemoreceptor trigger zone of the brain, producing postoperative nausea and vomiting.[16]
- Female gender, young age, nonsmoking status, longer duration of surgery, and history of nausea and vomiting are risk factors that increase a patient's risk of having postoperative nausea and vomiting.[16] Up to one-third of patients without prophylaxis would experience postoperative nausea and vomiting. Studies have found that the administration of prophylactic antiemetics can help reduce and treat postoperative nausea and vomiting.
- Patients report avoidance of postoperative nausea and vomiting as a greater concern than postoperative pain, and postoperative nausea and vomiting is the leading case of delay of discharge from the postanesthesia care unit.
- Additionally, postoperative nausea and vomiting can cause an aspiration risk, possible airway compromise, dehydration and electrolyte changes, and can cause increased central venous pressure, intracranial pressure, bleeding, or wound dehiscence.
- Patients are routinely given antiemetic prophylaxis during anesthesia care, and selection of antiemetic agents is based on patient characteristics, risk factors, and surgical procedure. The Apfel scoring system is commonly used to risk stratify patients at risk of postoperative nausea and vomiting to guide judicious use of antiemetic prophylaxis.
- Treatment for postoperative nausea and vomiting continues in the postanesthesia care unit, typically under the direction of the anesthesiologist. Postoperative nausea and vomiting may also be related to opioid use, and surgeons may prescribe antiemetics for use at home.

10.4.2 Malignant Hyperthermia

- Halogenated inhaled anesthetics and the muscle relaxant succinylcholine have been indicted in triggering malignant hyperthermia, a rare and potentially fatal hypermetabolic crisis. This can occur in patients with mutations in their ryanodine receptors that regulate calcium concentrations.

- When exposed to anesthetics, these patients release excessive amounts of calcium in skeletal muscles, which leads to the onset of a series of symptoms including muscle rigidity, hyperthermia, hyperkalemia, and metabolic imbalances.[6]
- The hypermetabolic rate also results in increased oxygen consumption, increased carbon dioxide production, severe lactic acidosis, arrhythmia, and risk of rhabdomyolysis.
- Malignant hyperthermia can be avoided or reduced by identifying risk factors in patients, such as family history or associated conditions, and avoiding the use of anesthetics that may increase risk in susceptible patients and nondepolarizing muscle relaxants.
- Treatment of malignant hyperthermia involves immediate discontinuous of triggering agents as well as administration of dantrolene. Management of hyperthermia and hyperkalemic states involves the use of ice packs, sodium bicarbonate, and calcium gluconate.

Expert Tip

Malignant hyperthermia is a rare and potentially fatal complication. Anesthesiologists may call the MHAUS (Malignant Hyperthermia Association of the United States) to report a case and to request resources.

10.4.3 Airway Injury

- During the insertion of airway devices such as endotracheal tubes, patients can receive minor injuries to different areas of the mouth, teeth, and upper airway tracts. Rarely can patients receive punctures and injuries to locations such as the vocal cords and esophagus.
- Sore throat and hoarseness are common side effects that arise in up to half of patients postoperatively as a result of trauma from intubation. Irritation or injury of the airway can also result in vocal cord dysfunction.[17]
- Patients with preexisting dental problems are at an increased susceptibility to injury during intubation; injuries can range from fractured or dislodged teeth to soft tissue damage of areas such as the lips, tongue, and gums.[18]
- Airway injuries can be proactively monitored by evaluating for indicators of airway difficulties such as limited neck mobility, small mouth opening, and other indicators.
- When airway injury does occur, it is important to provide supportive care for injuries such as swelling or minor injuries, as well as assessment of injuries that may indicate surgical intervention.

10.4.4 Hypothermia

- General anesthesia inhibits thermoregulation, placing patients at risk of hypothermia.
- Hypothermia can increase rates of infection, delay wound healing, and increase risk of surgical graft failure. This can be monitored and treated in the operating room by using active warming techniques such as forced-air warming blankets and warmed IV fluids.
- Further, it may induce a coagulopathy, leading to increased surgical blood loss and increased need for transfusion.
- Hypothermia also delays emergence from general anesthesia by prolonging the duration of action of many anesthetic agents.
- Hypothermia may also impair delivery of oxygen by left-shifting the oxygen–hemoglobin dissociation curve, have a negative effect on inotropy and chronotropy, induce dysrhythmias, and increase postoperative shivering.
- The American Society of Anesthesiologists guidelines note that temperature monitoring for patients receiving anesthesia is required when clinically significant changes in body temperature are intended, anticipated, or suspected. Hypothermic patients can be warmed using forced-air warmers, fluid warmers, or by raising the ambient temperature in the operating room.

10.4.5 Awareness under Anesthesia

- Awareness under anesthesia has an estimated incidence of 1 to 2 per 1,000 general anesthetic cases. Awareness is more common in high-risk procedures on unstable patients and may require early postoperative counseling.

10.4.6 Adverse Drug Reactions

- Adverse drug reactions may occur during general anesthesia. These allergic reactions can manifest as mild skin rashes or severe reactions, including life-threatening anaphylaxis leading to difficulty breathing, swelling, and shock.[19]
- Patients who experience a serious intraoperative allergic reaction may benefit from seeing an allergy specialist postdischarge to help elucidate the trigger for the allergic reaction.

10.4.7 Cognitive Dysfunction

- General anesthesia can lead to a range of short- and long-term cognitive effects in patients, impacting both memory and cognition. These effects can range from confusion, disorientation, and delirium immediately postoperatively or long-term memory issues and difficulty with higher-level cognitive skills such as planning, organizing, and problem-solving.[20] Measures can be taken to reduce the risk of cognitive dysfunction as a result of anesthesia, including limiting the duration of anesthesia and incorporating multimodal analgesia to reduce risk of postoperative delirium.
- These adverse effects are described in further detail in a later chapter and are outside the scope of this chapter.

10.5 Risk Profile of Anesthetic Techniques

- General anesthesia provides complete unconsciousness during a surgical operation. A combination of medications induces lack of awareness, analgesia, and muscle relaxation.
- Regional anesthesia encompasses the use of neuraxial and/or peripheral nerve blocks. Deposition of local anesthetic at target sites allows the anesthesiologist to numb specific areas of the body, providing complete surgical anesthesia and/or postoperative analgesia. If regional anesthesia is selected as the primary anesthetic technique, patients may be aware, alert, and comfortable during surgery.[21]
- Monitored anesthesia care is often seen as a middle ground between general anesthesia and being fully awake during an operation. Patients are in a relaxed and sedated state, but may have purposeful response to stimuli. Vigilant monitoring is required due to the potential need to manipulate the airway during the operation.[22]
- Regional anesthesia and monitored anesthesia care can be used for shorter procedures, facilitating fast-track recovery with decreased risks of perioperative complications.[23]
- General anesthesia can be associated with an increased risk of perioperative complications, though it is challenging to define this incidence.
- Ultimately the selection of an anesthetic type should be done after careful discussion of patient risk factors, surgical needs, and anesthetic considerations.

10.6 Conclusion

General anesthesia has a profound impact on the field of medicine and surgical practices while engaging the importance of patient-focused medicine. The development of modern anesthesia practices in the surgical operating room has played an important role in increasing patient safety and optimizing operating conditions; however, there are still inherent risks associated with the use of general anesthesia. Complications can range from minor adverse effects such as nausea and sore throat to severe complications.

References

[1] Robinson DH, Toledo AH. Historical development of modern anesthesia. J Invest Surg. 2012; 25(3):141–149

[2] Abhyankar RS, Jessop KM. From craft to profession: the development of modern anesthesiology—part II. Mo Med. 2022; 119(1):14–20

[3] Rosenberg M, Weaver J. General anesthesia. Anesth Prog. 1991; 38(4–5):172–186

[4] Lobo SA, Ojeda J, Dua A, Singh K, Lopez J. Minimum Alveolar Concentration. Treasure Island, FL: StatPearls Publishing; 2022

[5] Walsh CT. Propofol: milk of amnesia. Cell. 2018; 175(1):10–13

[6] Miller AL, Theodore D, Widrich J. Inhalational Anesthetic. Treasure Island, FL: StatPearls Publishing; 2023

[7] Barker SJ, Gamel DM, Tremper KK. Cardiovascular effects of anesthesia and operation. Crit Care Clin. 1987; 3(2):251–268

[8] Akata T, Warltier DC. General anesthetics and vascular smooth muscle: direct actions of general anesthetics on cellular mechanisms regulating vascular tone. Anesthesiology. 2007; 106(2):365–391

[9] Eis S, Kramer J. Anesthesia Inhalation Agents and Their Cardiovascular Effects. Treasure Island, FL: StatPearls Publishing; 2024

[10] Grayburn PA, Hillis LD. Cardiac events in patients undergoing noncardiac surgery: shifting the paradigm from noninvasive risk stratification to therapy. Ann Intern Med. 2003; 138(6):506–511

[11] Kwon CH, Kim SH. Intraoperative management of critical arrhythmia. Korean J Anesthesiol. 2017; 70(2):120–126

[12] Santer P, Wachtendorf LJ, Suleiman A, et al. Mechanical power during general anesthesia and postoperative respiratory failure: a multicenter retrospective cohort study. Anesthesiology. 2022; 137(1):41–54

[13] Bigatello L, Pesenti A. Respiratory physiology for the anesthesiologist. Anesthesiology. 2019; 130(6):1064–1077

[14] Petran J, Ansems K, Rossaint R, et al. Effects of hypercapnia versus normocapnia during general anesthesia on outcomes: a systematic review and meta-analysis. Braz J Anesthesiol. 2022; 72(3):398–406

[15] Chen F, Fang L, Feng K, Xu J. Respiratory tract infection after oral and maxillofacial surgery under general anesthesia and related factors. J Infect Dev Ctries. 2023; 17(7):979–985

[16] Shaikh SI, Nagarekha D, Hegade G, Marutheesh M. Postoperative nausea and vomiting: a simple yet complex problem. Anesth Essays Res. 2016; 10(3):388–396

[17] El-Boghdadly K, Bailey CR, Wiles MD. Postoperative sore throat: a systematic review. Anaesthesia. 2016; 71(6):706–717

[18] Kotani T, Inoue S, Kawaguchi M. Perioperative dental injury associated with intubated general anesthesia. Anesth Prog. 2022; 69(1):3–9

[19] Laguna JJ, Archilla J, Doña I, et al. Practical guidelines for perioperative hypersensitivity reactions. J Investig Allergol Clin Immunol. 2018; 28(4):216–232

[20] Lee YL, Wong J, Ng SY. Delirium in patients following general anaesthesia. Ann Acad Med Singap. 2022; 51(2):71–73

[21] Vail EA, Feng R, Sieber F, et al. Long-term outcomes with spinal versus general anesthesia for hip fracture surgery: a randomized trial. Anesthesiology. 2024; 140(3):375–386

[22] Ghisi D, Fanelli A, Tosi M, Nuzzi M, Fanelli G. Monitored anesthesia care. Minerva Anestesiol. 2005; 71(9):533–538

[23] Breen P, Park KW. General anesthesia versus regional anesthesia. Int Anesthesiol Clin. 2002; 40(1):61–71

11 Lessons from COVID-19 and Lower and Medium Income Countries—Egypt

Mohamed Fawzy Khattab

Abstract

Lumbar spine surgeries like diskectomy, microscopic lumbar spinal canal decompression, and lumbar fixation and fusion are most commonly performed under general anesthesia, which can be associated with several perioperative morbidities associated with prone positioning morbidities like posterior ischemic optic neuropathy, nausea, vomiting, atelectasis, pulmonary aspiration, prolonged postanesthesia recovery, and special complications for high-risk patients such as those with respiratory disease. It is possible that fewer complications may occur if the procedure is performed under neuroaxis anesthesia. Recently there has been an increased interest in regional or spinal anesthesia in spine surgery. These techniques are less expensive and may allow for faster recovery for patients and are not associated with the same possible complications as general anesthesia. However, there are some important considerations when using these techniques, including issues with redosing, ability to use neuromonitoring, and airway management when patients are prone. During the COVID-19 pandemic, there was a decrease in the available resources, such as ventilators, hence the role of awake spinal anesthesia in reducing cost and rationing resources for those with higher acuity medical conditions. This chapter aims to provide a comprehensive guide for health care professionals working in resource-limited settings, empowering them to perform spine surgeries safely and effectively using spinal anesthesia.

Keywords: spinal anesthesia, spine surgery, limited resources, awake spine surgery, Egypt, socioeconomic, COVID-19

Key Points

- Spine surgical intervention under awake spinal anesthesia has fewer major cardiopulmonary complications.
- No significant intraoperative complications that affected patient satisfaction underwent surgery with spinal anesthesia.
- Patients were able to eat immediately after the operation.
- Time to ambulation, time to hospital discharge, and rate of complications were satisfactory to both the patient and the surgeon.
- Awake lumbar spinal anesthesia is a safe and effective alternative to general anesthesia with increased patient and surgeon satisfaction.
- During the COVID-19 pandemic, there were variability among countries in response and preparedness to handling the situation during the early phase of the pandemic.
- The COVID-19 pandemic showed the vulnerability in health care systems with limited resources.
- Spinal surgery under spinal anesthesia plays an important role in spinal health care in the presence of future pandemics.

11.1 Introduction

- It is crucial to guarantee the safe, effective, and cost-efficient administration of anesthetic in spine surgeries.[1] General anesthesia (GA) is currently the most common type of anesthetic used in spine surgery. This is probably because in the past, spine surgery was linked to a significant amount of morbidity, such as blood loss, prone position complications, extended operating times, and the requirement for excellent airway control. Predicting the duration and degree of invasiveness of the procedure may have been challenging because of the significant variability in these factors. Spine surgery has been more regulated with the introduction of newer, minimally invasive procedures, growing understanding of spine pathology, and the presence of an efficient, well-trained spine surgery team.[2]
- In nations with limited resources, spine surgery presents particular difficulties because of limitations in resources, infrastructure,

equipment, and skilled workers. In certain situations, especially in the presence of respiratory, renal, cardiac, and hepatic pathologies, regional spinal anesthesia present a good substitute for GA. The ideas, advantages, and practical aspects of spine surgery under spinal anesthesia in resource-constrained settings have been examined previously in Egypt.[3]

11.2 COVID-19 and Spine Surgery

- In December 2019, an outbreak of severe lower respiratory tract infection was identified in Wuhan City, China. The outbreak was declared a global pandemic by the World Health Organization (WHO) on March 11, 2020. This resulted in an overwhelming burden on the health care system, medical resources, and staff. In addition, it created a global state of panic among populations, politicians, and health care providers.[4]
- Possible aerosolization of the virus from asymptomatic patients during intubation or extubation was a risk, in a negative flow operating theaters, as the virus might settle in the wind tunnel.[5]
- However, despite the pandemic, chronic illnesses such as back pain did not decrease. Thus, there is a need to be able to take care of these patients in an efficient manner and not use important resources such as ventilators or put patients at increased risk of contracting COVID-19. Spinal anesthesia may provide this.[6]

11.3 Egyptian Experience during the COVID-19 Pandemic

- Between 2019 and 2021, a case series of 250 patients admitted to our spine unit facility in Cairo, Egypt, for lumbar and lower thoracic spine surgeries. Informed consent was obtained before every procedure, and all operations were performed by the same surgical team. The breakdown of the 250 scheduled surgeries is as follows: revision of posterior spinal fusion in 27 patients, removal of instrumentation in 10 patients, vertebroplasty in 30 patients, soft transforaminal lumbar interbody fusion (TLIF) in 30 patients, posterolateral fusion in 33 patients, TLIF in 36 patients, lumbar decompression in 47 patients, diskectomy in 35 patients, and thoracic decompression and posterolateral fusion in 2 patients.
- The age of the patients ranged from 20 to 85 years, with the mean age was being 47.5 ± 19.3 years, and 129 (51.6%) patients were males and 121 (48.4%) patients were females.
- The mean estimated blood loss across all procedures was 395 ± 156 mL, and the operative time ranged from 45 to 310 minutes. Under spinal anesthesia, the patients were able to assist with their positioning in the beginning of surgery and were capable of intraoperative conversation and interaction. In nine cases, an injection of an extra dose of spinal anesthesia was necessary. In one case, a 5-hour, three-level revision, the patient was converted to GA after 3 hours under spinal anesthesia using laryngeal mask airway.
- Visual analog scale (VAS) score and Oswestry Disability Index (ODI) were assessed preoperatively, immediately postoperation, and 1 year after surgery. Patients demonstrated excellent postoperative pain relief, as measured by VAS and ODI, which was maintained and improved upon at the 1-year postoperative follow-up. Patient satisfaction was assessed with a simple questionnaire containing the following questions: (1) Would you recommend this type of anesthesia to other patients? (2) If you had the same condition again, would you accept the same type of anesthesia?
- In all, 207 patients (82.8%) were satisfied with spinal anesthesia and would recommend the anesthesia for other patients. Forty-three female patients (17.2%) were not satisfied with the spinal anesthesia although they were satisfied with the postoperative clinical and functional outcomes. These females underwent spinal fusion procedures.

Expert Tip

- *Spinal anesthesia is cost-effective when compared to GA.*[7]
- *It can be done for lumbar spine surgeries and lower dorsal spine surgeries.*[8,9]
- *A rapid, fast, and efficient surgical and anesthesia team is required to perform the procedure.*

- *Cooperative of the patient is required (see Chapter 9 on Patient Anxiety in Awake Spine Surgery).*
- *It is helpful in patients with comorbidities and those with risk of vision loss.*
- *Postoperative fatigue is reduced in patients with spinal anesthesia.*[10]
- *It can be done in simple primary cases and revision cases.*

11.4 Advantages of Spine Surgery under Spinal Anesthesia

- *Reduction in resource requirements:* Spinal surgeries like lumbar diskectomies, lumbar decompressions, lumbar fusion, and removal of implants can be done under spinal anesthesia. Spinal anesthesia necessitates fewer resources than GA, especially less reliance on advanced airway ventilators.[6]
- The cost of spinal anesthetic is generally lower than that of GA.[1]
- Spinal anesthesia is associated with lower risk of postoperative nausea and vomiting, deep venous thrombosis, and pulmonary complications.[3]
- Patients experience quicker postoperative recovery, which is crucial in settings with limited hospital stay durations.
- It is very useful when the patient has had a recent eye surgery or there is risk of vision loss.
- The patient can be cooperative and help in their positioning.[6]
- Some patients can interact during surgery.[3]

11.5 Limitations

- It is suitable only for lumbar spine surgery.
- It is not technically suitable for ankylosed patients.
- It is contraindicated in infection cases such as spondylodiskitis or anticoagulation.
- It requires a safe and efficient surgeon and anesthesia team.
- The surgical team should be aware of the limited time of the surgery.

Expert Tip

The highest level of surgery performed was at the dorsal T10, T11, and T12.

11.6 Preoperative Considerations

- Thorough preoperative assessment is crucial. Evaluate the patient's medical history, current health status, and suitability for spinal anesthesia.
- *Informed consent:* Clearly explain the procedure, benefits, and potential risks to the patient. Obtain informed signed written consent.

11.7 Equipment and Medications

- *Essential equipment:* Spinal needles, local anesthetic agents, sterile drapes, antiseptic solutions, and resuscitation equipment must be readily available.
- *Drug selection:* Long-acting local anesthetics like bupivacaine are preferred for prolonged surgeries. Adjuncts such as opioids or steroids may be used to enhance the duration of anesthesia.

11.8 Intraoperative Management

- Standard monitors of blood pressure, heart rate, respiratory rate, and oxygen saturation were applied to the patient in the operating theater and the patient was placed in a lateral position (▶ Fig. 11.1).

Expert Tip

Anesthesia consultants prefer the lateral position with flexion of the hip to open the interlaminar space.

- After sterile preparation and draping of the back, 3 to 4 mL of 2% lidocaine was injected subcutaneously into the third or fourth lumbar interspace. A 25-gauge Sprotte spinal needle was then introduced in the lumbar interspace until free flow of cerebrospinal fluid was visualized after removal of the spinal needle stylet (► Fig. 11.2).
- At this time, 3 mL (15 mg) of 0.5% spinal bupivacaine was injected into the spinal canal. The patient turned to the supine position and remained in this position with the head slightly elevated for 15 minutes, after which the patient helped in positioning himself or herself on the surgical frame (► Fig. 11.3).
- Patients receiving spinal anesthetic for lumbar surgery have also been shown to experience less blood loss. This has been attributed to a significant drop in intraoperative blood loss due to a significant reduction in both blood pressure and heart rate in patients administered a spinal anesthetic.

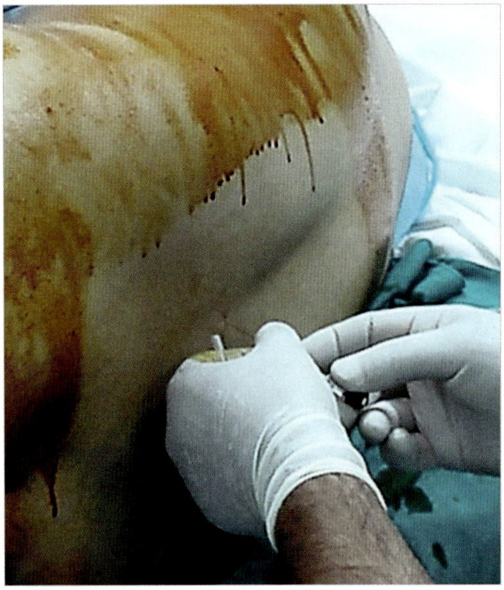

Fig. 11.1 Anesthesia was given while the patient was in the lateral position.

Expert Tip

The reduced blood loss was due to a combination of sympathetic blockade—producing vasodilation and relative hypotension—and lowered intrathoracic pressure experienced when patients are allowed to breathe spontaneously.

Expert Tip

The anesthesia team should be familiar with different anesthesia techniques and be prepared for managing complications such as the following:

- *Hypotension: Promptly treat hypotension with intravenous fluids and vasopressors if needed.*
- *Bradycardia: Administer atropine or other appropriate medications to manage bradycardia.*
- *High block: In case of an excessively high block, be prepared to convert to GA.*

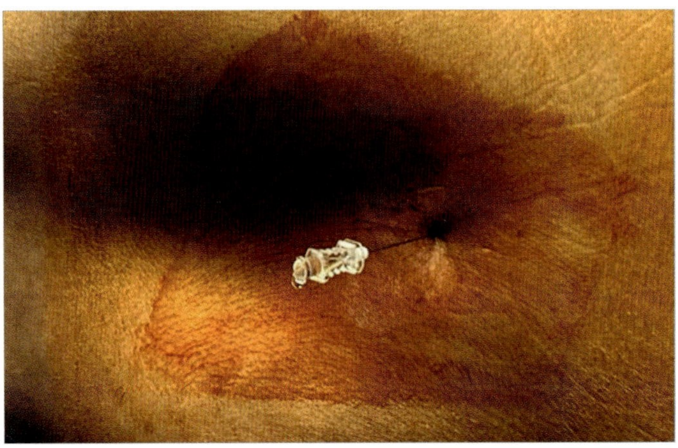

Fig. 11.2 Cerebrospinal fluid appears after removal of the spinal needle stylet.

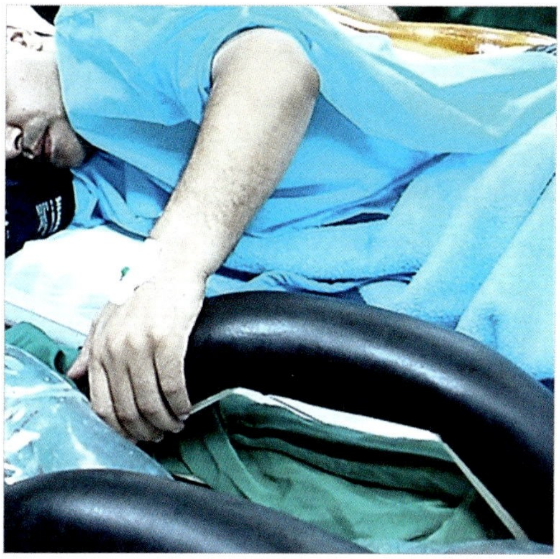

Fig. 11.3 The patient can help in their positioning.

11.9 Postoperative Care

- Postoperative pain relief was excellent with improvement in the VAS score. There was no incidence of postdural puncture headache. This technique avoided the deleterious physiological consequences of the prone position under GA. The maintenance of spontaneous ventilation resulted in less distension of the epidural veins and produced an excellent bloodless surgical field. Although spinal anesthesia has previously been reported for diskectomy[11,12,13,14] and is mentioned in anesthetic textbooks,[15] it is unclear exactly how widely the technique has been practiced.
- Patients were encouraged to mobilize early on the same day for diskectomy and decompression surgeries and the next day for lumbar fusion surgeries. This was to prevent complications such as deep venous thrombosis and to facilitate recovery.

11.10 Postoperative Recovery

- In the Egyptian experience, patients receiving a spinal anesthetic experienced less postoperative pain as well as fewer episodes of nausea and emesis. Both heart rate and mean arterial blood pressure were also more physiologically stable (approximating resting preoperative values), reflecting a lower level of systemic stress and pain. Improved postanesthetic comfort contributes to a high level of patient satisfaction, as documented in the literature.[16]

Expert Tip

From our experience, females, obese and overweight patients, diabetics do not prefer awake spinal anesthesia.

11.11 Perioperative Complications

- We had no intraoperative complications that affected patient satisfaction.
- If needed, patients with longer revision lumbar fusion surgery for adjacent segment disease can be converted to GA using a laryngeal mask in prone positioning.
- Redosing of the spinal anesthetic can be done easily by the surgeon due to the exposed dural sac.
- Only one patient had postoperative spondylodiskitis at the L3–L4 level 1 month after diskectomy. The patient's back pain improved with intravenous antibiotics.

11.12 Clinical Cases

11.12.1 Case 1

A 64-year-old woman with diabetes, hypertension, and ischemic heart disease presented with low back pain, right sciatica, and intermittent claudication. She had a history of posterolateral fusion performed 12 years ago (▶ Fig. 11.4).

A trial of spine injections and conservative treatment was attempted. The patient had unacceptable quality of life and walked with a flexed posture.

She underwent revision spine surgery with extension of fusion and removal of the previous construct, which were all done under spinal anesthesia (▶ Fig. 11.5).

The operative time was 150 minutes, and blood loss 500 mL.

Intraoperatively, the patient remained stable, and postoperative recovery was uneventful with early mobilization achieved on the first postoperative day.

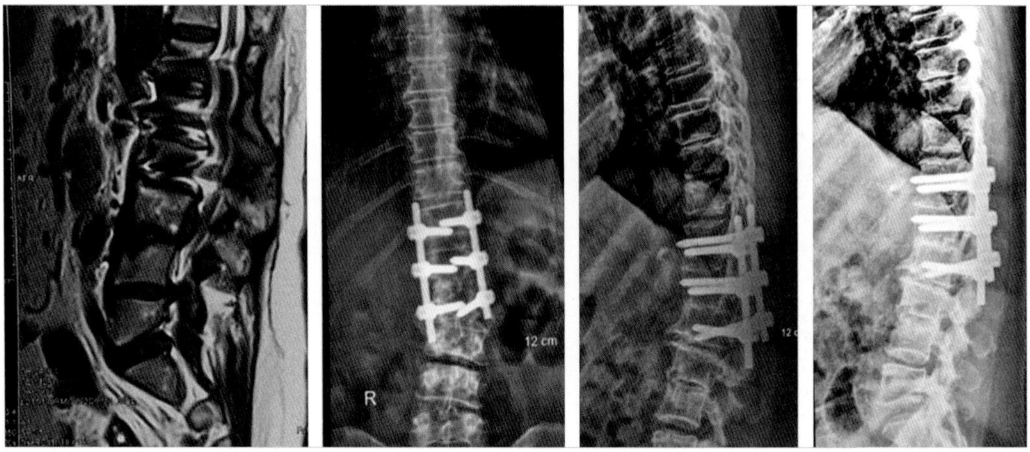

Fig. 11.4 Preoperative radiological investigations showed the adding on, degenerative coronal and sagittal malalignment. Previous posterolateral fusion and previous implant.

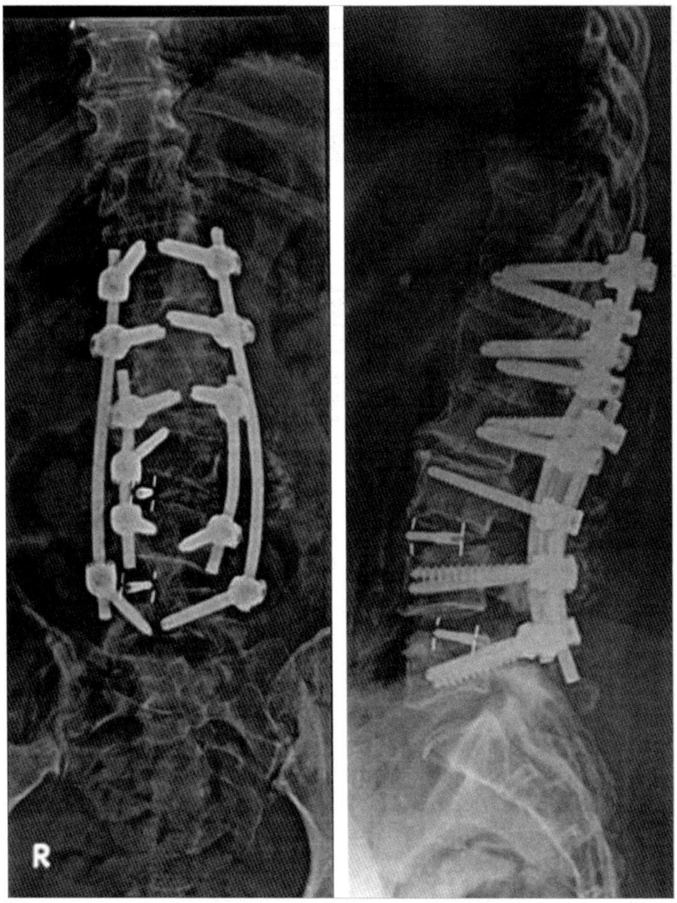

Fig. 11.5 Postoperative X-ray with correction of coronal and sagittal malalignment by the posterior-only approach under spinal anesthesia.

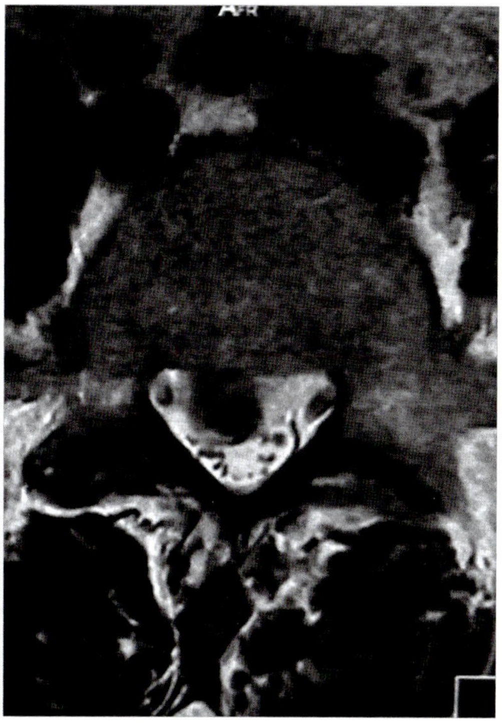

Fig. 11.6 Axial magnetic resonance imaging showing right disk prolapse.

Previous posterolateral fusion with retention of previous implant.

11.12.2 Case 2

A 48-year-old male patient with a history of monocular vision secondary to loss of an eye presented with lumbar disk herniation with right lower limb sciatica and weakness following failed conservative management (▸ Fig. 11.6, ▸ Fig. 11.7). The patient underwent an uneventful diskectomy with an awake spinal anesthesia. The procedure was done without any pressure on his remaining eye and he had interval recovery of his preoperative symptoms.

11.13 Conclusion

Spine surgery under spinal anesthesia is a viable and effective option in resource-limited countries. By understanding the principles and practical considerations, health care providers can optimize patient outcomes while efficiently utilizing available resources.

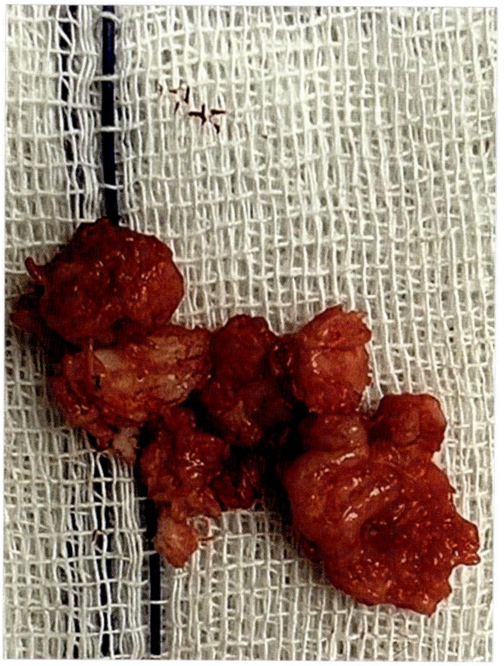

Fig. 11.7 Disk material after removal with uneventful surgery.

Spinal anesthesia not only offers cost-effective and safe anesthetic care but also contributes to faster recovery and better resource management in challenging environments.

References

[1] Agarwal P, Pierce J, Welch WC. Cost analysis of spinal versus general anesthesia for lumbar diskectomy and laminectomy spine surgery. World Neurosurg. 2016; 89:266–271

[2] Olmos M, Patel J, Kanter M, Karimi H, Kryzanski J. Evaluating the potential impact of spinal anesthesia use in lumbar surgery on global healthcare cost and climate change. Brain Spine. 2023; 3:101754

[3] Khattab M, El-Hawary Y, El-Ghamry S, Montasser A.. Spine surgery under spinal anaesthesia. Global Spine Journal. 2016; 6 1_suppl. DOI: 10.1055/s-0036-1582826

[4] Khattab MF, Abou-Madawi AM. Current effect of COVID-19 global pandemic on the professional and life profiles of the Egyptian spine surgeons. SICOT J. 2020; 6:31

[5] Khattab MF, Kannan TMA, Morsi A, et al. The short-term impact of COVID-19 pandemic on spine surgeons: a cross-sectional global study. Eur Spine J. 2020; 29(8):1806–1812

[6] Khattab MFM, Sykes DAW, Abd-El-Barr MM, et al. Spine surgery under awake spinal anesthesia: an Egyptian experience during the COVID-19 pandemic. Neurosurg Focus. 2021; 51 (6):E6

[7] Sarkar S, Banerji A, Chattopadhyaya A, Banerjee S. Lumbar spine instrumented fusion surgery under spinal anaesthesia

versus general anaesthesia: a retrospective study of 239 cases. J Clin Orthop Trauma. 2021; 18:205–208
[8] Jellish WS, Shea JF. Spinal anaesthesia for spinal surgery. Best Pract Res Clin Anaesthesiol. 2003; 17(3):323–334
[9] Wang AY, Liu P, Balonov K, Riesenburger R, Kryzanski J. Use of spinal anesthesia in lower thoracic spine surgery: a case series. Oper Neurosurg (Hagerstown). 2022; 23(4):298–303
[10] De Biase G, Gruenbaum SE, Quiñones-Hinojosa A, Abode-Iyamah KO. Spine surgery under spinal vs general anesthesia: prospective analysis of quality of life, fatigue, and cognition. Neurosurgery. 2022; 90(2):186–191
[11] Ditzler JW, Dumke PR, Harrington JJ, Fox JD. Should spinal anesthesia be used in surgery for herniated intervertebral disk. Anesth Analg. 1959; 38(2):118–124
[12] Rosenberg MK, Berner G. Spinal anesthesia in lumbar disc surgery. Review of 200 cases with a case history. Anesth Analg. 1965; 44:419–423
[13] Riegel B, Alibert F, Becq MC, Duckert I, Krivosic-Horber R. Hernie discale lombaire avec option chirurgicale: anesthésie générale versus anesthésie loco-régionale. Table ronde [Lumbar disk herniation with surgical option: general versus local anesthesia. Round table]. Agressologie. 1994; 34(Spec No 1):33–37
[14] Laakso E, Pitkänen M, Kyttä J, Rosenberg PH. Knee-chest vs horizontal side position during induction of spinal anaesthesia in patients undergoing lumbar disc surgery. Br J Anaesth. 1997; 79(5):609–611
[15] Drummond JC, Patel PM. Neurosurgical anesthesia. In: Miller RD, ed. Anesthesia, 5th ed. Philadelphia, PA: Churchill Livingstone; 2000:1928–1929
[16] McLain RF, Kalfas I, Bell GR, Tetzlaff JE, Yoon HJ, Rana M. Comparison of spinal and general anesthesia in lumbar laminectomy surgery: a case-controlled analysis of 400 patients. J Neurosurg Spine. 2005; 2(1):17–22

12 Lessons from COVID-19 and Lower and Medium Income Countries—India

Bhavana Kayarat, Punit Khanna, and Bhavuk Garg

Abstract

The use of spinal anesthesia for lumbar disk herniation was first described by Ditzler et al in 1959. But even after decades, lumbar spine surgery is usually performed under general anesthesia (GA). The major reasons for anesthesiologists' preference for GA over regional anesthesia (RA) are secured airway prior to placing the patient in the prone position, fear of complications requiring to turn the patient again on the back, and patient preference for sleep during surgery instead of remaining awake. However, over the last decade a new interest for the use of RA in this type of surgery has emerged owing to major improvements in anesthetic procedures, surgical techniques, and rehabilitation protocols. Although awake spine surgery (ASPS) with the help of RA is a relatively new concept with limited supporting evidence, it may prove to be highly effective in reducing postoperative hospital stays, in-hospital complications, and cost of surgery while at the same time expediting recovery and rehabilitation. Another impetus for ASPS was the COVID-19 pandemic. During this pandemic, there was limited availability of ventilators and hospital beds, which were being used to keep COVID-19 patients alive and thus limiting the available ventilators for elective surgeries.

Keywords: awake spine surgery, spinal anesthesia, TLIF

Key Points

- During the COVID-19 pandemic, awake spinal surgeries gained traction in India as a practical alternative to the traditional spine surgery. Core components include conscious sedation, endoscopic visualization, expandable interbody device, osteobiologics, long-acting local analgesia, and percutaneous instrumentation.
- Regional anesthesia in spinal surgery not only enhances patient safety and postoperative outcomes but also aligns with trends toward minimally invasive, cost-effective surgical care. These advantages make it an increasingly preferred anesthetic approach for spine surgeries, particularly in patients with comorbidities or when fast recovery and discharge are priorities.

12.1 Introduction

Wang and Grossman in 2016[1] pioneered an endoscopic approach for one of the first minimally invasive transforaminal lumbar interbody fusion (TLIF). Since then, multiple studies have described modifications to the technique as well as other types of awake spine surgeries. The commonly performed awake spine surgeries include the following:

- TLIF.
- Laminectomy/diskectomy.
- Dorsal column (DC) stimulator placement.

With clinical innovation and technological advancement, a wider range of conditions from single-level decompression to multistage extensive reconstruction are now being addressed.[2]

Awake endoscopic TLIF is a newer innovation, having become more popular during the COVID-19 epidemic. The core components include conscious sedation, endoscopic visualization, expandable interbody device, osteobiologics, long-acting local analgesia, and percutaneous instrumentation

During the COVID-19 pandemic, awake spinal surgeries gained traction in India as a practical alternative to the traditional spine surgery. Awake spine procedures, which use local or regional anesthesia instead of general anesthesia, offered several benefits that addressed challenges posed by the pandemic. First, they reduced the risk of respiratory complications associated with general anesthesia, an important factor given COVID-19's impact on respiratory health. Additionally, these surgeries facilitated shorter hospital stays and faster recovery times, helping alleviate strain on hospital resources and reduce potential viral exposure for both patients and health care staff. As a result, many spine centers across India adopted awake techniques, not only to meet pandemic-era demands but also to offer a safer, efficient option for spine care in a resource-limited setting. This period marked a significant shift toward minimally invasive and general anesthesia–sparing methods in spinal surgery across the country.

12.2 Advantages of Regional Anesthesia in Spine Surgery

General anesthesia is usually preferred for all kinds of surgical procedures involving the spine due to better patient tolerance, secure airway, and better surgical exposure under muscle relaxants. However, with the feasibility of minimally invasive surgical procedures of the spine, regional anesthesia offers the following benefits (▶ Table 12.1):

- **Reduction in respiratory complications:** Regional anesthesia eliminates the need for endotracheal intubation and airway manipulation, significantly decreasing the risk of respiratory complications, especially relevant in patients with compromised pulmonary function.
- **Hemodynamic stability:** Compared to general anesthesia, regional techniques often maintain more stable hemodynamics, which can be beneficial for patients with cardiovascular comorbidities. Reduced sympathetic response and stress associated with regional anesthesia contribute to fewer intraoperative fluctuations in blood pressure and heart rate, enhancing intraoperative safety.[3]
- **Enhanced recovery and mobilization:** Patients receiving regional anesthesia can experience accelerated recovery with faster postoperative mobilization. This is due to fewer side effects from sedatives and narcotics, allowing for early ambulation. Rapid mobilization also reduces the risk of thromboembolic events and other complications associated with prolonged immobility.[4]
- **Superior analgesia and opioid-sparing effects:** Regional anesthesia can provide prolonged analgesia postoperatively through the use of long-acting local anesthetics or adjuncts, decreasing the need for systemic opioids and their associated side effects, such as respiratory depression, nausea, and constipation. This opioid-sparing effect is particularly important in spine surgery, where effective pain management is crucial for patient satisfaction and functional outcomes.
- **Blunted surgical stress response:** By blocking afferent nerve transmission, regional anesthesia mitigates the neuroendocrine stress response triggered by surgical trauma. This leads to a decrease in stress hormones, which in turn can reduce postoperative complications, particularly

Table 12.1 Advantages and disadvantages of various modes of anesthesia in spine surgery

Surgery	Mode of anesthesia	Advantages	Disadvantages
Endoscopic transforaminal lumbar interbody fusion (TLIF)	Conscious sedation	Lesser surgical duration, decreased blood loss, decreased duration of hospital stay	Nausea and vomiting
Lumbar diskectomy and laminectomy	Regional anesthesia (spinal and epidural)	Better analgesia, decreased blood loss, decreased rise in intraocular pressure in the prone position	Not suitable in anticipated difficult airway, severe spinal stenosis, coagulopathy, skin infections May hamper postoperative neurological examination
Conditions not suitable for conscious sedation or regional anesthesia	General anesthesia	Secured airway, improved patient tolerance, early postoperative examination feasible without the confounding results from conventional regional anesthetic agents	Increased morbidity in patients with poor cardiopulmonary function

in high-risk patients with diabetes or cardiovascular disease.[3]

- **Suitability for ambulatory surgery:** The minimal sedation and rapid recovery associated with regional techniques facilitate outpatient spine surgeries, allowing same-day discharge. This has economic benefits and minimizes hospital stay, reducing exposure to nosocomial infections—a valuable consideration in both pandemic and nonpandemic contexts.
- **Cost-effectiveness:** Regional anesthesia is often associated with shorter surgical times, reduced need for postanesthesia care, and shorter hospital stays, all of which contribute to cost savings for health care facilities. This is particularly relevant in high-volume centers and resource-constrained settings.

Sekerak et al[6] in their retrospective comparative study between spinal anesthesia and general anesthesia in one- and two-level lumbar TLIF surgeries, noted that spinal anesthesia significantly reduced the time in the operating room, postoperative recovery room time, and time under anesthesia. Postoperative pain scores and opioid requirement were also less in the spinal anesthesia group. The complications and operative costs were not different between the two groups. Spinal and regional anesthesia protocols combined with Enhanced Recovery After Surgery (ERAS) principles has led to awake spinal fusion gaining popularity in the last few years.

12.3 Preoperative Concerns of Awake Spinal Surgery

Preoperatively thorough assessment of the airway and respiratory, cardiovascular, musculoskeletal, and neurologic systems is mandatory.

- **Airway:** Airway management in upper thoracic or cervical spine surgery is challenging. The presence of osteoarthritis, rheumatoid arthritis, ankylosing spondylitis, neuromuscular disorders, and previous radiation of the head or neck makes the situation more demanding for selection of intubation technique.
- **Pulmonary evaluation:** Significant spinal deformity results in restrictive respiratory physiology, with a reduction in vital capacity and total lung capacity. It may even lead to pulmonary hypertension and cor pulmonale.[6] Significant displacement or rotation of the trachea or main stem bronchi may also occur, leading to mechanical airway obstruction. Clinically the most significant change is abnormal gas exchange, due to ventilation–perfusion mismatch. Routine preoperative respiratory assessment through pulmonary function testing, chest X-ray, and room air arterial blood gas analysis is necessary before complex spine procedures.
- **Cardiovascular evaluation:** The majority of the spine surgeries are performed in the prone position, which causes a reduction in cardiac index by 12 to 24%, in comparison to the supine position. Thus, the presence of preexisting cardiac dysfunction makes the scenario more complex. Both patient-related factors and the extensiveness of the proposed surgery are taken into consideration for preoperative cardiac evaluation. An electrocardiogram (ECG) is a minimum requirement, while echocardiography may be deferred in patients with good exercise tolerance.
- **Musculoskeletal evaluation:** Preexisting limitation in range of motion of the joints in patients undergoing spine surgery makes surgical positioning challenging. Detailed skin examination, presence of bruise, or other signs of injury should be documented preoperatively. Neuromuscular evaluation and identification and documentation of preexisting motor and sensory neurologic deficits are essential for accurate surveillance and diagnosis of new postoperative deficits. It significantly impacts the selection of both neuromuscular blocking agents and the site of assessment for neuromuscular blockade.
- Preexisting comorbidities and extensiveness of the surgical procedure dictate preoperative laboratory evaluation. Baseline hemoglobin, platelet count, serum creatinine, electrolytes, and cross-matching of blood group for surgical procedures that involve more than two vertebral levels may be required prior to surgery.

12.4 Intraoperative Concerns

12.4.1 Blood Loss

- Major spine surgery is usually associated with significant blood loss. The complexity of surgery, instrumentation at multiple levels, and revision surgeries increase the risk. Without any preventive measures, blood loss can substantial, with transfusion rates as high as 81%.

- Three antifibrinolytic agents, tranexamic acid (TXA), epsilon aminocaproic acid (EACA), and aprotinin, are being evaluated for their effectiveness in preventing blood loss and reducing blood transfusion rates in spine surgery. A systematic review has found TXA to be a more effective tool than placebo for reducing intraoperative as well as postoperative and total blood loss along with lower transfusion rates. The subgroup analysis has shown no differences in terms of blood loss reduction with low-dose TXA (bolus of up to 10 mg/kg followed by up to 10 mg/kg/h) and high-dose TXA (bolus of 10–100 mg/kg followed by infusion > 10 mg/kg/h).
- Aprotinin reduces intraoperative blood loss but is not effective for perioperative loss. Owing to concerns over increased renal and cardiovascular toxicity, it is no longer approved by the Food and Drug Administration (FDA).
- Suboptimal prone positioning may increase the intra-abdominal and intrathoracic pressure, leading to a rise in transmitted venous pressure to the inferior vena cava and epidural veins, thereby causing unexpected surgical bleeding. The mean blood loss per level was found to be significantly lower in the wide width chest support in comparison to the narrow width chest support on a Wilson frame for patients undergoing posterior lumbar spine fusion surgery.

12.4.2 Position-Related Complications

Despite adequate precautions, position-related injuries are quite frequent ranging from minor skin and soft tissue lesion to postoperative visual loss, peripheral nerve injury (PNI), spinal cord injury, and rhabdomyolysis. Simulation-based training of surgeons, anesthetists, and nursing staffs and implementation of an ERAS spine protocol will be beneficial for alleviating these position-related complications.

12.4.3 Peripheral Nerve Injury

- With the use of somatosensory evoked potential during neurosurgical procedures, 15% of patients are found to develop unusual signals due to mispositioning. A recent anesthesia closed claim study reported that spine surgery accounted for 14% of patients with PNI. However, the majority of the injuries are self-limiting.[7]
- An integrated team approach, careful selection of equipment, and utilization of checklists for careful positioning, padding, and periodic assessment reduce position-related complications.

12.4.4 Pain Management

Complex spine surgery is ranked as one of the most painful procedures. Poor pain control is associated with delayed wound healing, prolonged hospital stays, morbidity, and higher expenditures.

12.4.5 Epidural Anesthesia

A meta-analysis of 938 patients from 17 randomized controlled trials (RCTs) has demonstrated a reduction in visual analog scale (VAS) score on postoperative day 1 and lesser opioid consumption in the first 24 hours with a 15 times increased risk (relative risk [RR]: 15.07 [2.04, 111.34]) of motor blockade, which may affect the neurological assessment.[8]

12.4.6 Intrathecal Morphine

In a meta-analysis of 8 RCTs of 393 patients has found intrathecal morphine with doses from 0.1 to 1 mg reduces VAS scores and morphine equivalent consumption. However, the incidence of pruritus (OR: 4.09 [1.84, 9.11]) and respiratory depression (OR: 3.48 [0.41, 29.32]) was high.[9]

12.4.7 Epidural Steroid

A meta-analysis has found the use of epidural steroids at closure during lumbar surgery reduces VAS scores at 24 hours and decreases opioid consumption. However, it did not comment on wound healing and infection.[10]

12.4.8 Erector Spinae Block

Bilateral ultrasound-guided erector spinae plane block has been found to be effective for reducing postoperative opioid requirement and provide better patient satisfaction in comparison to conventional analgesia in lumbar spine surgery.[11]

12.4.9 Pharmacological Agents

- Paracetamol is frequently used in the perioperative period. Although it has not been found to be effective for reducing opioid consumption in the first 24 postoperative hours.
- Selective cyclooxygenase-2 (COX-2) inhibitors are found to be an effective tool to reduce postoperative pain and opioid consumption in spine surgeries. However, the risk of nonunion and bleeding is debatable.
- Pregabalin and gabapentin have emerged as an effective tool for reducing VAS scores and opioid consumption up to 48 hours postoperatively without significant side effects.
- A meta-analysis from 14 RCTs has found that ketamine, used as either bolus (0.2–1 mg/kg) or infusion (1–4 mg/kg/min), reduces pain score and morphine equivalent consumption without any unpleasant dreams, dysphoria, hallucinations, postoperative nausea and vomiting, and sedation.[9]
- Tramadol continues to be the cornerstone for postoperative pain management due to its strong potency. It reduces both the VAS score and opioid consumption up to 6 hours after surgery

12.5 Enhanced Recovery after Surgery Protocol in Spine Surgery

- ERAS pathway is a set of evidence-based interventions that are carried out in the perioperative period that lead to faster recovery of patients.
- The goal of ERAS remains improvement of patient outcomes by preoperative optimization, preemptive analgesia, opioid-sparing multimodal anesthesia, early mobilization and nutrition, etc., in an attempt to prevent catabolism and immune dysfunction.
- The interventions can be divided into preoperative, intraoperative, and postoperative measures (▶ Table 12.2). ▶ Table 12.3 highlights the recommendations endorsed by the ERAS Society for perioperative care in lumbar spine fusion surgeries.

Expert Tip

Proper patient counseling and preemptive analgesia are paramount for ASPS. Patients should be explained in detail about the various advantages of ASPS and simultaneously should be assured of remaining comfortable and pain free throughout the procedure. It generally involves preoperative administration of nonopioid agents in order to reduce narcotics consumption. Commonly used nonopioids analgesics are gabapentinoids, acetaminophen, dexamethasone, and nonsteroidal anti-inflammatory drugs (NSAIDs).

Preemptive analgesia plan may include a multimodal analgesia regimen using dexamethasone (0.2 mg/kg) intravenous (IV) in 100 mL normal saline over a period of 30 minutes

Table 12.2 Components of the ERAS protocol in spine surgeries

Preoperative measures	Intraoperative measures	Postoperative measures
1. Preoperative education and counseling	1. Prophylactic antibiotics and surgical preparation	1. Postoperative analgesia
2. Preoperative optimization of nutrition and anemia	2. Standardized anesthesia protocol and multimodal analgesia	2. Postoperative nausea and vomiting care
3. Cessation of smoking and alcohol	3. Maintenance of normothermia and euvolemia	3. Early mobilization
4. Preemptive analgesia	4. Use of minimally invasive surgical techniques	
	5. Opioid-free analgesia	
	6. Early removal of urinary catheters and drains	

and a combination of paracetamol 1 g IV and NSAIDs such as ketorolac 30 mg IV before performing regional anesthesia.

Various regional anesthesia techniques can be considered for spine surgeries. These include fascial plane blocks, local infiltration, and neuraxial anesthesia (▶ Table 12.3*). The thoracolumbar interfascial plane and erector spinae plane blocks are interfascial plane blocks that target the dorsal rami and are beneficial in minimally invasive spine (MIS) surgeries. Spinal anesthesia is a rationale choice for MIS and open spinal surgeries like laminectomies and TLIF surgeries. At our institution, the subarachnoid block is often used, together with IV dexmedetomidine infusion for sedation. In the operating room, the procedure is performed over a shifting trolley. Patients receive spinal anesthesia one or two level above the intended level of surgery, using 12.5 to 15 mg of hyperbaric bupivacaine with 25 µg of fentanyl. We target to achieve dense block up to the level of T8–T10. High levels of motor block are poorly tolerated due to lack of abdominal muscle strength and inability to breathe deeply against increased abdominal pressure. For these reasons, surgery above the T10 level is not recommended under neuraxial anesthesia. Our sedation protocol includes midazolam 1 mg IV and fentanyl 20 to 30 µg IV before prone positioning and IV dexmedetomidine infusion (0.5–0.7 µg/kg/h) after prone positioning. Long-acting benzodiazepines or opioids are avoided, in order to promote a rapid recovery.*

12.6 Lessons from COVID-19: Our Experience with Awake Spine Surgeries

- In the last 2 years from 2022 to 2024, 50 (approximately) patients underwent single-level TLIF surgery under spinal anesthesia. All surgeries remained uneventful, except three patients, two of whom required general anesthesia before proning for surgery due to inadequate effect and one female patient needed ketamine boluses because of pain on instrumentation during surgery. Thirty patients were discharged on the same day, 15 patients on postop day 1, and 5 on postop day 2.
- Awake spinal surgery is a promising technique that can be highly effective in reducing postoperative stay, expediting recovery, and decreasing the cost of surgery. This can be a part

Table 12.3 Recommendations from ERAS Society: perioperative care in lumbar spine fusion

Preoperative	Intraoperative	Postoperative
Optimization	**Stress minimization**	**Protocolized normalization**
Preoperative education and counseling	Standard anesthetic protocol	Early mobilization
Patient optimization: • Smoking • Alcohol • Anemia	Local anesthetic techniques	Early oral nutrition
Preoperative nutritional evaluation and supplementation	Multimodal opioid-sparing techniques	Management of drains
Optimization of medications	Intraoperative hypothermia prevention	Antithrombotic prophylaxis treatment
	PONV prevention	
	Optimal fluid management	
	Antimicrobial prophylaxis	

Abbreviations: ERAS, Enhanced Recovery After Surgery; PONV, postoperative nausea and vomiting.

of the ERAS protocol that may be implemented for better patient care. Patient counseling and optimal regional anesthesia techniques along with careful sedation are of prime importance in awake spine surgeries. Good-quality randomized, prospective, and multicenter trials are required to demonstrate the safety, efficacy, and cost-effectiveness of this technique.

References

[1] Wang MY, Grossman J. Endoscopic minimally invasive transforaminal interbody fusion without general anesthesia: initial clinical experience with 1-year follow-up. Neurosurg Focus. 2016; 40(2):E13

[2] Navarro-Garcia de Llano JP, Fuentes-Fernandez Cueto M, Roberts AP, et al. Spinal anesthesia for multilevel awake minimally invasive transforaminal lumbar interbody fusion: single-center experience. Oper Neurosurg (Hagerstown). 2025; 28(6):855–861

[3] Hahnenkamp K, Herroeder S, Hollmann MW. Regional anaesthesia, local anaesthetics and the surgical stress response. Best Pract Res Clin Anaesthesiol. 2004; 18(3): 509–527

[4] Zixuan L, Chen W, Li Y, et al. Incidence of deep venous thrombosis (DVT) of the lower extremity in patients undergoing surgeries for ankle fractures. J Orthop Surg Res. 2020; 15(1):294

[5] Sekerak R, Mostafa E, Morris MT, Nessim A, Vira A, Sharan A. Comparative outcome analysis of spinal anesthesia versus general anesthesia in lumbar fusion surgery. J Clin Orthop Trauma. 2020; 13:122–126 Published 2020 Nov 27. doi:10.1016/j.jcot.2020.11.017

[6] Wang Y, Wang D, Zhang G, et al. Effects of spinal deformities on lung development in children: a review. J Orthop Surg Res. 2023; 18(1):246

[7] Chui J, Murkin JM, Posner KL, Domino KB. Perioperative Peripheral Nerve Injury After General Anesthesia: A Qualitative Systematic Review. Anesth Analg. 2018; 127(1): 134–143

[8] Meng Y, Jiang H, Zhang C, et al. A comparison of the postoperative analgesic efficacy between epidural and intravenous analgesia in major spine surgery: a meta-analysis. J Pain Res. 2017; 10:405–415

[9] Pendi A, Acosta FL, Tuchman A, et al. Intrathecal morphine in spine surgery: a meta-analysis of randomized controlled trials. Spine. 2017; 42(12):E740–E747

[10] Wilson-Smith A, Chang N, Lu VM, et al. Epidural steroids at closure after microdiscectomy/laminectomy for reduction of postoperative analgesia: systematic review and meta-analysis. World Neurosurg. 2018; 110:e212–e221

[11] Singh S, Chaudhary NK. Bilateral ultrasound guided erector spinae plane block for postoperative pain management in lumbar spine surgery: a case series. J Neurosurg Anesthesiol. 2019; 31(3):354

[12] Pendi A, Field R, Farhan S-D, Eichler M, Bederman SS. Perioperative ketamine for analgesia in spine surgery: a meta-analysis of randomized controlled trials. Spine (Phila Pa). 2018; 43(5):E299–E307

13 Developing an Outpatient Awake Spine Surgery Program

Alok Sharan

Abstract
The transition of spine surgery cases to outpatient centers is expected to increase markedly over the next decade. There has already been a shift of minor cases, such as laminectomies, diskectomies, and anterior cervical surgeries, out of the hospital and toward outpatient centers. As protocols and learning improve, there will be a greater shift in lumbar fusions toward the outpatient setting. Achieving this transition requires more than a change in the site of service. It requires the implementation of protocols to medically optimize a patient, proper education, change in anesthesia protocols, and increasing communication between the provider and the patient after surgery. With the expected increase in spine surgeries due to an aging population, there will be a greater need for shifting these cases toward lower-cost centers.

Keywords: spine surgery, ambulatory surgery, outpatient surgery, rapid recovery

Key Points

- There has been a trend toward performing spine surgery in an outpatient setting.
- Doing so requires optimization of the patient's health and expectations prior to surgery.
- Preoperative education along with nutrition is critical to performing safe outpatient spine surgeries.
- Transitioning from general to spinal anesthesia helps reduce the length of stay.
- Paraspinal blocks help reduce pain after surgery.
- Performing outpatient spine surgery requires more touch points with the patient after surgery.
- Developing protocols, along with an interdisciplinary team, helps develop a consistent outpatient spine program.

13.1 Introduction

Spine surgery has undergone major advancements in the past two decades. Many surgeries that were traditionally performed in the hospital setting are now safely being performed in outpatient surgery centers. The traditional length of stay for a spinal fusion has moved from 1 to 2 days to 4 hours in certain centers.[1]

Achieving an outpatient discharge requires the coordination of many parts to the whole system. Once a patient has decided to undergo spine surgery, they have to be optimized to undergo a procedure to produce the best results.

In this chapter, we will discuss the three phases of care in outpatient spine surgery: preoperative, intraoperative, postoperative. Each phase has unique considerations.

13.2 Definition

- According to the Medicare claims manual, there are two broad categories of outpatient spine surgeries.[2]
  - A patient can undergo a spine surgery and be discharged within 4 to 6 hours.
  - Alternatively, a patient who undergoes surgery may have to be observed for an extended period of time (< 23 hours).
- These two subtypes of outpatient surgery are typically reimbursed differently by payors.

13.3 Preparing the Patient for Outpatient Spine Surgery

- Patient selection:
  - American Society of Anesthesiologists (ASA) class I or II:
    - There is no consensus on what types of patients are suitable for spine surgery.
    - Generally, patients who are healthier with minimal comorbidities are ideally suited for outpatient spine surgery (ASA I or II).[3]
    - Even patients with certain comorbidities (e.g., hypertension, diabetes) that are under

  control can undergo same-day spine surgery.
- The patient wants to go home the same day:
  - Patients should be asked if they want to go home the same day.
  - Critical to them is asking if they have proper social support at home.[3]
- Age:
  - Patients undergoing laminectomies and microdiskectomies can go home the same day.
  - Spinal Fusion patients with age < 75 can consider going home the same day.
- Comorbidities:
  - Patients with multiple comorbidities should be admitted overnight.

- Patient safety:
  - Incumbent upon discharging a patient home the same day is making sure they are safe.
    - Office staff should understand what type of support the patient will have afterward at home.
    - Ultimately the goal is to prevent readmission after surgery.
- Preoperative education:
  - Patient education is paramount in performing outpatient spine surgery.
  - Traditionally when patients were admitted to the hospital, the few days that they were admitted allowed the providers to answer any questions and go over specific instructions with the patient.
  - For ambulatory surgery, these instructions have to be given prior to surgery.
  - Ideally a family member or another caregiver should accompany the patient to an office visit as the information can be overwhelming. This helps ensure that no information is lost.
- Patient communication:
  - It is important for all members of the team to have consistent messaging.
    - Consistent messaging from all members of the care team (i.e., physician, office staff, nurses, physical therapists) ensures that the patient has confidence in their ability to go home.
    - The patient should understand the benefit of outpatient spine surgery.
      Faster mobilization.
      Less risk of developing deep vein thrombosis (DVT).
      Sleep in their own bed.
- Consider the use of technology to ensure protocol compliance.
  - Some providers have begun to use app technology to deliver this information. Having the information readily available when the patient needs allows for better compliance.
- Preoperative nutrition:
  - There has been an increasing awareness that surgery is a catabolic event and thus it is important to load patients with proper nutrition prior to surgery.[4]
  - This has been demonstrated to help in the postoperative recovery process and in some instances leads to a more rapid recovery after surgery.
  - In addition, many patients have improper nutrition going into surgery. Helping improve their nutritional status can also help in the recovery process.
  - Much of the literature regarding nutritional optimization comes from the total joint replacement literature.[5]
    - There has been an increasing amount of evidence of the role of essential amino acids to help maintain and improve muscle mass.
    - In addition, patients are encouraged to take carb loading prior to surgery to give a proper energy boost.
      This has been shown to help reduce inflammation and boost muscle mass prior to surgery.
- Mobility (prehab):
  - Some studies suggest that prehab can help patients prior to outpatient spine surgery.[6]
    - While evidence is not clear, it does make sense that a patient should have proper mobility prior to surgery.
    - Many patients with spinal disorders use a cane or a walker to maintain a forward flexed posture.
    - If they are not independent prior to surgery, they will have increasing dependency once they have pain from the incision/surgery.
    - Educating the patient prior to surgery on how to get out of bed, how to rise from a chair, etc., can be helpful.
- Ask the patients to pick up their medicine prior to surgery.
  - Prescribe their postop meds preoperatively.

- It will prevent them from scrambling the day of surgery.
- Give the patients an ice pack prior to surgery to use on their back.
- Make sure their home is safe.
  - Patients should be able to climb stairs after surgery.
    - If there is any issue, patients should be counseled to set up their first floor with a bedroom to minimize how much they need to go up or down the stairs.

Expert Tip

For any outpatient spine surgery program to be successful, patient safety has to be the number 1 priority. Achieving success requires more touch points with the patient. This includes proper education on what to anticipate for surgery. Preparing the patient for surgery includes optimizing their nutrition, making their home safe, and asking them to pick up their medicine before surgery. Every surgeon should develop their own criteria for which patient should undergo spine surgery.

13.4 Intraoperative Considerations

- Regional anesthesia:
  - Spinal versus general.
    - Benefits:
      - There have been numerous published studies that have demonstrated that spinal anesthesia can reduce the length of stay when compared to general anesthesia in spine surgery.[7]
      - Patients experience less postoperative nausea and vomiting with spinal anesthesia.
      - In the elderly population, general anesthesia can lead to delirium, which delays their discharge.[8]
      - Medicine to be used for spinal anesthesia:
      - The choice of medicine to use for the spinal is important.
      - The duration of anesthesia is important.
      - Even more important is the ability for the medicine to wear off in a timely manner.
      - Prolonged anesthesia can affect the return of bladder and motor function.
      - Food and Drug Administration (FDA) approved medicine for spinal anesthesia:
        - Bupivacaine.[9]
        - Chloroprocaine.
        - Mepivacaine.
        - Ropivacaine.
        - Each of these medicines has a variable amount of duration.
  - Paraspinal blocks:
    - Regional blocks can be an effective method to minimize pain after surgery. Long-acting bupivacaine has been demonstrated to provide enduring pain relief after surgery.
- Factors that lead to discharge delays after surgery:
  - There are a variety of factors that can lead to a delay in discharge after surgery.
  - When possible, these factors should be addressed prior to surgery.
    - Blood pressure (hyper- or hypotension).
    - Oversedation.
    - Postoperative urinary retention.
    - Postoperative nausea and vomiting.
    - Pain.
    - Social support at home.

Expert Tip

The use of spinal anesthesia has been demonstrated to lead to a shorter length of stay when compared to general anesthesia. The addition of regional blocks can help with pain relief postoperatively. Understanding the factors that can lead to a delayed discharge can help anticipate challenges for performing an outpatient surgery.

13.5 Aftercare for Patient after Outpatient Spine Surgery

- Day of surgery:
  - Every hospital has different criteria for discharge.
  - Outpatient surgery centers should develop their own criteria.

 - The patient should be able to ambulate independently.
 - The patient can urinate.
- Need more touch points:
 - Typically need to call the patient on postoperative days 1 and 2.
- Can travel on a plane after 5 days (risk of DVT):
 - Many patients are traveling for their spine surgery.
 - We typically ask the patients not to do extended traveling for more than 5 days. The risk of developing a DVT is highest within the first 48 hours.
 The pressure changes from an airplane travel can put a patient at risk of DVT formation.

Expert Tip

Outpatient spine surgery requires more touch points. The surgeon should either call the patient or have an assistant communicate with the patient after surgery. Specific criteria should be established to determine if a patient can be discharged the same day. Travel should be restricted for 5 days after surgery.

13.6 Protocol Development

- As the outpatient spine program evolves, developing standardized protocols can help.
- Protocols should be developed for the following needs:
 - Education.
 - Medical optimization.
 - Nutritional optimization.
 - Anesthesia protocol.
 - Postop pain protocol.
 - Postop physical therapy.

13.7 Conclusion

Developing an outpatient spine program is a complex, multifaceted endeavor that requires careful planning, strategic thinking, and a commitment to excellence. By understanding the evolving landscape of spine care, assessing the needs of your target population, and designing a program that prioritizes patient-centered care, you can establish a successful outpatient spine program that delivers high-quality care, enhances patient outcomes, and drives growth and sustainability in the years to come.

References

[1] Djurasovic M, Kiskaddon E, Bratcher K, et al. Determinants of hospital length of stay in patients undergoing lumbar spinal fusion. The Spine Journal. 2014; 14(11):S103–S104

[2] Centers for Medicare & Medicaid Services. Medicare Claims Processing Manual, Chapter 4, Section 290.2.2. Accessed May 29, 2025 at: https://www.cms.gov/Regulations-and-Guidance/Guidance/Manuals/downloads/clm104c04.pdf

[3] Chan F, Stelma S, Cho W, Krystal J, Sharan AD. Analysis of surgeon experience and impact of comorbidities on early discharge after mini-open transforaminal lumbar interbody fusion. Curr Orthop Pract. 2016; 27(4):382–387

[4] Khalooeifard R, Oraee-Yazdani S, Keikhaee M, Shariatpanahi ZV. Protein supplement and enhanced recovery after posterior spine fusion surgery: a randomized, double-blind, placebo-controlled trial. Clin Spine Surg. 2022; 35(3):E356–E362

[5] de Souza Borges JH, Junior PL, de Brito FF, et al. Effects of amino acid supplementation on muscle mass, muscle performance and functional capacity in subjects undergoing total knee arthroplasty: a systematic review of randomized clinical trials. Eur J Orthop Surg Traumatol. 2024; 34(3):1717–1729

[6] Bogaert L, Thys T, Depreitere B, et al. Rehabilitation to improve outcomes of lumbar fusion surgery: a systematic review with meta-analysis. Eur Spine J. 2022; 31(6):1525–1545

[7] Lu VM, Brusko GD, Urakov TM. Defining the time benefit of awake versus general anesthesia for single-level lumbar spine surgery. World Neurosurg. 2022; 158:e793–e798

[8] American Society of Anesthesiologists. Age. Accessed May 29, 2025 at: https://madeforthismoment.asahq.org/preparing-for-surgery/risks/age/?utm_source=chatgpt.com

[9] Food and Drug Administration (FDA). Marcaine™ Spinal: bupivacaine hydrochloride in dextrose injection, USP. Accessed May 29, 2025 at: https://www.accessdata.fda.gov/drugsatfda_docs/label/2018/018692s020lbl.pdf?utm_source=chatgpt.com

Part II

Intraoperative Considerations

II

14 Advances in Minimally-Invasive Techniques—A Brief Introduction

Arnav Sharma, Peter N. Drossopoulos, and Muhammad M. Abd-El-Barr

Abstract

The evolution of spine surgery toward increasingly minimally invasive techniques has allowed for complex procedures to be performed while minimizing "surgical footprint." On an overarching level, improvements in technology have allowed for improved preoperative planning and operative modifications aimed at minimizing surrounding tissue damage; the interplay of pre- and intraoperative imaging with perioperative planning is especially seen in optimizations being made to the transforaminal lumbar interbody fusion (TLIF). Beyond surgical planning and anatomical approach, the emergence of awake surgeries using regional anesthetic techniques has allowed for another method to minimize surgical footprint. An awake technique has allowed for seamless yet innovative modifications in current surgical technologies, such as robotic and endoscopic surgery, and current techniques, such as lateral lumbar interbody fusion and TLIF. Altogether, these advances indicate synergistic technological and procedural growth in the future that will continue to expand both applicability and accessibility of minimally invasive spine surgery.

Keywords: awake spine surgery, minimally invasive spine surgery, robotic spine surgery, transforaminal lumbar interbody fusion, endoscopic spine surgery, lateral lumbar interbody fusion

Key Points

- Among advances in minimally invasive approaches to spine surgery, awake surgery has demonstrated significant promise in enhancing preoperative accessibility for patients and improving patient outcomes and satisfaction.
- Robotic spine technology has burgeoned since its inception in 2004 and has been used primarily in lumbar fusion approaches, though advancements have made percutaneous lumbar interbody fusion and S2 alar-iliac screw placement possible as well. Awake robotic surgery is still being explored with no further complications being described in the literature when compared to asleep robotic surgery.
- In addition to innovation involving awake surgery, TLIF procedures have shown significant interplay with imaging technology as a means to decrease surgical footprint. Emerging spine segmentation technology allows for improved preoperative planning and determination of safer anatomical corridors.
- Innovations in endoscopic spine surgery have especially flourished over the last 15 years. Awake endoscopic surgeries show significant promise in improved patient outcomes and provide a natural progression in the advancement of an already prominent cornerstone of minimally invasive surgery.
- Described for the first time in literature, awake lateral lumbar interbody fusion (LLIF) procedures may provide notable benefits over traditional LLIF procedures.

14.1 Introduction to Minimally Invasive Spine Surgery

As minimally invasive spine surgery techniques have further developed over the last few decades, surgeons have been able to perform complex spinal procedures through smaller incisions, with less trauma to overlying muscles and tissue and, thus, advancing the pursuit of minimizing surgical footprint on the patient. Evidence continues to support the transition toward minimally invasive techniques within spine surgery, as they have been associated with reduced blood loss, tissue dissection, operative time, and opioid consumption, and earlier hospital discharges.[1,2] Besides surgical techniques, the use of awake surgery and other regional anesthetic techniques is another method to minimize the "surgical footprint." Preoperatively, awake options allow for previously poor surgical candidates to be viable for spine surgery[3] while also allowing for surgeries to be conducted in an outpatient settings. Peri- and postoperatively, spinal anesthesia–based awake surgeries have shown shorter operative times, decreased blood loss, less hypertension, less postoperative nausea and vomiting, shorter postanesthesia care unit stays, overall shorter lengths of stay, less opioid use, and faster ambulation.[4,5] Corresponding developments in technologies and techniques have played a pivotal role in increasing the accessibility and efficacy of awake spine surgeries; in this and the following chapters, we aim to introduce and elaborate on some of the most notable advancements that have furthered the goal of reducing surgical footprint.

14.2 Awake Robotic Surgery

14.2.1 Emergence

- Robotic spine surgery commenced as an advancement in the field following the introduction of the Mazor SpineAssist in 2004. Since then, the field has grown significantly, with multiple multimillion and billion dollar companies investing in furthering development.
- Today, multiple robotic systems have been approved by the U.S. Food and Drug Administration, with the most current including the ExcelsiusGPS, Mazor X Stealth Edition, and ROSA ONE Spine. As of now, few comparisons of efficacy exist between these devices due to significant cost and time associated with implementation.[6]

14.2.2 Indications

- Robotic systems have become further ubiquitous in augmenting pedicle screw placement accuracy, as malposition can cascade into downstream neurologic and vascular complications.[6]
- Robotic technology has been used in both percutaneous and open pedicle screw fixation; the most common procedures for robotic fixation have included lumbar fusion procedures, anterior lumbar interbody fusions, lateral lumbar interbody fusion (LLIF) procedures, and transforaminal lumbar interbody fusion (TLIF) procedures.[6]
- Novel advancements have led to increased feasibility of surgical approach through Kambin's triangle; as freehand approaches require superior articular process drilling, the increased precision offered by a robotic approach allows for improved disk space access through the limited-size corridor with avoidance of adjacent structures, allowing viability for a more minimally invasive percutaneous interbody fusion in more patients.[7,8,9]
- Novel advancements have also led to robotic-assisted S2 alar-iliac screw placement and percutaneous screw fixation.[7,10,11,12]

14.2.3 Pros

- One prospective study reported on 10 single-level robotic minimally invasive TLIF (MIS-TLIF) procedures performed with the Mazor X robot. Significant improvements in pros were reported at 1-month and 1-year follow-ups (median back pain 7.8 preop, 1.5 at 1-month follow-up, 0 at 1-year follow-up). This study concluded that awake robotic surgery provided the benefits of both awake surgery (shorter operative and total operating room [OR] times, improved postoperative pain control, and decreased time to ambulation and fatigue) and robotic surgery (improved precision).[13]
- Dalton et al conducted a 10-patient retrospective study on robotic-assistant percutaneous lumbar interbody fusion (percLIF) through access to Kambin's triangle. Of the 10 surgeries, 4 were conducted as awake surgeries. No perioperative or postoperative complications were reported, alongside no postoperative motor or sensory deficits. As such, awake robotic assistance was shown to be feasible in percLIF procedures.[9]
- Robotic approaches have shown potential to be combined with endoscopic approaches, allowing for an approach that could theoretically combine the precision of robotic assistance with the limited invasiveness of endoscopy and further augment the transition of minimally invasive spine surgery toward outpatient/ambulatory surgical center care.

14.2.4 Cons

- De Biase et al identified the potential for movement as a major concern in awake patients undergoing robotic-assisted fusions. In the study, anxiolytic sedation and judicious patient

selection were marked as mediums to avoid large movements prior to screw placement; following screw placement, patients were allowed to adjust position for comfort. These solutions allowed avoidance of large movements in the awake surgeries documented.[13]
- Contradicting results exist regarding the accuracy of pedicle screw placement with robots versus freehand, with a meta-analysis comparing freehand versus robotic pedicle screw application determining no statistically significant difference in accuracy.[7,14]
- Awake robotic spine surgery is still a relatively emerging field with little literature out on efficacy. However, given the promising results of conventional general anesthetic robotic surgery, there exists viability for awake robotic surgery as an alternative.

Expert Tip

Robotic surgery has seen a dramatic increase in scope of usage. Limited data on this new field show that improvements in auxiliary surgical technology combined with an awake technique highlight a synergistic effect that preserves the benefits of both robotic and awake surgeries.

14.3 Next-Generation Transforaminal Lumbar Interbody Fusions

14.3.1 Emergence

- TLIF has evolved significantly since its origins. Initially, Cloward, Briggs, and Milligan introduced the posterior lumbar interbody fusion in 1943 by way of "bone chip fusion"; however, it faced significant limitations.[15]
- The advent of TLIF and the later minimally invasive variant thereof by Foley and Lefkowitz in 2006 marked a shift toward minimizing the surgical footprint while maintaining patient safety and surgical efficacy.[16]
- Most recently, large-scale advancements in operative technology and industry in the realm of intraoperative visualization, namely computed tomography (CT) navigation, robotics, and neurosegmentation, have been made, which continue to minimize the surgical footprint and provide excellent outcomes.

14.3.2 Indications

- The seminal descriptions of spine segmentation technology aimed to facilitate reduced risk of iatrogenic injury to nerve roots during percutaneous TLIF procedures.[17] Its applications have since broadened to include identifying boundaries of Kambin's triangle and facilitating interbody placement via the transfacet.[17]
- Tabarestani et al demonstrated this in a case series by measuring Kambin's triangle and transfacet volumes bilaterally and selecting the safest entry point based on the largest, safest corridors.[18] This group also identified that higher-order spondylolisthesis rescues the safe zone for percutaneous access to the disk space through Kambin's triangle but increased safe zone volume of the transfacet corridor.

14.3.3 Pros

- Leveraging three-dimensional neurosegmentation for surgical planning has numerous advantages. Although its novelty precludes large-scale study, there are several theoretical advantages as well as examples of such benefits in smaller studies.[18,19]
- By segmenting a patient's anatomy preoperatively, a surgeon may identify variant anatomy, like conjoined nerve roots, and determine the appropriateness or suitability, and laterality of a given arthrodesis technique (like comparing percutaneous trans-Kambin's triangle TLIF to transfacet TLIF and selecting the more favorable trajectory that allows for the passage of the desired cage size and lordosis).[18,19]
- TLIF procedures have also shown viability as awake surgeries; De Biase et al describe a series of 10 patients undergoing awake TLIF that demonstrated no intraoperative complications and a mean hospital stay of 1.3 ± 0.46 days.[20] A more recent prospective study from De Biase et al showed an even more improved mean length of stay of 16.5 hours.[13]
- A retrospective review of all single-level awake MIS-TLIF procedures performed at Mayo Clinic from 2016 to 2019 found similar results, with

no complications and a mean hospital stay of 1.4 ± 1.381 days, less than the general anesthesia cohort, which had a mean of 3 ± 2.274 days.[21]

- A study from Duke compared 10 patients undergoing asleep one- or two-level lumbar interbody fusions under general anesthesia versus 10 awake one- or two-level fusions under spinal anesthesia using a matched cohort analysis. Awake fusions were found to yield significantly shorter hospital lengths of stay ($p = 0.001$), lower postoperative opioid use ($p = 0.006$), and shorter time to ambulation ($p = 0.022$). Procedure duration was found to be nonsignificantly reduced in spinal anesthesia patients ($p = 0.089$). In addition to broadly improved patient outcome metrics, awake fusions yielded no 90-day readmissions.[5]

14.3.4 Cons

- Although these advances are commendable and represent significant strides made to decrease the surgical footprint, they are not without notable limitations.
- Inherent to the minimally invasive nature of these TLIF adaptations, percutaneous and microscopic approaches to the disk space through Kambin's triangle and the transfacet corridor face challenges, balancing reduced direct visualization with radiation exposure.[22] This radiation burden, if significant, is associated with many long-term morbidities to the operative team.[22,23]
- As anticipated, these techniques are associated with a learning curve, demonstrating that operative times improve as surgeons become more proficient. However, it is important to note that outcomes and complications remain stable throughout the learning curve.[24,25]

Expert Tip

Next-generation TLIF procedures benefit from enhanced imaging technology and show considerable potential in optimizing postoperative outcomes through a combination of improved preoperative planning and awake spine protocol recovery.

14.4 Awake Endoscopy

14.4.1 Emergence

- Endoscopy use in spine surgery first emerged in percutaneous endoscopic diskectomy. In 1988, a paper by Parvin Kambin et al was the first to demonstrate the endoscopic view of a herniated nucleus pulposus.[26] The first report of a modified arthroscope into the intervertebral disk space was first written about by Forst and Hausman in 1983.[27] Since, and especially within the last 15 years, innovations in endoscopic spine surgery have broadened applications and promoted ubiquity, especially in the context of awake surgeries.[24]
- Original uses for endoscopic spine approaches were in treatments of vertebral disk herniation in the lumbar spine through natural windows such as the intervertebral foramen or interlaminar window; with the advent of the endoscopic burr and bone reamer, foraminoplasty and laminotomy are able to be conducted to increase accessibility to the spinal canal.[28,29]

14.4.2 Indications

- Today, endoscopic approaches are used at all three levels of the spine with varying modifications.
- Lumbar full endoscopic approaches are used for herniated intervertebral disks, lumbar spinal stenosis, infective spondylodiskitis, revision surgeries, and spondylolisthesis.
- Thoracic full endoscopic approaches are used for herniated vertebral soft disks, thoracic spinal stenosis, and infective spondylodiskitis.
- Cervical full endoscopic approaches are limited to anterior or posterior approaches to minimize muscle trauma and risk of injury to vessels and esophagus. Indications include herniated intervertebral soft disks, cervical spinal stenosis, and infective spondylodiskitis.[28]
- Endoscopic approaches have been used to access Kambin's triangle.

14.4.3 Pros

- As a whole, endoscopic spine surgeries have demonstrated higher patient satisfaction rates,

reduced lengths of stay, and lower opioid usage while maintaining a high degree of safety.[7,30]
- A 2023 meta-analysis demonstrated that awake endoscopic spine surgeries showed reduced likelihoods of encountering postoperative complications (95% confidence interval [CI]: 0.22–4.41), surgical complications (95% CI: 0.08–2.69), and major medical complications (95% CI: 0.03–2.12).[31,32]
- As such, the ability to conduct endoscopic surgeries awake has led to procedures to be conducted in ambulatory surgical centers, allowing for procedural accessibility in patients who may ordinarily have been ordinarily unable to undergo traditional general anesthesia–based surgery.
- One study comparing traditional endoscopic approaches to MIS-TLIF has demonstrated significantly decreased operative blood loss ($p < 0.001$) as well as significantly lower postoperative low back and leg pain, and Oswestry Disability Index (ODI) decrease ($p < 0.05$) while demonstrating identical fusion rates and a 0% complication rate.[32,33,34]
- Similarly positive results have been demonstrated when comparing endoscopic surgery to traditional techniques in treating degenerative cervical spine disorders.[37,38]
- Viability exists for future innovation regarding a combination of endoscopic, CT-navigated, and robotic surgery. Recent studies examining endoscopic CT-navigated spine surgery have yielded positive results in both short- and long-term analyses.[39,40] The few studies on robotic-endoscopic approaches demonstrate similar favorability, though these studies are primarily retrospective studies and consist of limited sample sizes. For example, Wang et al found lower intraoperative blood loss and a similar complication profile in robotic-endoscopic lumbar diskectomy. Nonetheless, potential clearly exists for further innovation within endoscopic approaches.[41]
- Endoscopic rhizotomy (ER) has emerged as an alternative to lumbar interbody fusion for chronic low back pain caused by facet joint pathology. Studies have demonstrated 50% pain reductions in patients with an average duration of pain relief of 7.3 to 9.0 months following a single intervention. ER can provide long-term relief of chronic low back pain following previous spinal instrumentation and can additionally treat sacroiliac joint pain.[28,42,43,44]

14.4.4 Cons

- Endoscopic approaches in cases of high-grade spondylolisthesis or severe bilateral radiculopathy are contraindicated, as contralateral indirect decompression will not ameliorate the pathology.[7]
- However, broadly, endoscopic approaches allow an efficient and accessible minimally invasive approach that could serve as the foundation for significant advancement in conjunction with increasingly ubiquitous technology, including robotics.

Expert Tip

Modern endoscopic approaches can be used at any vertebral level, offering one of the most minimally invasive approaches possible with limited sacrifice to versatility. Awake endoscopy allows for wider surgical accessibility for patients in terms of both preoperative selection and health care setting of procedure.

14.5 Awake Lateral Fusions

14.5.1 Emergence

- Although substantial literature exists on LLIF since its inception in 2006, LLIF as an awake spine surgery has not been significantly addressed.
- In Chapter 18, awake LLIF indications, surgical/anesthetic technique, and postoperative management are described.

14.5.2 Pros

- Awake LLIF procedures share the same advantages as traditional asleep LLIF procedures. In brief, this includes limiting damage to the paravertebral muscles and anterior and posterior longitudinal ligaments, restoring sagittal/coronal alignment, and allowing for more accessible revision surgeries compared to posterior approaches.

- In addition, the awake aspect provides further benefits of reduced sedation time, OR times, lengths of hospital stay, and increased patient satisfaction.
- The prospective single-surgeon case series in Chapter 19 includes 15 awake LLIF procedures and concludes that, in conjunction with epidural anesthesia, lower complications, shorter hospitalizations, reduced costs, and significant improvement in surgery-related experience are achievable.

14.5.3 Cons

- With limited numbers of awake LLIF procedures having been conducted, drawbacks are not yet well established.

Expert Tip

Awake LLIF procedures will continue improving in operative time and outcomes as a standardized protocol is defined. Data, though limited, show the likelihood of robust patient outcomes, high patient satisfaction, and wide procedural accessibility due to early postoperative mobilization.

14.6 Conclusion

The goal of reducing "surgical footprint" through surgical and anesthetic techniques remains at the forefront of consideration in improving patients' postoperative outcomes. Within spine surgery, minimally invasive approaches have demonstrated continued improvements in pre-, intra-, and postoperative metrics while contributing to increased patient satisfaction. As novel technologies are developed and corresponding techniques optimized, previously esoteric approaches, including the broader category of awake spine surgery, will continue to grow in accessibility and efficacy. In the following few chapters, we aim to further explore the techniques previously highlighted and how they will impact care in the near future.

References

[1] Choi JY, Park SM, Kim HJ, Yeom JS. Recent updates on minimally invasive spine surgery: techniques, technologies, and indications. Asian Spine J. 2022; 16(6):1013–1021

[2] Liounakos JI, Wang MY. The endoscopic approach to lumbar discectomy, fusion, and enhanced recovery: a review. Global Spine J. 2020; 10(2) Suppl:65S–69S

[3] Sykes DAW, Tabarestani TQ, Salven DS, et al. Awake spinal anesthesia facilitates spine surgery in poor surgical candidates: a case series. Neurochirurgie. 2023; 69(3):101444

[4] Urick D, Sciavolino B, Wang TY, Gupta DK, Sharan A, Abd-El-Barr MM. Perioperative outcomes of general versus spinal anesthesia in the lumbar spine surgery population: a systematic review and meta-analysis of data from 2005 through 2021. J Clin Orthop Trauma. 2022; 30:101923

[5] Sykes DAW, Tabarestani TQ, Chaudhry NS, et al. Awake spinal fusion is associated with reduced length of stay, opioid use, and time to ambulation compared to general anesthesia: a matched cohort study. World Neurosurg. 2023; 176: e91–e100

[6] Farber SH, Pacult MA, Godzik J, et al. Robotics in spine surgery: a technical overview and review of key concepts. Front Surg. 2021; 8:578674

[7] Drossopoulos PN, Sharma A, Ononogbu-Uche FC, et al. Pushing the limits of minimally invasive spine surgery: from preoperative to intraoperative to postoperative management. J Clin Med. 2024; 13(8):2410

[8] Hoshide R, Feldman E, Taylor W. Cadaveric analysis of the Kambin's triangle. Cureus. 2016; 8(2):e475

[9] Dalton T, Sykes D, Wang TY, et al. Robotic-assisted trajectory into Kambin's triangle during percutaneous transforaminal lumbar interbody fusion-initial case series investigating safety and efficacy. Oper Neurosurg (Hagerstown). 2021; 21 (6):400–408

[10] Lee NJ, Khan A, Lombardi JM, et al. The accuracy of robot-assisted S2 alar-iliac screw placement at two different healthcare centers. J Spine Surg. 2021; 7(3):326–334

[11] Laratta JL, Shillingford JN, Lombardi JM, et al. Accuracy of S2 alar-iliac screw placement under robotic guidance. Spine Deform. 2018; 6(2):130–136

[12] Park C, Crutcher C, Mehta VA, et al. Robotic-assisted percutaneous iliac screw fixation for destructive lumbosacral metastatic lesions: an early single-institution experience. Acta Neurochir (Wien). 2021; 163(11):2983–2990

[13] De Biase G, Akinduro OO, Garcia D, et al. Awake robotic minimally invasive transforaminal lumbar interbody fusion under spinal anesthesia: a prospective study with 1-year follow-up. World Neurosurg. 2024; 189:e941–e947

[14] Peng YN, Tsai LC, Hsu HC, Kao CH. Accuracy of robot-assisted versus conventional freehand pedicle screw placement in spine surgery: a systematic review and meta-analysis of randomized controlled trials. Ann Transl Med. 2020; 8(13): 824–824

[15] Cloward RB. The treatment of ruptured lumbar intervertebral discs by vertebral body fusion. I. Indications, operative technique, after care. J Neurosurg. 1953; 10(2):154–168

[16] Schwender JD, Holly LT, Rouben DP, Foley KT. Minimally invasive transforaminal lumbar interbody fusion (TLIF): technical feasibility and initial results. J Spinal Disord Tech. 2005; 18 Suppl:S1–S6

[17] Tabarestani TQ, Sykes DAW, Kouam RW, et al. Novel approach to percutaneous lumbar surgeries via Kambin's triangle-radiographic and surgical planning analysis with nerve segmentation technology. World Neurosurg. 2023; 177:e385–e396

[18] Tabarestani TQ, Drossopoulos PN, Huang CC, et al. The importance of planning ahead: a three-dimensional analysis of the novel trans-facet corridor for posterior lumbar interbody

fusion using segmentation technology. World Neurosurg. 2024; 188:e247–e258

[19] Drossopoulos PN, Ononogbu-Uche FC, Tabarestani TQ, et al. Evolution of the transforaminal lumbar interbody fusion (TLIF): from open to percutaneous to patient-specific. J Clin Med. 2024; 13(8):2271

[20] De Biase G, Bechtle P, Leone B, Quinones-Hinojosa A, Abode-Iyamah K. Awake minimally invasive transforaminal lumbar interbody fusion with a pedicle-based retraction system. Clin Neurol Neurosurg. 2021; 200:106313

[21] Abode-Iyamah K, Ghaith AK, Bhandarkar AR, et al. Single-level awake transforaminal lumbar interbody fusion: a Mayo Clinic institutional experience and national analysis. Neurosurg Focus. 2021; 51(6):E4

[22] Kim CH, Lee CH, Kim KP. How high are radiation-related risks in minimally invasive transforaminal lumbar interbody fusion compared with traditional open surgery?: a meta-analysis and dose estimates of ionizing radiation. Clin Spine Surg. 2016; 29(2):52–59

[23] Chou LB, Lerner LB, Harris AHS, Brandon AJ, Girod S, Butler LM. Cancer prevalence among a cross-sectional survey of female orthopedic, urology, and plastic surgeons in the United States. Womens Health Issues. 2015; 25(5):476–481

[24] Son S, Ahn Y, Lee SG, et al. Learning curve of percutaneous endoscopic transforaminal lumbar discectomy by a single surgeon. Medicine (Baltimore). 2021; 100(4):e24346

[25] Ransom NA, Gollogly S, Lewandrowski KU, Yeung A. Navigating the learning curve of spinal endoscopy as an established traditionally trained spine surgeon. J Spine Surg. 2020; 6 Suppl 1:S197–S207

[26] Forst R, Hausmann B. Nucleoscopy–a new examination technique. Arch Orthop Trauma Surg (1978). 1983; 101(3):219–221

[27] Kambin P, Schaffer JL. Percutaneous lumbar discectomy. Review of 100 patients and current practice. Clin Orthop Relat Res. 1989(238):24–34

[28] Chen KT, Kim JS, Huang APH, Lin MHC, Chen CM. Current indications for spinal endoscopic surgery and potential for future expansion. Neurospine. 2023; 20(1):33–42

[29] Choi G, Lee SH, Lokhande P, et al. Percutaneous endoscopic approach for highly migrated intracanal disc herniations by foraminoplastic technique using rigid working channel endoscope. Spine. 2008; 33(15):E508–E515

[30] Kwon JW, Park Y, Lee BH, et al. Ten-year outcomes of minimally invasive versus open transforaminal lumbar interbody fusion in patients with single-level lumbar spondylolisthesis. Spine. 2022; 47(11):773–780

[31] Hussain I, Hofstetter CP, Wang MY. Innovations in spinal endoscopy. World Neurosurg. 2022; 160:138–148

[32] Jadczak CN, Vanjani NN, Pawlowski H, et al. The current status of awake endoscopic surgery: a systematic review and meta-analysis. World Neurosurg. 2023; 180:e198–e209

[33] Ao S, Zheng W, Wu J, et al. Comparison of Preliminary clinical outcomes between percutaneous endoscopic and minimally invasive transforaminal lumbar interbody fusion for lumbar degenerative diseases in a tertiary hospital: is percutaneous endoscopic procedure superior to MIS-TLIF? A prospective cohort study. Int J Surg. 2020; 76:136–143

[34] Kang MS, You KH, Choi JY, Heo DH, Chung HJ, Park HJ. Minimally invasive transforaminal lumbar interbody fusion using the biportal endoscopic techniques versus microscopic tubular technique. Spine J. 2021; 21(12):2066–2077

[35] Lv Y, Chen M, Wang SL, et al. Endo-TLIF versus MIS-TLIF in 1-segment lumbar spondylolisthesis: a prospective randomized pilot study. Clin Neurol Neurosurg. 2022; 212:107082

[36] Kim JE, Yoo HS, Choi DJ, Park EJ, Jee SM. Comparison of minimal invasive versus biportal endoscopic transforaminal lumbar interbody fusion for single-level lumbar disease. Clin Spine Surg. 2021; 34(2):E64–E71

[37] Ma W, Peng Y, Zhang S, et al. Comparison of percutaneous endoscopic cervical keyhole foraminotomy versus microscopic anterior cervical discectomy and fusion for single level unilateral cervical radiculopathy. Int J Gen Med. 2022; 15:6897–6907

[38] Clark JG, Abdullah KG, Steinmetz MP, Benzel EC, Mroz TE. Minimally invasive versus open cervical foraminotomy: a systematic review. Global Spine J. 2011; 1(1):9–14

[39] Gong J, Huang X, Luo L, et al. Radiation dose reduction and surgical efficiency improvement in endoscopic transforaminal lumbar interbody fusion assisted by intraoperative O-arm navigation: a retrospective observational study. Neurospine. 2022; 19(2):376–384

[40] Quillo-Olvera J, Quillo-Reséndiz J, Quillo-Olvera D, Barrera-Arreola M, Kim JS. Ten-step biportal endoscopic transforaminal lumbar interbody fusion under computed tomography-based intraoperative navigation: technical report and preliminary outcomes in Mexico. Oper Neurosurg (Hagerstown). 2020; 19(5):608–618

[41] Wang Z, Tan Y, Fu K, Meng Z, Wang L. Minimally invasive trans-superior articular process percutaneous endoscopic lumbar discectomy with robot assistance. BMC Musculoskelet Disord. 2022; 23(1):1144

[42] Du R, Xu G, Bai X, Li Z. Facet joint syndrome: pathophysiology, diagnosis, and treatment. J Pain Res. 2022; 15:3689–3710

[43] Smuck M, Crisostomo RA, Trivedi K, Agrawal D. Success of initial and repeated medial branch neurotomy for zygapophysial joint pain: a systematic review. PM R. 2012; 4(9): 686–692

[44] Lee JH, Chen KT, Chang KS, Chen CM. How I do it? Fully endoscopic rhizotomy assisted with three-dimensional robotic C-arm navigation for sacroiliac joint pain. Acta Neurochir (Wien). 2021; 163(12):3297–3301

15 Awake Robotic Surgery

Maya Blasingame, Kingsley Abode-Iyamah, and Elird Bojaxhi

Abstract

Robotic surgery has been gaining popularity in various specialties, most notably in urologic surgery. From the improved outcome noted in that field, there has been an increase in the interest in the use of robotic assistance in spinal surgery. There has now been adoption of robotic assistance during awake spine surgery. The adoption of robotic assistance in awake spine surgery is not surprising given we look at the overall evaluation of spine surgery from development of pedicle screws, minimally invasive procedures, and imaging technology. In this chapter, we explore the evaluation that has led to the adoption and benefits of robotic assistance in awake spine surgery.

Keywords: robotic, robotic awake spine surgery, minimally invasive spine surgery, awake spine surgery

Key Points

- Awake robotic spine surgery is a natural evolution of minimally invasive awake spine surgery.
- Awake robotic spine surgery allows the surgeon to combine the benefits of the MIS approach with the accuracy of robotics while minimizing anesthesia by using regional anesthesia.
- Awake robotic screw placement is safe and maintains the accuracy of robotic screw placement with minimum radiation.
- Robotic arm use in awake spine surgery allows for optimization of space utilization in the OR, especially when considering equipment around an awake patient.

15.1 History of Spinal Fusion Surgery

Spinal fusion surgery was introduced during a time when patients with spine-related disorders and pathologies suffered from poor quality of life and prognoses.[1] With the lack of viable alternative treatment for debilitating disorders such Pott's disease, scoliosis, and spinal instability, physicians of the time sought innovative treatment options.[2] The goal of spinal fusion was to allow the stabilization of spinal injuries, aid in the treatment of patients suffering from spinal deformities, and stabilize spinal curvatures.[2] This early period of innovation and expansion of the knowledge of spinal stability is a testament to the relentless pursuit by physicians to alleviate pain, find effective treatment modalities, and expand on the knowledge of the spine in the field of neurosurgery and orthopaedic surgery.[2] By the end of the 19th century, physicians began to develop the concept of modern spinal fusion techniques using techniques that involved bone grafts to fuse vertebrae.

In 1891, Dr. Berthold Ernest Hadra was one of the first to use wiring to stabilize cervical vertebrae, wrapping around the spinal column to fuse the sixth and seventh vertebrae.[1] This became one of the earliest successful fusions in a patient with progressive cord injury resulting from a fracture dislocation. Shortly after, Dr. Fritz Lange became the first physician to develop a technique to straighten the spine using celluloid bars, steel, and wiring, operating on patients with scoliosis.[1] This was followed by the work of Drs. Russell Hibbs and Fred Albee in the early 1900s, who developed novel techniques to enhance the success of spinal fusion surgery. Hibbs and Albee became pivotal figures in refining techniques for spinal arthrodesis, placing bone grafts along the decorticated surfaces to allow fusion of two vertebrates. Hibbs' technique of using a bone graft over a fusion bed became one of the first forms of fusion without instrumentation. However, this technique required long bouts of bed rest, which was associated with its own complications.[1] In the middle of the 19th century, the Milwaukee brace technique was developed by Drs. Walker Blount and Albert Schmidt, which was originally designed as a casting technique to stabilize pediatric patients after an operation.[2] The use of casts for postoperative immobilization and stabilization continued into the 1950s with the development of the localizer cast by Dr. Joseph Risser. This cast involved the use of a rigid frame that applied pressure to the rib cage in order to aid in postoperative surgical corrective maintenance.[2] Soon after the implementation of the localizer cast, the Harrington rod was developed by Paul Harrington, which took an individualized approach to patient care by using celluloid bars, steel, and wires to realign the curvature of a patient's spine to stabilize the spine.[2] The 1970s were filled with advancements in instrumentation, such as the Luque implant by Dr. Eduardo Luque who utilized flexible rods and wires to achieve fixation of the spine. Then finally in the late 1960s pedicle screws were developed by Dr. Raymound Roy-Camille to improve fusion rates postoperatively and three-column fixation of the vertebrae body. In the late 1980s, Dr. Yves Cotrel and Dr. Jean Dubousset developed a system that involved the use of several hook and contourable, bilateral rods.[3] Then the 1990s saw the development of interbody fusion with posterior lumbar interbody fusion (PLIF) and transforaminal lumbar interbody fusion (TLIF) techniques. These techniques involved an incision in the dorsal portion of the annulus and removal of the intervertebral disk, allowing for interbody fusion by placement of bone graft and/or cage in disk space to help promote bone growth, fusion, and spine stabilization.[4]

Over the decades, advancements in surgical techniques, instrumentation, and materials have refined spinal fusion surgery, making it a safer and more effective procedure. Currently, spinal fusion has played an important role in providing a source of treatment of pain that results from degeneration of vertebrae; with increasing development of minimally invasive approaches, spinal fusion surgery is moving toward a future with improved outcomes and faster recovery times.

15.2 History of Intraoperative Imaging

15.2.1 Intraoperative X-ray

Intraoperative imaging has also evolved almost in tandem with surgical fusion and represents a remarkable shift in surgical practice that has played a significant role in enhancing precision and patient safety in fusion surgery. Early attempts at intraoperative imaging date back to the 19th century with the implementation of X-ray technology by Wilhelm Conrad Roentgen in 1895.[5] This imaging modality was used for operative planning as well as intraoperative and postoperative evaluation. Unfortunately, this technique was limited by the bulky machine, ease of availability of the machine, and high breach rate as reported by Odgers et al.[6]

In the 1950s, the advancement of X-ray fluoroscopy allowed for the use of real-time imaging during surgery.[7] This was a groundbreaking achievement for its time and served the role of allowing surgeons to visualize anatomical structures and surgical instruments in a dynamic fashion.[8] Fluoroscopy involves the use of X-ray beams to pass through the body, with the transmitted radiation detected by a fluoroscope, which converts X-ray transmission into visible images that are displayed on a monitor.[9] Fluoroscopy provides invaluable use as a diagnostic procedure when used in conjunction with other procedures. While this modality provided the benefits of its promptness in intraoperative imaging, multiplanar imaging was lacking for providing real-time anatomical imaging and it still had the incidence of significant breach rate posing risk of injury to patients.[10] Although an efficient technique, the use of fluoroscopy does involve radiation and therefore exposes the patient and surgeon to more radiation than usual. As more awareness arose about the risks of radiation and its prevalence in society, scientists and physicians began to unearth novel techniques that involved the use of intraoperative imaging while attenuating the adverse effects of such tools.[11]

15.2.2 Intraoperative Ultrasound

The evolution of intraoperative imaging also involved ultrasound.[12] The rise of intraoperative ultrasound (IOUS) began in the 1960s, which provided immediate and dynamic imaging, giving surgeons insight into assessment of the anatomy, lesions, and precise surgical interventions. This technique provided significant advances in neurosurgical procedures, allowing for precise delineation of tumor margins and vascular structures.[13] While this imaging technique was useful for tissue delineation and tumor identification, it served a minimal role in spinal instrumentation and fusion.[13] Although its role in the evolution of other intraoperative techniques cannot be overlooked. As the need for detailed imaging of soft tissues, bones, and blood vessels arose, techniques of intraoperative imaging began to involve the use of computed tomography (CT).[13]

15.2.3 Intraoperative CT and Image Guidance

The 1970s saw the advent of CT and magnetic resonance imaging (MRI) to offer three-dimensional (3D) visualization of internal structures, providing a pivotal transition in guiding complex surgeries in an accurate and efficient manner.[14] Advancements in CT technology involved the development of portable CT scanners that provided efficient use during surgery, including the development and integration of 3D navigation into the "C-arm."[15] This device provided significant progression in imaging during neurosurgical procedures by obtaining detailed images of the brain during surgery, facilitating precise localization of tumors and abnormalities.[16] The use of intraoperative imaging in percutaneous pedicle screw placement has been a vital step in the field of minimally invasive spinal surgeries.[16] The use of CT-guided technology has allowed the field to overcome obstacles that were found by traditional use of fluoroscopy as a form of intraoperative imaging. In a study published in the *European Spine Journal* that looked at the placement of thoracolumbar pedicle screws in over 1,000 patients, it was found that the use of intraoperative CT-guided imaging during screw placement allowed for a statistically significantly higher accuracy of screw placement (96.4% using CT navigation compared to 93.9% with fluoroscopy), without affecting operation time. A meta-analysis published in *Medicine* found that the use of intraoperative imaging in combination with robotic-assisted techniques led to increased accuracy and improved pedicle screw placement.[16] It was found that the navigation guidance provided by CT imaging helps provide greater confidence for the placement of larger diameters and longer screws, providing more efficient ways to identify the trajectory needed for screw placement. This is also paramount in deformity surgery where the anatomy may be significantly distorted, making it difficult to place screws traditionally.[17]

Intraoperative imaging provides accurate imaging that guides surgeons and physicians during a procedure with real-time, accurate information. In recent years, the integration of intraoperative imaging has been used in collaboration with navigation systems and robotics, revolutionizing new surgical approaches to spinal procedures. These new advances have allowed for the onset of minimally invasive procedures involving instrument guidance.

15.3 Evolution of Robotic Surgery

The evolution of robotic surgery has led to significant advancements in the field of surgery and patient care. It has now become a common application to surgery and is often requested by patients albeit it remains in its infancy in spine surgery. In the 1980s, early experiments began with the use of robotic-assisted surgery using the PUMA 560 robotic surgical arm in neurosurgical procedures.[18] In the late 1990s, the rise of the da Vinci Surgical System provided a novel development within minimally invasive surgeries. This technique involved the use of robotic arms that were controlled from a console that allowed for highly precise movements with increased dexterity during complex surgeries. The use of robotic surgery became vital in improving patient care and patient outcome following urologic surgery and has since expanded to various areas of general surgery. This improvement of outcome in general and urologic surgery has sparked a keen interested in the use of robotic surgery in spine procedures. Within the field of spinal surgery, robotic surgery provided a lens in which there was a fixed trajectory, increased accuracy, and decreased operating room (OR) time with screw placement with the use of both semiautonomous and autonomous devices.[19] In 2004, the first robotic instrumentation device "SpineAssist" was approved by the Food and Drug Administration (FDA) for use in humans. Since that time, there have been drastic advancements with availability of spine robotic systems for screw placement.

Currently, robotics in spine surgery primarily involves pedicle screw placement, with a robotic arm providing a fixed trajectory through which screws are placed. The two most used systems are the Medtronic Mazor system and the Globus Excelsius system. Both systems use a fixed arm with a preselected trajectory whose accuracy is based on registration and a fixed reference point. When used correctly, these devices provide accurate screw placement, avoiding screw malplacement even in the most difficult pedicle screw trajectories, allowing surgeons to avoid screw misplacement, which can lead to various injuries (e.g., nerve root, vascular, cerebrospinal fluid leak) that may require revision surgery. This is typically accomplished through a small incision through a fixed trajectory through which the pedicle can be cannulated and screws can be placed. While improving the screw accuracy, robotic-assisted screw placement has also helped in transitioning to a more minimally invasive surgery, leading to patient experiences with less spine manipulation, less blood loss, less tissue damage, and faster recovery.

15.4 Awake Robotic Spine Surgery

As instrumentation, intraoperative imaging, and robotic screw placement have evolved, so has the modality of anesthetic used for spine surgery. While the use of spinal anesthesia for spinal fusion is relatively new in spine treatment, the use of spinal anesthesia for spine surgery in the form of decompression surgery is not. In 1959, John Ditzler first reported on the use of spinal anesthesia for spinal decompression surgery. He compared 766 cases under spinal anesthesia versus 333 cases under general anesthesia between 1937 and 1957 for herniated intervertebral disk surgery. He concluded that spinal anesthesia was an acceptable method of anesthesia for spinal surgery. More recently, the use of spinal anesthesia for spine surgery has gained popularity and has shown promise in also improving the current practice of spinal surgery. The benefits of spinal anesthesia for spine fusion include avoiding the side effects of a general anesthesia and thus allowing a more rapid recovery. Just as minimally invasive surgery allows the surgeon to perform surgery with minimal tissue damage, spinal anesthesia allows surgery to be performed while avoiding the collateral damage of general anesthesia.

The benefits of awake spine surgery include the reduction of operative time, minimization of postoperative opioid use, and decrease in postoperative nausea and vomiting. Furthermore, patients were found to experience decreased hospital stays and had increased satisfaction.[20] Postoperative benefits such as decrease in postoperative fatigue also suggest long-term benefits of awake spine surgery to patients compared to general anesthesia. As awake spine surgery continues to evolve, improving patient selection, enhancing patient comfort, and expanding this novel technique to more patients and procedures remain a major driving force.

One such advancement of awake spine surgery is the integration of robotics in awake surgery for an awake robotic spinal fusion. Awake robotic transforaminal interbody fusion (ARTLIF) is a novel procedure that uses a robotic arm for assistance in performing a TLIF. This procedure was first reported by Abode-Iyamah et al in 2021 in a case involving a 78-year-old woman who required a TLIF.[21] The previously mentioned significant benefits of the use of robotic-assisted screw placement in the spine naturally drove the evolution of incorporation of this technology in awake spine surgery.

15.4.1 General Benefits

Expert Tip

It is important to ask patients to minimize movement during screw placement. Watch for any large movement by the patient. Any such movement should lead to re-registration.

Like awake spinal fusion, robotic awake spinal fusion offers similar benefits. These benefits are attributed to awake surgery itself and are not decreased with the use of robotic assistance during these procedures. These benefits include the following:

- *Decreased operating time and overall OR time:* The benefits of decreased OR time noted in awake spine surgery are maintained in robotic awake spine surgery. This suggests that the registration time does not significantly increase overall OR time with robotic-assisted screw placement.
- *Decreased visual analog scale (VAS) score and opioid use immediately postoperatively:* There is an increase in pain control with spinal fusion and a decrease in opioid use in patients undergoing fusion via spinal versus general anesthesia.
- Increased time to ambulation.
- Increased patient and surgeon overall satisfaction.

- *Decreased fatigue:* There is decreased fatigue in patients undergoing spinal fusion compared to general anesthesia.
- Decreased radiation exposure to operating theater (OT) staff and surgeons.

15.4.2 Specific Benefits

- *Increased accuracy of instrumentation placement using robotic assistant:* The fixed trajectory for screw placement in robotic-assisted screw placement may also increase the accuracy of screw placement in patients under spinal anesthesia. A study by De Biase et al reported on the outcomes of 10 patients who underwent a robotic TLIF. The study reported good outcome in all patients without any intraoperative or perioperative complications. There was a screw placement accuracy of 99%.[22]
- *Decrease in VAS score:* Those undergoing robotic awake spine surgery experience decreased pain compared to their preoperative score at both 1 month and 12 months postoperatively in a study by De Biase et al.
- *OR space utilization:* One notable benefit they reported was the OR space utilization that the robotic system provided. This is compared to the O-arm, which is significantly bulkier. Additionally, the low-profile nature of the robotic arm compared to the C-arm or O-arm may also make it more feasible and beneficial to use around patients undergoing surgery under conscious sedation.
- *Patient comfort:* There may be increased patient comfort with robotic screw placement compared to stealth screw placement. The drilling used in ARTLIF for preparation of the pilot hole compared to the hammering involved in other techniques for screws placement may also serve an additional benefit for patients undergoing awake spine surgery. While this may not play a role in the overall safety of the techniques, it no doubt increases patient comfort during screw placement.

Expert Tip

Optimize patient comfort prior to starting the procedure, and maintain good communication with anesthesiology team. The anesthesiology team should routinely check on the patient.

- *Awake robotic patients can ambulate early following surgery:* The average time to first mobilization in a patient after robotic awake spine surgery was approximately 280 minutes after the procedure. Also, half of the patients with robotic awake spine surgery could be discharged on the same day.

Expert Tip

Patients with a history of opioid use prior to surgery are more likely to require readmission and should therefore not be discharged the same day of surgery.

15.4.3 Limitation

Of course, robotic-assisted awake spinal fusion is not without some concerns. There are some concerns of the natural breathing decreasing the accuracy of screw placement. These concerns are alleviated by the report from De Biase et al who, in their cohort of patients involving 100 pedicle screw placement with 33% of screws placed with robotic assistance, found a 99% accuracy rate. Other limitations of awake robotic spinal fusion include the following:

- *Cost of robotic arm:* The cost of the robotic device cannot be ignored as a hinderance to transitioning to awake robotic surgery. This is especially true in outpatient surgery facilities. While the cost of these devices can reach millions, there are less costly robotic assistance in addition to programs to limit the upfront cost of obtaining a device.
- *Screw restriction:* Another limitation is the requirement by the companies to use their instrumentation compatible only with their specific robotic arm.
- *Learning curve:* The learning curve of adopting to the use of robotics may also limit the adoption of robotic awake spinal fusion.

Expert Tip

It is important to become proficient in robotic spinal fusion under general anesthesia before switching to awake surgery.

15.5 Conclusion

Spinal fusion has continued to evolve since its inception in the late 1900s. This advancement addressed the method of fixation to pedicle screws, intraoperative imaging modalities for screw placement, and ultimately anesthetic technique for surgery for spinal fusion. Although awake spinal fusion is in its early stage, the integration of robotic assistance for screw placement in awake spinal fusion is a natural evolution of these procedures. The addition of robotic assistance to awake spinal fusion not only adds all the previously known benefits of awake spinal fusion (decreased OR time, improved pain control, increased patient satisfaction, increased time to ambulation, and more) but also adds additional benefits such as increased accuracy of screw placement, improved OR space utilization, and increased patient comfort during the procedure. As the role of robotics in spinal surgeries increases, it is clear it may also have an increasing role in awake spinal fusion.

References

[1] Virk S, Qureshi S, Sandhu H. History of spinal fusion: where we came from and where we are going. HSS J. 2020; 16(2): 137–142

[2] Tarpada SP, Morris MT, Burton DA. Spinal fusion surgery: a historical perspective. J Orthop. 2016; 14(1):134–136

[3] Walker CT, Kakarla UK, Chang SW, Sonntag VKH. History and advances in spinal neurosurgery: JNSPG 75th anniversary invited review article. J Neurosurg Spine SPI. 2019; 31 (6):775–785

[4] Eisenstein SM, Balain B, Roberts S. Current treatment options for intervertebral disc pathologies. Cartilage. 2020; 11(2):143–151

[5] Nimsky C, Carl B. Historical, current, and future intraoperative imaging modalities. Neurosurg Clin N Am. 2017; 28(4): 453–464

[6] Odgers CJ , IV, Vaccaro AR, Pollack ME, Cotler JM. Accuracy of pedicle screw placement with the assistance of lateral plain radiography. J Spinal Disord. 1996; 9(4):334–338

[7] Upadhyay UM, Golby AJ. Role of pre- and intraoperative imaging and neuronavigation in neurosurgery. Expert Rev Med Devices. 2008; 5(1):65–73

[8] Helm PA, Teichman R, Hartmann SL, Simon D. Spinal navigation and imaging: history, trends, and future. IEEE Trans Med Imaging. 2015; 34(8):1738–1746

[9] Khan A, Soliman MAR, Lee NJ, et al. CT-to-fluoroscopy registration versus scan-and-plan registration for robot-assisted insertion of lumbar pedicle screws. Neurosurg Focus. 2022; 52(1):E8

[10] Soriano-Sánchez JA, Ortega-Porcayo LA, Gutiérrez-Partida CF, et al. Fluoroscopy-guided pedicle screw accuracy with a mini-open approach: a tomographic evaluation of 470 screws in 125 patients. Int J Spine Surg. 2015; 9:54

[11] Narain AS, Hijji FY, Yom KH, Kudaravalli KT, Haws BE, Singh K. Radiation exposure and reduction in the operating room: perspectives and future directions in spine surgery. World J Orthop. 2017; 8(7):524–530

[12] Makuuchi M, Torzilli G, Machi J. History of intraoperative ultrasound. Ultrasound Med Biol. 1998; 24(9):1229–1242

[13] Ganau M, Syrmos N, Martin AR, Jiang F, Fehlings MG. Intraoperative ultrasound in spine surgery: history, current applications, future developments. 2018; 8(3):261–267

[14] Mislow JM, Golby AJ, Black PM. Origins of intraoperative MRI. Neurosurg Clin N Am. 2009; 20(2):137–146

[15] De Silva T, Punnoose J, Uneri A, et al. Virtual fluoroscopy for intraoperative C-arm positioning and radiation dose reduction. J Med Imaging (Bellingham). 2018; 5(1): 015005

[16] Ashraf M, Choudhary N, Hussain SS, Kamboh UA, Ashraf N. Role of intraoperative computed tomography scanner in modern neurosurgery: an early experience. Surg Neurol Int. 2020; 11:247

[17] Al-Naseem AO, Al-Muhannadi A, Ramadhan M, et al. Robot-assisted pedicle screw insertion versus navigation-based and freehand techniques for posterior spinal fusion in scoliosis: a systematic review and meta-analysis. Spine Deform. 2024; 12(5):1203–1215

[18] Theodore N, Arnold PM, Mehta AI. Introduction: the rise of the robots in spinal surgery. Neurosurg Focus. 2018; 45 VideoSuppl1:Intro

[19] Shah J, Vyas A, Vyas D. The history of robotics in surgical specialties. Am J Robot Surg. 2014; 1(1):12–20

[20] Fiani B, Reardon T, Selvage J, et al. Awake spine surgery: an eye-opening movement. Surg Neurol Int. 2021; 12:222

[21] De Biase G, Chen S, Akinduro O. Quinones-Hinojosa A, Abode-Iyamah K. Awake Robotic Minimally Invasive L4-5 Transforaminal Lumbar Interbody Fusion. World Neurosurg. 2021; 148:93

[22] De Biase G, Bechtle P, Leone B. Quinones-Hinojosa A, Abode-Iyamah K. Awake minimally invasive transforaminal lumbar interbody fusion with a pedicle-based retraction system. Clin Neurol Neurosurg. 2021; 200:106313

16 Next Generation TLIFs

Alyssa M. Bartlett, Peter N. Drossopoulos, and Muhammad M. Abd-El-Barr

Abstract

Transforaminal lumbar interbody fusion (TLIF) has significantly evolved from traditional open surgery to a minimally invasive procedure under awake anesthesia, enhancing patient outcomes and recovery. Initially, TLIF was performed through a large open incision, which involved significant muscle dissection and manipulation of spinal structures. This traditional method often resulted in substantial postoperative pain, longer hospital stays, and a higher risk of complications such as infection and blood loss. The evolution toward minimally invasive TLIF began with the development of specialized instruments and techniques that allowed surgeons to perform the procedure through smaller incisions. This approach minimized tissue damage and preserved muscle integrity, leading to reduced postoperative pain and faster recovery times. The use of tubular retractors and percutaneous screw placement further refined the technique, allowing for a more precise and less invasive operation. In recent years, there has been a shift toward performing minimally invasive TLIF under awake anesthesia. This innovative approach utilizes regional anesthesia and conscious sedation, avoiding the risks associated with general anesthesia. Awake TLIF results in patients experiencing fewer side effects from anesthesia, less postoperative pain, and a quicker return to normal activities. Additionally, regional anesthesia may allow for real-time patient feedback, which can help reduce the risk of positional nerve damage and improve surgical accuracy. The combination of minimally invasive techniques and awake anesthesia has marked a significant advancement in spinal surgery, offering patients a safer and more comfortable surgical experience.

Keywords: awake TLIF, minimally invasive TLIF, minimally invasive spine surgery, trans-Kambin TLIF, transfacet lumbar interbody fusion, awake anesthesia

Key Points

- Transforaminal lumbar interbody fusion (TLIF) was developed in 1952 by Harms and Rolinger, improving upon earlier techniques like posterior lumbar interbody fusion (PLIF) by minimizing muscle damage and neural manipulation.
- The procedure involves a midline skin incision with extensive bony resection for nerve root access and decompression, followed by diskectomy, endplate preparation, and placement of interbody cages.
- Open TLIF has risks such as durotomy, neural injury, increased blood loss, and longer hospital stays. Unilateral nerve root retraction also limits contralateral decompression, often requiring additional procedures.
- MIS-TLIF and trans-Kambin TLIF reduce muscle damage through smaller incisions and minimize blood loss, though they require advanced technology and skills, and have steeper learning curves.
- Awake TLIF under spinal anesthesia has been trialed and offers a viable option for patients unsuitable for general anesthesia.

16.1 Introduction

Transforaminal lumbar interbody fusion (TLIF) is a cornerstone in treating degenerative spinal conditions, offering patients relief from debilitating back and leg pain. Since its inception, TLIF has undergone a remarkable evolution, shaped by advancements in surgical technology and techniques and a deepened understanding of spinal anatomy and pathology. From its roots as a safer approach compared to posterior lumbar interbody fusion (PLIF), TLIF is now a pioneering, adaptive technique, ranging from open to minimally invasive to patient-specific approaches (▶ Fig. 16.1). Recent advances include an increased interest in using regional anesthesia for TLIF, giving the advantage of less postoperative opioid utilization, decreased operative time, and increased patient satisfaction.[1] These emerging trends may further refine and expand the capabilities of TLIF, offering the prospect of further enhanced patient outcomes. This chapter will outline a brief history and overview of the PLIF and open TLIF before expounding on the innovations of minimally invasive TLIF and awake anesthesia.

16.2 Open Transforaminal Lumbar Interbody Fusion

16.2.1 History and Innovation

- Although anterior lumbar interbody fusion was first described in the 1930s, the first

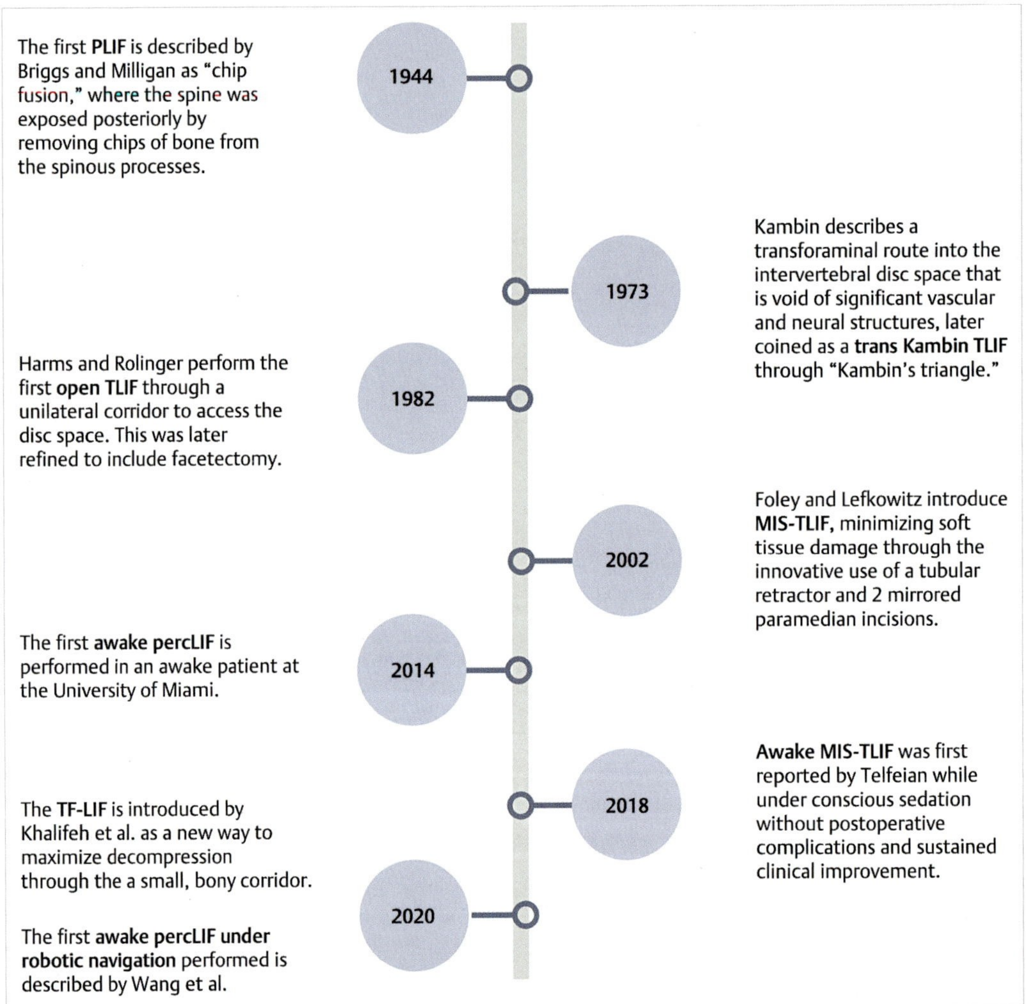

Fig. 16.1 A timeline of the evolution of lumbar interbody fusion from 1944 to 2020. Abbreviations: PLIF, posterior lumbar interbody fusion; TLIF, transforaminal lumbar interbody fusion; MIS-TLIF, minimally invasive transforaminal lumbar interbody fusion; percLIF, percutaneous transforaminal lumbar interbody fusion; TF-LIF, transfacet lumbar interbody fusion.

posterolateral approach to accessing the intervertebral space was described by Briggs and Milligan in 1944.[2] In this initial iteration of PLIF, a bone peg was used as a precursory interbody device rather than modern mainstays.

- The advent of TLIF technique, first described by Harms and Rolinger in 1982, represented a significant advancement over its PLIF predecessor, addressing many of its shortcomings related to inherent paravertebral muscle damage, increased manipulation of surrounding neural structures, and epidural damage.[3]
- Notably, TLIF, compared to PLIF, requires only unilateral bony resection and unilateral nerve root retraction and achieves similar bilateral neuroforaminal decompression and stabilization.

16.2.2 Key Steps

- Through a midline skin incision, subcutaneous tissue is dissected down to the fascia and exposed using retractors before cauterizing the fascia overlying the spinous processes.
- Subperiosteal dissection of the lamina is performed cranially to caudally before exposing the facet capsule using a Cobb elevator.
- After dissecting to the transverse process, a laminectomy is performed by removing the spinous processes of the operative levels with rongeur and subsequently removing the lamina. The ligamentum flavum is then resected to allow for decompression.
- To perform decompression, the pedicle is located and exposed with care taken to avoid exiting nerve root injury.
- Pedicle screws are inserted at the intersection of the facet and transverse process and contoured rods are placed.
- Complete facetectomy and disk preparation were performed via an approach from the side of maximal pain indicated by the patient. An osteotome is used to expose the superior vertebra's inferior articular process before dissecting the inferior vertebra's superior articular process from the ligamentum flavum. After resecting the pars and facet joint, a diskectomy is performed.
- Interbody implants are trialed with size confirmed via fluoroscopy before final anterior placement into the disk space. Finally, the construct is secured with connectors spanning the previously inserted pedicle screws, and the incision is closed in a retrograde, layered fashion and dressed at the discretion of the operative team.

16.2.3 Limitations

- As previously mentioned with the PLIF, and inherent to any large, open spinal procedure requiring extensive muscular dissection and retraction, iatrogenic injury to the paraspinal musculature is unavoidable.
- The midline access to the disk space, which requires extensive, and complete bony ligamentous resection and neural retraction, introduces a significant risk for durotomy and iatrogenic neural injury.
- The disadvantages of TLIF such as incomplete removal of the intervertebral disk and vertebral endplate, and potential occult injury to exiting nerve root are uncommon under experienced hands. TLIF, being a unilateral transforaminal approach, is also unable to decompress the opposite nerve root. This may require contralateral laminotomy, which is a straightforward procedure.[4]

16.3 Minimally Invasive Transforaminal Lumbar Interbody Fusion

16.3.1 History and Innovation

- Innovators Drs. Kevin Foley and Michael Lefkowitz introduced the concept of minimally invasive TLIF (MIS-TLIF) in 2002 to minimize soft tissue injury that may promote paraspinal muscle denervation.[5,6] Their technique utilized two mirrored 1-inch paramedian incisions, allowing access to the bilateral facet joints for diskectomy, implant placement, and bone grafting through a tubular retractor. Further percutaneous fixation could occur via these incisions, reducing disruption of the soft tissue.[7]
- The emergence of the MIS approach to lumbar interbody fusion promoted advances in interbody implants, namely through expandable interbody cages. These are designed with a narrow profile and then expanded once in the evacuated disk space to acquire the ideal fit between vertebral endplates with reduced

nerve root contraction required for insertion. As a result, expandable interbody cages allow for indirect contralateral decompression and a lower risk of cage subsidence.[8,9]

- Awake MIS-TLIF was first reported by Telfeian in 2018, where a patient with lumbar radiculopathy underwent L4–S1 MIS-TLIF with endoscopy while under conscious sedation without postoperative complications and sustained clinical improvement at 1 year.[10]

16.3.2 Key Steps

- Patients are positioned in a prone "superman" position on a Jackson table with the neck in neutral alignment. To avoid iatrogenic nerve injury, the shoulders are placed at no more than 90 degrees; the axillae, medial elbow, and bony prominence of the anterior superior iliac spine are padded; and the abdomen is hanging free.
- Pre- and/or intraoperative computed tomography (CT) scans can be utilized for navigation, with intraoperative imaging providing real-time information on spinal alignment. Typically, the operating microscope will be placed at the cranial end of the table with the associated viewing screen across from the surgeon and the intraoperative guidance at the caudal end. Anatomical landmarks are then verified with the navigation probe and the trajectory for placement of pedicle screws and tubular retractor is planned.
- Through paramedian incisions 4 to 5 cm from the midline, soft tissue is bluntly dissected to facilitate the placement of a mounted tubular retractor. Pedicle screws are often placed at this point. Completely percutaneous access can be done, especially on the side contralateral to the interbody side.
- Once the inferior articular process can be visualized, the facet capsule is entered, and the inferior and superior facets are resected on the symptomatic side or the side with worse radiculopathy using a high-speed drill. The ligamentum flavum can then be resected to visualize the disk in the floor of the spinal canal.
- The disk space is then prepared by mobilizing the thecal sac and creating a window into the disk space before performing a complete diskectomy. A bone graft of choice is then packed into the anterior portion of the diskectomy site.
- The appropriate size of the interbody implant is trialed and confirmed with fluoroscopy before packing with additional morselized bone graft and implanting into the empty disk space.
- A high-speed burr is used to remove additional lamina, transverse processes, and facet joints before tightening pedicle screws and placing rods.

16.3.3 Outcomes

- Several retrospective studies have consistently found similar rates of reoperation and other long-term complications and commensurate changes to patient-reported outcomes for both open TLIF and MIS-TLIF.[11,12] This was ultimately supportive in a 2023 multicenter cohort study of 297 patients comparing peri- and postoperative outcomes of MIS-TLIF and open TLIF; the two patient cohorts had similar blood loss and complication rates, as well as long-term improvement in disability and pain despite a longer operative time.[13]
- In this cohort study, patients undergoing MIS-TLIF also experienced significantly less blood loss and comparable length of stay.[13] However, these results are not consistently supported in the literature.
- While some have found that MIS-TLIF is associated with shorter lengths of stay, many studies report no significant differences.[11,13] The inconsistencies may be the result of patient expectations, surgeon preference, or even surgical skill.[13] Further, the setting in which MIS-TLIF is performed may influence the length of stay. For example, in a retrospective comparison of patients undergoing TLIF in a hospital versus outpatient setting, those who received inpatient care had a median length of stay that was 15 times greater than that for ambulatory patients (23.9 vs. 1.6 hours; $p = 0.001$).[14]
- Similar variability is found in published reports of operative time for MIS-TLIF. In a meta-analysis of 32 studies (total $n = 2{,}385$ patients), there was no significant difference in operative time between open TLIF and MIS-TLIF.[15] However, there is a known learning curve to attain surgical proficiency in MIS-TLIF, especially with minimally invasive advances being relatively novel in spine surgery. For example, a meta-analysis of nine studies

examining the learning curve of MIS-TLIF showed a gradual decrease in the length of operations, confirming that surgeons may become more efficient with increased experience.[16]
- MIS-TLIF may also elicit more changes to spinopelvic parameters when compared to open TLIF. According to a 2022 propensity score–matched comparison of open TLIF and MIS-TLIF patients, MIS-TLIF patients experienced significantly larger improvements in anterior disk height and sacral slope, though there is variability in the literature.[17]
- Although awake MIS-TLIF is relatively novel, reported outcomes so far are robust and positive. In a 2021 retrospective case control study, patients undergoing MIS-TLIF under spinal anesthesia had significantly shorter operative times, lower immediate postoperative pain scores, and decreased time to ambulation compared to those who received general anesthesia.[18]

16.3.4 Limitations

- An inherent disadvantage of minimally invasive surgery is the lack of direct visualization of the surgical anatomy and field, often necessitating the use of fluoroscopy and CT navigation during surgery and increasing the risk associated with radiation exposure. A study of radiation-related risks in MIS-TLIF versus open TLIF found that patients undergoing MIS-TLIF had a 2.4-fold increase in radiation exposure.[19]
- As MIS-TLIF is heavily dependent on available technology, especially with the increasing use of CT intraoperative navigation and surgical robotics, there is a concern about increased costs to use and maintain these additional tools. Although some studies have shown that MIS-TLIF is more cost-effective than open TLIF, there is no consensus in the current literature.[19]

Expert Tip

Awake Anesthesia for TLIF

- *Awake TLIF is an ideal option for patients with comorbidities that increase the risk of general anesthesia, such as geriatric or frail patients. Awake TLIF may be more challenging for patients with complex spinal deformities and severe central canal stenosis due to the need for extensive decompression and longer operative times; therefore, the decision should be left to the surgeon's discretion.*
- *For spinal anesthesia, bupivacaine is appropriate for sensory and motor blockade below T4.*
- *During positioning, continuously check for signs of discomfort or pain and communicate to ensure they remain comfortable, as an uncomfortable position may lead to increased movement during surgery.*
- *Remain vigilant for signs of discomfort, especially during manipulation of nerve roots, interbody device placement, or decompression. If the patient experiences discomfort, anesthesia or surgical technique will need to be reassessed or adjusted accordingly.*

One of the key benefits of performing awake TLIF is the likelihood of faster postoperative recovery. Encourage early ambulation to aid in mobility.

16.4 Trans-Kambin's Triangle Lumbar Interbody Fusion

16.4.1 History and Innovation

- Kambin's triangle, first described by its namesake Dr. Parviz Kambin in the 1970s, is defined by the exiting nerve root, the superior articular process of the inferior vertebrae, and the superior endplate of the inferior vertebral body.[20,21] As this area is devoid of important neural and vascular structures, this is considered a "safe space" for access to the spine.
- In early utilizations of this anatomical corridor, Kambin's triangle was used as a path for percutaneous nerve root decompression by aspirating herniated lumbar disks.[20] However, this technique has been modified as a means for alleviating spinal stenosis and interbody fusion with minimal electrocautery and drilling, coined as percutaneous transforaminal lumbar interbody fusion (percLIF). This technique can be further adapted by adding the use of endoscopy for direct intraoperative visualization known as percutaneous endoscopic transforaminal lumbar interbody fusion (PETLIF).

- The first percLIF was performed in an awake patient in 2014 using only local bupivacaine and moderate doses of ketamine and propofol with overall positive results and minimal conversion to general anesthesia. Since then, awake percLIF procedures have been successfully performed with erector spinae plane blocks with similarly positive results.[22]

16.4.2 Key Steps

- Spinal anesthesia is induced at the L3/L4 or L4/L5 level by inserting a larger 20-gauge introducer needle followed by a 25-gauge Quincke needle between the spinous processes. The needle is advanced into the interspinous ligament and into the thecal space, where the desired anesthetic is placed to induce complete loss of sensation and paresis below T4.
- Similar to other TLIF variations, patients are placed prone with the arms in the "superman" position with strategic pad placement to protect pressure points.
- Two stab incisions are made over the left and right posterior superior iliac spines for placement of the reference frame. Once the C-arm fluoroscopy is brought into the operative field and planned trajectories are confirmed, additional stab incisions are made overlying entry sites for the screws before placing pilot holes, taps, and pedicle screws into the pedicles of interest.
- Next, the trajectory into Kambin's triangle is planned. Ideally, this will be the farthest caudal from the superior pedicle to ensure the greatest distance from the exiting nerve root, decreasing the likelihood of iatrogenic nerve injury.
- Diskectomy is then facilitated using successive dilation until the introduction of a portal or working channel is allowed. Diskectomy is then performed using drill brushes, pituitary rongeurs, and curettes to prepare the endplate for subsequent fusion.
- Bone morphogenic protein is then placed anteriorly into the disk space before hammering the expandable cage and obturator into the disk space with a mallet. Upon expansion to the appropriate size, the obturator is removed. Finally, pedicle screws are tightened and the final placement of pedicle screws and cage is confirmed with intraoperative CT before proceeding with closure.

16.4.3 Outcomes

- Tabarestani et al found significant improvement in anterior and posterior disk height as well as spondylolisthesis in 16 patients who had undergone single-level percLIF for grade 1 lumbar spondylolisthesis.[23] Moreover, these effects were maintained at the 12-month follow-up with additional significant improvement in the Oswestry Disability Index.
- These findings were echoed by a 2023 retrospective review of patients who underwent percLIF via Kambin's triangle that found significant improvement in spondylolisthesis and disk height as well as lumbar lordosis, sacral slope, and pelvic tilt.[23] These patients had a 94.4 and 87.5% postoperative fusion rates at 1 and 2 years, respectively.
- Compared to MIS-TLIF, a meta-analysis found that percLIF reduces blood loss and length of hospitalization and is associated with less postoperative pain.[24] A retrospective review from Shalita et al also showed that percLIF is associated with less opioid utilization postoperatively although the relationship was not significant.[25]
- While general anesthesia is still the standard modality of analgesia for endoscopic TLIF, an increasing number of studies have examined the operative and clinical outcomes of those undergoing percLIF under spinal anesthesia. In 10 patients undergoing PETLIF under spinal anesthesia, Wang and Grossman demonstrated notable reductions in patient-reported disability and health-related quality of life.[26] A matched cohort study by Sykes et al also showed that percLIF under spinal anesthesia had significantly lower opioid utilization compared to those who were under general anesthesia.[27]

16.4.4 Limitations

- The limitations of trans-Kambin TLIF are not unlike other minimally invasive spine surgery techniques, namely that the technique compromises direct visualizes and suffers from increased utilization of radiation compared to open approaches. However, endoscopic approaches have a noteworthy learning curve.
- In a retrospective review of patients undergoing trans-Kambin TLIF, the operative time significantly decreased as the surgeon progressed along the learning curve.[28] The same study also found

less favorable amounts of the remnant disk and a greater rate of exiting nerve root injury in patients undergoing surgery in less experienced surgeons. However, disease recurrence remains stable on the learning curve.

- An additional limitation is that trans-Kambin TLIF may only be suitable for select cases. For example, patients with a history of osteoporosis may not be appropriate candidates as indirect compression relies on applying pressure on the vertebral endplates. Further, severe central canal stenosis may not be sufficiently treated as indirect compression can only achieve a limited amount of central canal enlargement.

16.5 Transfacet Lumbar Interbody Fusion

16.5.1 History and Innovation

- Transfacet LIF (TF-LIF), an alternative to MIS-TLIF, was reported by Khalifeh et al in 2020.[29] The technique maximizes direct and indirect decompression through the bony "working access corridor," creating a safe and precise method of treating low-grade spondylolisthesis and degenerative disk disease (▶ Fig. 16.2).
- Although this novel technique is still in its infancy, adaptations have already enhanced the potential impacts of the TF-LIF. One such instance is the use of an "in-parallel" TF-LIF under spinal anesthesia to facilitate awake surgery beyond one- to two-level decompression and fusion.[30] In addition, augmented reality has been used to improve workflow.[31,32]

16.5.2 Key Steps

- The patient is placed prone on a Jackson table in a kyphotic flexion of 35 degrees. This facilitates greater access to the disk space.
- Once the correct levels are identified using fluoroscopy to examine vertebral anatomy, the skin is marked for entry for pedicle targets. Bilateral linear 2- to 3-cm paramedian skin incisions are made approximately 2 cm off midline. After dissecting subcutaneous tissue to the lumbar fascia, an incision is made along the extent of the exposed fascia. Tubular dilators are inserted for sequential dilation to expose the bilateral facet complexes.
- The pedicles are cannulated using K-wires and Jamshidi needles. Pedicle screws are inserted at the superior articular processes with care to avoid rostral facet joints.
- On the working side, the 8- to 12-mm working corridor is defined as the rostral aspect of the disk space, the rostral aspect of the caudal pedicle, and 0.5- to 1-cm medial to the caudal pedicle screw. The high-speed drill is then used to access the disk space without interfering with the traversing or exiting nerve roots. On the

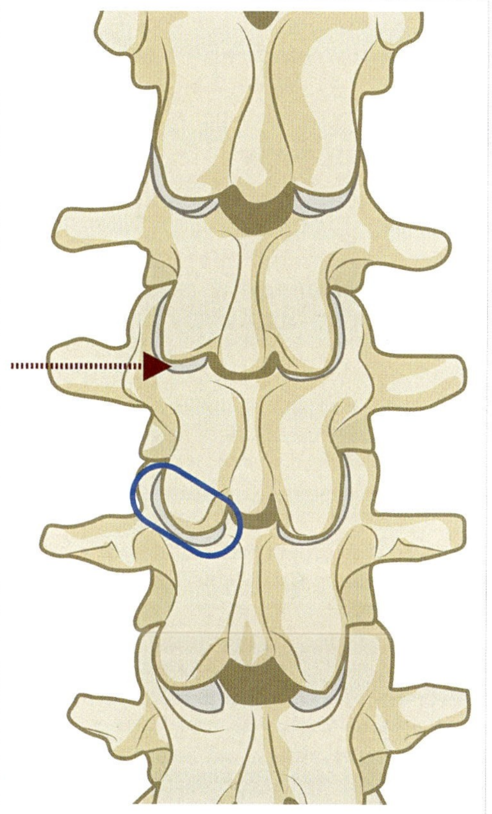

Fig. 16.2 Depiction of the entry sites for transfacet and trans-Kambin lumbar interbody fusion. The area encompassed by the *blue oval* represents the facet joint, the site of entry for transfacet lumbar interbody fusion (TF-LIF). The *red dashed arrow* is pointing to the corridor of Kambin's triangle, which is unable to be visualized in this view. (Reproduced from Drossopoulos PN, Ononogbu-uche FC, Tabarestani TQ, Huang C-C, Paturu M, Bardeesi A, Ray WZ, Shaffrey CI, Goodwin CR, Erickson M, et al. Evolution of the Transforaminal Lumbar Interbody Fusion (TLIF): From Open to Percutaneous to Patient-Specific. *Journal of Clinical Medicine*. 2024; 13(8):2271.Open access article distributed under the terms of the Creative Commons Attribution License (CC BY 4.0).)

asymptomatic side, the facet joint is decorticated using a high-speed drill. This partial facetectomy of the contralateral facet provides sufficient access for indirect compression and interbody implant expansion. The disk is then removed, and the vertebral endplates are prepared for fusion.
- Much like in other TLIF variations, the interbody implant is trialed using fluoroscopy. Once the appropriate size is found, both the device and disk space are packed with morselized bone graft. The interbody implant is then inserted into the anterior disk space before expanding to provide maximum improvement in disk height.

16.5.3 Outcomes

- Given its novelty, there is a paucity of long-term results of TF-LIF. However, early investigations provide robust evidence of improved spinopelvic parameters and patient-reported outcomes. In the largest prospective study thus far, Khalifeh et al reported significant improvements in disability and back pain scores among its 68 patients. Accordingly, they also found improvements in disk height, lumbar lordosis, and segmental lordosis with over 94% of patients illustrating fusion at 12 months postoperatively.[33] However, they also report subsidence in 8.1% of patients, although this is similar to rates of subsidence in MIS-TLIF.[34]
- Awake TF-LIF has also begun to receive some attention. A 2023 report describes the successful use of a one-level TF-LIF performed concurrently with a two-level decompression under erector spinae plane block and spinal anesthesia by two independent surgeons.

16.5.4 Limitations

- As the TF-LIF ultimately uses a similar approach to the disk space as MIS-TLIF and trans-Kambin TLIF, the techniques share the same limitations, such as increased reliance on intraoperative radiation.
- An additional limitation is the restriction of its use due to anatomy. Namely, the working corridor must be large enough to safely prepare endplates for fusion and pass an interbody device.

Expert Tip: TLIF Technique

- *For pedicle screw insertion in MIS-TLIF, consider a trajectory that starts more lateral on the side of the facetectomy to allow for more space for retractor and cage placement.*
- *For tubular retractor trajectory in MIS-TLIF, the trajectory should be angled medially directly over the facet joint and lead into the intervertebral disk space.*
- *Entry points for screws in MIS-TLIF are generally chosen based on the intersection of the transverse process, the mamillary process, and the lateral surface of the superior articular facet.*
- *While assembling the pedicle screw and rod construct, the Jackson table can be turned into a neutral 0-degree position for interbody implant insertion to increase operating room efficiency.*
- *To ensure clear visualization of the disk space during diskectomy and interbody implant placement, modular screws may be used on the ipsilateral side of the target disk space with standard pedicle screws used on the contralateral side. The ipsilateral screws may provide a landmark for the boundaries of the space.*

16.6 Conclusions

TLIF, whether open, minimally invasive, or otherwise modified, remains a hallmark of the treatment of degenerative disk disease and spondylolisthesis and is poised for significant advancements driven by emerging innovations. As minimally invasive techniques become more refined, reducing patient recovery times and minimizing tissue damage, the integration of robotic-assisted surgery, augmented reality, and bioengineered materials and implants promises increased precision, allowing for more accurate placement of implants and reducing the risk of complications. However, the use of spinal and local anesthesia for TLIF continues to gain attention, offering the hope of minimizing complications, reducing length of hospitalization, and hastening time to ambulation. Further, awake TLIF can allow for patients who may otherwise be poor general anesthesia candidates due to frailty or comorbidity to receive quality-of-life-altering surgery. As research continues to support the efficacy and safety of spinal anesthesia in TLIF, its use is likely to increase, offering a promising alternative for both patients and surgeons.

References

[1] Lee JK, Park JH, Hyun SJ, Hodel D, Hausmann ON. Regional anesthesia for lumbar spine surgery: can it be a standard in the future? Neurospine. 2021; 18(4):733–740

[2] Briggs H, Milligan PR. Chip fusion of the low back following exploration of the spinal canal. J Bone Jt Surg. 1944; 26(1):125–130

[3] Harms J, Rolinger H. A one-stager procedure in operative treatment of spondylolistheses: dorsal traction-reposition and anterior fusion (author's transl). Z Orthop Ihre Grenzgeb. 1982; 120(3):343–347

[4] Humphreys SC, Hodges SD, Patwardhan AG, Eck JC, Murphy RB, Covington LA. Comparison of posterior and transforaminal approaches to lumbar interbody fusion. Spine. 2001; 26 (5):567–571

[5] Foley KT, Lefkowitz MA. Advances in minimally invasive spine surgery. Clin Neurosurg. 2002; 49:499–517

[6] Dave BR, Marathe N, Mayi S, et al. Does conventional open TLIF cause more muscle injury when compared to minimally invasive TLIF?: a prospective single center analysis. Global Spine J. 2024; 14(1):93–100

[7] Schwender JD, Holly LT, Rouben DP, Foley KT. Minimally invasive transforaminal lumbar interbody fusion (TLIF): technical feasibility and initial results. J Spinal Disord Tech. 2005; 18 Suppl:S1–S6

[8] Hiyama A, Katoh H, Sakai D, Sato M, Tanaka M, Watanabe M. Comparison of radiological changes after single-position versus dual-position for lateral interbody fusion and pedicle screw fixation. BMC Musculoskelet Disord. 2019; 20(1):601

[9] Macki M, Hamilton T, Haddad YW, Chang V. Expandable cage technology-transforaminal, anterior, and lateral lumbar interbody fusion. Oper Neurosurg (Hagerstown). 2021; 21 Suppl 1:S69–S80

[10] Telfeian AE. An awake, minimally-invasive, fully-endoscopic surgical technique for treating lumbar radiculopathy secondary to heterotopic foraminal bone formation after a minimally invasive transforaminal lumbar interbody fusion with BMP: technical note. J Spine Surg. 2018; 4(1):162–166

[11] Kwon JW, Park Y, Lee BH, et al. Ten-year outcomes of minimally invasive versus open transforaminal lumbar interbody fusion in patients with single-level lumbar spondylolisthesis. Spine. 2022; 47(11):773–780

[12] Hu W, Yang G, Wang H, et al. Which is better in clinical and radiological outcomes for lumbar degenerative disease of two segments: MIS-TLIF or OPEN-TLIF? J Pers Med. 2022; 12 (12):1977

[13] Chan AK, Bydon M, Bisson EF, et al. Minimally invasive versus open transforaminal lumbar interbody fusion for grade I lumbar spondylolisthesis: 5-year follow-up from the prospective multicenter Quality Outcomes Database registry. Neurosurg Focus. 2023; 54(1):E2

[14] Schlesinger SM, Gelber BR, Gerber MB, Lorio MP, Block JE. Comparison of transforaminal lumbar interbody fusion in the ambulatory surgery center and traditional hospital settings, part 1: multi-center assessment of surgical safety. J Pers Med. 2023; 13(2):311

[15] Hammad A, Wirries A, Ardeshiri A, Nikiforov O, Geiger F. Open versus minimally invasive TLIF: literature review and meta-analysis. J Orthop Surg Res. 2019; 14(1):229

[16] Shuman WH, Baron RB, Neifert SN, et al. MIS-TLIF procedure is improving with experience: systematic review of the learning curve over the last decade. Clin Spine Surg. 2022; 35(9):376–382

[17] Dibble CF, Zhang JK, Greenberg JK, et al. Comparison of local and regional radiographic outcomes in minimally invasive and open TLIF: a propensity score-matched cohort. J Neurosurg Spine. 2022; 37(3):384–394

[18] De Biase G, Gruenbaum SE, West JL, et al. Spinal versus general anesthesia for minimally invasive transforaminal lumbar interbody fusion: implications on operating room time, pain, and ambulation. Neurosurg Focus. 2021; 51(6):E3

[19] Kim CH, Lee CH, Kim KP. How high are radiation-related risks in minimally invasive transforaminal lumbar interbody fusion compared with traditional open surgery?: a meta-analysis and dose estimates of ionizing radiation. Clin Spine Surg. 2016; 29(2):52–59

[20] Kambin P, Sampson S. Posterolateral percutaneous suction-excision of herniated lumbar intervertebral discs. Report of interim results. Clin Orthop Relat Res. 1986; 207:37–43

[21] Fanous AA, Tumialán LM, Wang MY. Kambin's triangle: definition and new classification schema. J Neurosurg Spine. 2019; 32(3):390–398

[22] Wang TY, Mehta VA, Sankey EW, et al. Single-position prone transpsoas fusion for the treatment of lumbar adjacent segment disease: early experience of twenty-four cases across three tertiary medical centers. Eur Spine J. 2022; 31(9):2255–2261

[23] Tabarestani TQ, Wang TY, Sykes DAW, et al. Two-year clinical and radiographic outcomes for percutaneous lumbar interbody fusion with an expandable titanium cage Through Kambin's triangle without facetectomy. Int J Spine Surg. 2023; 17(6):760–770

[24] Ao S, Zheng W, Wu J, et al. Comparison of Preliminary clinical outcomes between percutaneous endoscopic and minimally invasive transforaminal lumbar interbody fusion for lumbar degenerative diseases in a tertiary hospital: is percutaneous endoscopic procedure superior to MIS-TLIF? A prospective cohort study. Int J Surg. 2020; 76:136–143

[25] Shalita C, Wang T, Dibble CF, et al. Percutaneous lumbar interbody fusion results in less perioperative opioid usage compared to minimally invasive transforaminal lumbar interbody fusion: a single institution, multi-surgeon retrospective study. J Spine Surg. 2024; 10(2):190–203

[26] Wang MY, Grossman J. Endoscopic minimally invasive transforaminal interbody fusion without general anesthesia: initial clinical experience with 1-year follow-up. Neurosurg Focus. 2016; 40(2):E13

[27] Sykes DAW, Tabarestani TQ, Chaudhry NS, et al. Awake spinal fusion is associated with reduced length of stay, opioid use, and time to ambulation compared to general anesthesia: a matched cohort study. World Neurosurg. 2023; 176:e91–e100

[28] Son S, Ahn Y, Lee SG, et al. Learning curve of percutaneous endoscopic transforaminal lumbar discectomy by a single surgeon. Medicine (Baltimore). 2021; 100(4):e24346

[29] Khalifeh JM, Dibble CF, Stecher P, Dorward I, Hawasli AH, Ray WZ. Transfacet minimally invasive transforaminal lumbar interbody fusion with an expandable interbody device-

part II: consecutive case series. Oper Neurosurg (Hagerstown). 2020; 19(5):518–529

[30] Chan AK, Gnaedinger A, Ayoub C, Gupta DK, Abd-El-Barr MM. The "in-parallel" technique for awake, bilateral simultaneous minimally invasive transforaminal lumbar interbody fusion and multilevel lumbar decompression. Oper Neurosurg (Hagerstown). 2023; 24(3):e160–e169

[31] Bardeesi A, Tabarestani TQ, Bergin SM, et al. Using augmented reality technology to optimize transfacet lumbar interbody fusion: a case report. J Clin Med. 2024; 13(5):1513

[32] Sommer F, Hussain I, Kirnaz S, et al. Augmented reality to improve surgical workflow in minimally invasive transforaminal lumbar interbody fusion: a feasibility study with case series. Neurospine. 2022; 19(3):574–585

[33] Khalifeh JM, Dibble CF, Stecher P, Dorward I, Hawasli AH, Ray WZ. Transfacet minimally invasive transforaminal lumbar interbody fusion with an expandable interbody device-part I: 2-dimensional operative video and technical report. Oper Neurosurg (Hagerstown). 2020; 19(5):E473–E479

[34] Subramanian T, Merrill RK, Shahi P, et al. Predictors of subsidence and its clinical impact after expandable cage insertion in minimally invasive transforaminal interbody fusion. Spine. 2023; 48(23):1670–1678

17 Awake Endoscopic Spine Surgery

Devin St. Clair and Raymond Gardocki

Abstract

Awake endoscopic spine surgery represents a paradigm shift in spinal surgical approaches, offering patients a less morbid option with potentially reduced recovery times and complications. This chapter explores the principles, techniques, indications, and outcomes associated with awake endoscopic spine surgery.

Keywords: awake surgery, endoscopic surgery, conscious sedation, minimally invasive spine surgery

Key Points

- Less morbidity and delirium.
- Fewer anesthesia side effects and postop complications.
- Potential to treat sicker patients who may not be candidates for general anesthesia (higher-risk patients).
- Less need for postoperative narcotics.
- The potential to move higher-risk patients with more comorbidities to a lower-cost outpatient environment.[1]
- Overall, higher patient satisfaction scores.[2]

17.1 Introduction

Awake endoscopic spine surgery represents a paradigm shift in spinal surgical approaches, offering patients a less invasive option with potentially reduced recovery times and complications.[1,3,4,5,6,7,8,9,10] While this chapter explores the principles, techniques, indications, and outcomes associated with awake endoscopic spine surgery, these methods can be applied to other minimally invasive spine procedures as well.

Performing surgery while awake allows for several perceived and established benefits, many of which have been demonstrated within the literature.[3,4] Awake spine surgery lends itself to minimally invasive (MIS) or endoscopic surgical techniques. These techniques are associated with shorter surgical durations, reduced blood loss, and decreased length of stay when compared to open surgical techniques.[5] It has been well established that performing surgical procedures, specifically endoscopic spine procedures, under conscious sedation allows for improved hemodynamic stability intraoperatively, decreased pain both intraoperatively and acutely postoperatively, and significantly decreased anesthesia complications.[6,7] Neuraxial anesthesia is also thought to decrease plexus bleeding through peripheral vasodilation.[8]

There are several other benefits of performing surgery on a patient that is not deeply sedated. With the patient easily arousable, often we find the staff in the room are more focused on the procedure at hand. Background conversations and distractions are kept to a minimum, and efficiency and quality of care are improved as a result.

Expert Tip

With an awake patient, the staff are more alert and focused on the task at hand. Background conversation and distractions are kept to a minimum.

When the patient avoids general anesthesia, they are quicker to recover from the anesthetic medication. This results in a quicker discharge from the surgery center/hospital. This also decreases the side effects of anesthetic medication, including prolonged delirium, postoperative nausea and vomiting, and urinary retention.[6] There is also a cost to keeping patients in the postanesthesia care unit (PACU), which is minimized with awake surgery. This is facilitated by a decreased time to ambulation.[11]

In addition, performing surgery on an awake patient allows the patient to give feedback intraoperatively. Real-time feedback can be obtained directly from the patient including symptom improvement/worsening and pain location. With the patient able to give immediate feedback intraoperatively, this negates the need for neuromonitoring to protect the dorsal root ganglion (DRG) in transforaminal endoscopic approaches.[9] Traditionally, neuromonitoring is instituted to alert the surgeon if the DRG is injured, but it is important to note that neuromonitoring only becomes abnormal after the DRG is compromised. Intraoperative feedback from the patient during awake spine surgery allows immediate recognition if the DRG is being compressed, with the theoretical benefit of avoiding actual damage.

In addition, there may be further benefits from avoiding general anesthesia as it relates to cognitive decline, especially in the elderly population.[12,13] We frequently have elderly patients requesting to avoid general anesthesia due to prior prolonged recovery and postop delirium.

Another unintended benefit is the ability to allow the patient to position themselves on the operating room (OR) table and transfer themselves off the table after surgery. Not having to manually lift and position patients is a benefit that may reduce occupational hazards and potential patient injury.

Awake spine surgery has also enabled us to care for patients with increased comorbidities at increased risk with general anesthesia in a lower-cost outpatient environment while avoiding hospital admission.

Expert Tip

Awake surgery allows for real-time feedback and recognition of DRG irritation in real time. The patient will react if the nerve is compressed as it is happening, negating the need for neuromonitoring and potentially avoiding neural injury.

There are some downsides to awake spine surgery. The biggest hurdle one will face is establishing interest and active involvement from the anesthesia team. Patients undergoing awake surgery require constant and consistent coverage, more intense involvement from the anesthesia team, and a more nuanced approach that requires far greater attention. With the right team, however, this could be considered a strength, as a more innately involved anesthesia team will likely result in decreased anesthetic administration overall.

Another barrier to awake spine surgery is the timing and duration limit that it imposes on the surgeries. Our team tries to limit surgeries to no longer than 3 hours. This is an arbitrary limitation with no substantial data to support it. However, we found that our team can control the light sedation and narcotic administration far better with the patient in a prone position if the surgery duration is less than 3 hours. Longer duration surgeries require further attention and administration of anesthetic and can be more difficult to time the lightening of the patient to allow for feedback at appropriate points in the case. When spinal/epidural anesthetic is provided, this may need to be redosed if procedure duration extends past 3 hours.

As opposed to general anesthesia, the same dose of medication does not apply to every patient. The amount of narcotic and anesthetic medication given in these cases is highly variable and must be tailored to each patient. In addition to this, not every patient tolerates conscious sedation/awake surgery. Specific examples of this include patients with a history of psychiatric illness and psychosis. This also includes patients who cannot tolerate lying prone without being sedated. This is not an absolute contraindication because some cases can still be done in the lateral decubitus position; it should be noted that this can make the procedure more difficult as these patients often require more medication and can be difficult to arouse for feedback at appropriate times throughout the case. One advantage of the lateral decubitus position is the ability to perform a straight leg raise when performing a lumbar diskectomy. The other subset of patients that may find it difficult to have successful awake surgery are those with a history of heavy drug/opiate use. These patients often require higher doses of opiate medication, placing them at higher risk of respiratory depression intraoperatively, and may be safer approached with general anesthesia.

17.2 Pros

- Engaged staff.
- Fewer anesthetic complications.
- Patients can self-transfer.
- Quicker discharge from PACU.
- Intra-op feedback, which can guide surgery and prevent DRG injury without the need for neuromonitoring.
- May be able to shift some higher-risk patients to the lower-cost environment of an outpatient center while avoiding hospital admission.

17.3 Cons

- Cannot be done in patients with psychosis.
- Adequate sedation can be difficult in patients with heavy narcotic or drug use history.
- Surgery duration is somewhat limited without general anesthesia.

17.4 Indications

- The clearest indication for awake endoscopic spine surgery is with the transforaminal approach. This holds true in both the thoracic and lumbar spine.
  - We advocate for these lumbar procedures to be performed awake 100% of the time to adequately protect the DRG. Awake surgery results in the least expensive and most reliable way to protect the DRG, as feedback intraoperatively is immediate, more sensitive, and invaluable when it occurs. When these surgeries are performed with neuromonitoring, one may only detect changes in signals once damage/injury has already occurred. Some thoracic procedures with significant cord compression benefit from general anesthesia and neuromonitoring.
- For interlaminar approaches, we advocate for conscious sedation when this approach is applied for lumbar decompressions or diskectomies, when there are potential benefits for the patient. These cases are typically performed with a one-shot epidural adjunct. We have not yet implemented an awake protocol for the cervical spine or for thoracic interlaminar approaches due to the location of surgery. At this time, we believe that the risk may outweigh the benefit, but with time and as the field continues to push the boundaries of awake spine surgery, this may change in the future.
- For longer cases, such as in a unilateral laminectomy with bilateral decompression (ULBD), we recommend an epidural one to two levels cephalad to the target level. This allows for more time for decompression with less sedation to the patient, allowing for quicker recovery and decreased pain postoperatively. It also results in fewer anesthetic issues as less medication is administered intraoperatively.
- For instrumented fusions, such as endoscopic interbody fusions, we prefer spinal anesthetic with the duration matched to the potential duration of the surgery. The ideal dose results in motor function return in the lower extremities right as the wound is being closed. If underdosed, intraoperative redosing (spinal or epidural) can be performed by the surgeon. Caution must be used however, as excessive dosing can result in an extended PACU recovery/observation or even hospital admission due to extended motor blockade, if performed in the outpatient setting.

17.5 Methods

- We have established a protocol within our institution for these procedures.
- ▸ Table 17.1 demonstrates our protocol for transforaminal endoscopic cases utilizing conscious sedation.
- ▸ Table 17.2 demonstrates our protocol for spinal anesthesia, typically utilized for fusions.
- ▸ Table 17.3 demonstrates our general anesthesia protocol provided for reference.
- These protocols are displayed in the OR for easy reference.

17.6 Patient Positioning

- If spinal anesthetic is to be utilized, it is administered in the standard fashion per anesthesia protocol/preference.
- A Foley catheter can be placed at this time if needed but it is rarely used unless the patient has baseline incontinence.
- The patient is then allowed to roll into a prone position and settle into a comfortable position.
- Adequate head support should be provided with a foam pillow and a towel/blanket (▸ Fig. 17.1).
- Once the patient has settled into a comfortable position, surgical preparation of the surgical site can be pursued.

17.7 Airway Management

- The patient is positioned prone with the airway managed, and spontaneous breathing is maintained with mild sedation.
- A nasal cannula is utilized for oxygen delivery.
- Once the patient is positioned prone and the airway is confirmed stabilized, a propofol infusion is begun per anesthesia preference.
- The anesthesia team should be able and prepared to manage the airway prone if needed

Table 17.1 Transforaminal monitored anesthesia care (MAC) protocol

Transforaminal MAC for spine procedures		
Preop	**Intraop**	**Postop**
No gabapentin unless the surgeon orders Versed: as needed TXA: per surgeon orders, oral vs. IV	Preinduction "test dose" Propofol: < 50 mg Precedex: < 10 µg Maintenance Precedex: 0.4 µg/kg/h Propofol: start at 50 mg/kg/min; titrate as needed Propofol bolus as needed TXA IV dosing: bolus 1 g over 15 min, then 2nd bag at 3 mg/kg/h Fentanyl: as needed Decadron: 10 mg 1 L IVF unless contraindicated to aid voiding post op - For trocar placement, run deeper • For initial instrument placement, run lighter to monitor Nerve Root Contact	At closing of surgery • If the surgeon wants to talk to the patient, pause all infusions Ancef redose • 1 g: no hardware • 2 g: hardware Zofran: 4 mg Toradol: if the surgeon approves
Patient interview • Interview the patient on pain characteristics to aid with intra-op wake-up and surgeon questioning • Coach the patient on procedure: positioning, sedation level, awake as needed		Postop • Awake as possible to aid early ambulation
Patient positioning • Prone • Pillow(s) under the chest • Gel roll under the forehead • Head/neck neutral • Bilateral arm boards, superman position		Tips • Limit pain masking narcotics • Robaxin in the PACU for muscle spasms • Surgeon communication is key

Table 17.2 Spinal monitored anesthesia care (MAC) protocol

Epidural spinal MAC spines		
Preop	**Intraop**	**Postop**
No gabapentin unless the surgeon orders Versed: as needed TXA: surgeon orders, oral vs. IV Patient positioning • Prone • Pillow(s) under the chest • Gel roll under the forehead • Head/neck neutral • Bilateral arm boards, superman position	Induction Epidural 1% lidocaine PF: 15–25 mL Spinal 2% mepivacaine: 3 mL Maintenance Propofol: 50 mg/kg/min and bolus as needed TXA IV dosing: bolus 1 g over 15 min, then 2nd bag at 3 mg/kg/h Fentanyl: as needed Precedex: as needed Decadron: 10 mg Zofran: 4 mg 1 L IVF unless contraindicated to aid in voiding postop	At closing of surgery Ancef redose: • 1 g: no hardware • 2 g: hardware Zofran: 4 mg Toradol: if the surgeon approves Postop • Awake as possible to aid early ambulation

Table 17.3 General anesthesia protocol provided for reference

General spines		
Preop	**Intraop**	**Postop**
No gabapentin unless the surgeon orders	Induction ETT with LTA	At closing of surgery Ancef redose: • 1 g: no hardware • 2 g: hardware
Versed: as needed	Maintenance NDMR: as needed	Zofran: 4 mg
TXA: surgeon orders, oral vs. IV		Toradol: if the surgeon approves
Patient positioning • Prone • Head in helmet with form padding • Bilateral arm boards for lumbar (superman) • Arms tucked for cervical	TXA IV dosing: bolus 1 g over 15 min, then 2nd bag at 3 mg/kg/h Fentanyl or Dilaudid: as needed • Usually induction only Propofol infusion: as needed Decadron: 10 mg 1 L IVF unless contraindicated to aid in voiding postop	Postop • Awake as possible to aid early ambulation

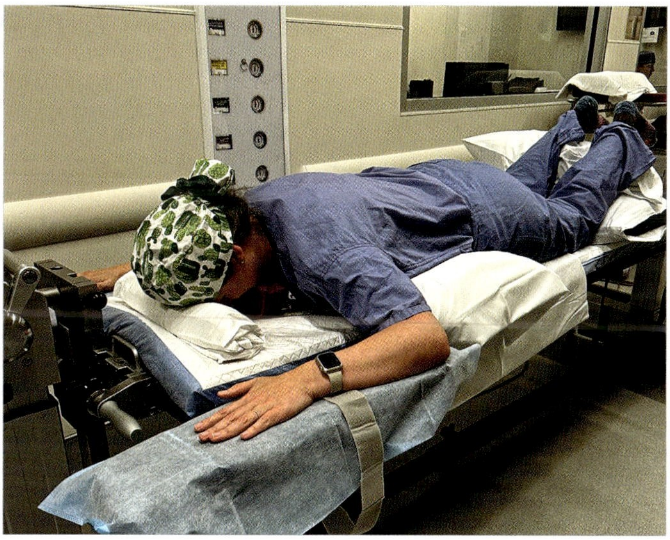

Fig. 17.1 Positioning on a Jackson flat OR bed with demonstration of face positioning. Notice a foam pillow is utilized for the chin and a rolled towel or blanket for the forehead.

in an emergency. This includes having available a laryngeal mask airway (LMA) and video laryngoscopy equipment available to allow for transition to general anesthesia, if needed.[14]

17.8 Anesthesia Protocol

- Our anesthesia team begin with applying a test dose of IV anesthetic while prepping the patient. This gauges if the patient will be a "low"- or "high"-requirement patient.
- The mainstay of anesthetic medication includes propofol and versed with minimal narcotic administration, if at all possible.
- The experience for the patient mimics a routine colonoscopy.
- Precedex can be used, but with caution. Precedex can cause hypotension in elderly or atherosclerotic patients.[15]

- We have found that a propofol drip is the most reliable as it can be titrated to need and easily bolused if sedation is needed. It dissipates quickly if patient input is required at a certain point in the surgery. Most importantly, it does all of this while maintaining amnesia.

17.9 Adjuncts

- We provide several preemptive analgesics intraoperatively to aid in pain control.
- Preemptive analgesia includes IV dexamethasone (8 mg IV).
- We always use local anesthesia into the surgical corridor. This consists of 10 mL of 1% lidocaine in the trajectory of the endoscope, with 5 mL injected into the landing spot and the other 5 mL injected as the needle is withdrawn to provide anesthesia to the tissues within the surgical corridor.
- Field blocks are an excellent adjunct that we routinely utilize. Specifically, we utilize erector spinae plane (ESP) blocks, administered one to two levels cephalad to the targeted level (typically at the L3 transverse process or higher). Delivering an ESP block at L5 or at the level of a short L4 transverse process can result in an inadvertent lumbar plexus block.
- We will utilize an 18-gauge spinal needle inserted down to the transverse process of the preidentified level. Our preferred injectate includes either lysosomal bupivacaine with bupivacaine or ropivacaine 0.20% plus dexamethasone 1 mL (10 mg) + clonidine 1 mL (100 µg). Lysosomal bupivacaine is not available at our institution, so we utilize ropivacaine, which has been found to be slightly less cardiotoxic than bupivacaine but does not last as long.[16]
- Clonidine is added to our cocktail as it is an alpha-2 agonist for its vasoconstriction properties and extends the effect of the peripherally metabolized ropivacaine.
- For transforaminal cases, we utilized 2 to 3 mL 1% lidocaine directly into Kambin's triangle, which decreases the DRG sensitivity, but does not result in a full motor block.
- We recommend avoiding use of sedating medications during the pre- and postoperative stages, especially the use of gabapentin/Lyrica. We found that these medications make arousal from anesthesia and quick discharge from the hospital/ASC more unreliable and prolonged and add little immediate postop benefit when utilizing an endoscopic approach.

17.10 Postoperative

- With the adjuncts listed above, patients often experience a gradual onset of postoperative pain, which often results in an easier control of postoperative pain.
- We employ every effort to avoid narcotics in these cases, and reserve these for severe pain or for those patients with high opiate tolerance or chronic opiate use.
- We do not routinely prescribe narcotic medication for postoperative pain control for endoscopic spine surgery patients as there is rarely a need when performed with the adjuvant blocks listed above.

17.11 Conclusion

While performing awake endoscopic spine surgery requires significant input from our anesthesia colleagues and arguably more attentiveness and focus from the OR staff, there are several perceived and established benefits as discussed above. With decreased anesthetic and narcotic administration, fewer anesthesia complications can result, including decrease in nausea/vomiting postoperatively, decrease in postoperative delirium, and decreased urinary retention. We also routinely see a much quicker discharge from our PACU/ASC. These patients also require significantly less postoperative narcotics when fusion is performed and typically require none with a decompression alone.[5,10] At our institution, we do not routinely prescribe narcotics after endoscopic diskectomies or decompressions.

Negating the need for neuromonitoring results in significant cost benefits, not only by not requiring their services but also by increased efficiency within the OR by not requiring neuromonitoring setup time.

With a patient that is awake and could potentially hear and respond to verbal cues, we often find that our OR staff have improved focus on the case at hand. This results in a more efficient and productive OR experience for the team.

Finally, and arguably most importantly, we have found a reliable way to decrease risk to the DRG in transforaminal approaches without adding cost.

We believe we are just now scratching the surface of the applications of awake endoscopic spine surgery, but believe that the complication reduction, cost benefits, and overall improvement to care provided to the patient are well worth the implementation of awake spine surgery for the appropriate cases with a committed spine team.

References

[1] Garg B, Ahuja K, Mehta N, Sharan AD. Awake spinal fusion. JBJS Rev. 2021; 9(6):e20.00163

[2] Dagher C, Naccache N, Narchi P, Hage P, Antakly MC. Regional anesthesia for lumbar microdiscectomy. J Med Liban. 2002; 50(5–6):206–210

[3] Drossopoulos PN, Sharma A, Ononogbu-Uche FC, et al. Pushing the limits of minimally invasive spine surgery-from preoperative to intraoperative to postoperative management. J Clin Med. 2024; 13(8):2410

[4] Waguia R, Touko EK, Sykes DAW, et al. How to start an awake spine program: Protocol and illustrative cases. IBRO Neurosci Rep. 2022; 13:69–77

[5] Eckman WW, Hester L, McMillen M. Same-day discharge after minimally invasive transforaminal lumbar interbody fusion: a series of 808 cases. Clin Orthop Relat Res. 2014; 472(6):1806–1812

[6] Garg B, Ahuja K, Sharan AD. Regional anesthesia for spine surgery. J Am Acad Orthop Surg. 2022; 30(17):809–819

[7] Jadczak CN, Vanjani NN, Pawlowski H, et al. The current status of awake endoscopic surgery: a systematic review and meta-analysis. World Neurosurg. 2023; 180:e198–e209

[8] De Rojas JO, Syre P, Welch WC. Regional anesthesia versus general anesthesia for surgery on the lumbar spine: a review of the modern literature. Clin Neurol Neurosurg. 2014; 119: 39–43

[9] Alexander N, Gardocki R. Awake transforaminal endoscopic lumbar discectomy in an ambulatory surgery center: early clinical outcomes and complications of 100 patients. Eur Spine J. 2023; 32(8):2910–2917

[10] Rivkin A, Rivkin MA. Perioperative nonopioid agents for pain control in spinal surgery. Am J Health Syst Pharm. 2014; 71 (21):1845–1857

[11] Fiani B, Reardon T, Selvage J, et al. Awake spine surgery: an eye-opening movement. Surg Neurol Int. 2021; 12:222

[12] Lessing NL, Edwards CC , II, Brown CH , IV, et al. Spinal anesthesia in elderly patients undergoing lumbar spine surgery. Orthopedics. 2017; 40(2):e317–e322

[13] Lessing NL, Edwards CC , II, Lin C, Brown CH , IV. Complex lumbar spine fusion for an elderly patient under spinal anesthesia. Orthopedics. 2017; 40(5):e915–e917

[14] De Biase G, Bechtle P, Leone B, Quinones-Hinojosa A, Abode-Iyamah K. Awake minimally invasive transforaminal lumbar interbody fusion with a pedicle-based retraction system. Clin Neurol Neurosurg. 2021; 200:106313

[15] Gerlach AT, Blais DM, Jones GM, et al. Predictors of dexmedetomidine-associated hypotension in critically ill patients. Int J Crit Illn Inj Sci. 2016; 6(3):109–114

[16] Bourne E, Wright C, Royse C. A review of local anesthetic cardiotoxicity and treatment with lipid emulsion. Local Reg Anesth. 2010; 3:11–19

18 Awake Lateral Fusion

Georgios Bakaloudis, Alice Baroncini, Michele Bochicchio, Lorenzo D'Apice, Alessandra Isidori, and Angelo Mazzarino

Abstract

Awake spine fusion (ASF) is an increasingly used operative method that enables surgeons to perform surgical interventions under spinal anesthesia. While this technique is particularly useful for older, comorbid patients who cannot otherwise undergo general anesthesia, it is also more frequently used for younger patients as it allows for a speedy recovery, shorter hospital stay, and potentially less overall hospital costs. The implementation of ASF when performing lateral lumbar interbody fusion has not yet been thoroughly described in the literature. The aim of this chapter is to illustrate the authors' surgical technique and clinical experience in this setting.

Keywords: awake spine fusion, lumbar fusion, lumbar degeneration, lateral lumbar interbody fusion

Key Points

- Awake spine fusion enables surgeons to perform surgical interventions under spinal anesthesia.
- Awake spine fusion allows for a speedy recovery, shorter hospital stay, and potentially less overall hospital costs.
- Awake spine fusion is safe and effective even when a lateral interbody fusion is performed.
- A standardized surgical, step-by-step, procedure should be followed.
- When epidural anesthesia is performed, real-time intraoperative motor neurologic examination can be performed.

18.1 Introduction

With the increasing aging of the population, the incident of patients requiring lumbar fusion for disk degeneration is naturally on the rise. At the same time, however, older patients present with more comorbidities that can render open fusion under general anesthesia risky or not possible.

Newer surgical techniques such as minimally invasive spine surgery (MISS) and ASF aim to provide high-level patient care while minimizing the intra- and perioperative risks for the patients. This allows surgeons to provide care for a wider range of pathologies with increased safety and effectiveness.[1,2,3,4,5] The use of ASF also ensures a reduced sedation time and, in turn, a reduced operating room time,[6] along with a shorter length of hospital stay.[7,8] It is important to highlight that, beyond the perioperative advantages, ASF can warrant an improved patient satisfaction and a better quality of life 1 month after surgery.[9,10]

Interestingly, in a surgical team that is familiar with MISS techniques, adoption of ASF is not connected with a prolonged learning curve[11] and ASF can thus be easily implemented in hospitals or ambulatory surgery centers that routinely perform both spinal anesthesia and MISS.

Expert Tip

The advantages of MISS modern surgical techniques implemented with awake anesthesia protocols include significantly reduced perioperative time and costs, along with an acceptable team learning curve.

Most available literature focusses on the use of ASF for decompressions (including endoscopic) and single-level posterior fusion with TLIF. However, in our experience, the use of ASF can be extended to lumbar lateral fusion as well, with encouraging results. The aim of this chapter is to illustrate the experience of the authors with ASF in lumbar lateral interbody fusion (LLIF), highlighting surgical and anesthesiologic techniques and protocols, and reporting preliminary obtained results.

Expert Tip

Spine surgical teams with well-established awake spine programs can implement their daily procedures not only with decompression and/or diskectomy but also with fusion (posterior and lateral).

18.2 Indications

Since Ozgur et al[12] first reported on lateral LLIF, it has become a standard surgical technique for the treatment of multiple degenerative spine conditions.

The advantages, and consequent indications, of this truly MISS technique include the following[13,14,15,16,17,18,19]:

- Indirect decompression of the neural elements, leaving the anterior and posterior longitudinal ligaments intact (mild single/multilevel lumbar stenosis, I°-II° spondylolisthesis, mild degenerative scoliosis; see Case Example).
- Restoration of the sagittal and coronal alignment of the spine (mild degenerative scoliosis, postdiskectomy/laminectomy syndrome, adjacent level disease.)
- A lower subsidence rate because of larger footprint of cages (osteopenic or revision cage insertion).
- No damage caused to the paravertebral muscles compared to the conventional open posterior arthrodesis and direct decompression techniques (revision cases/sarcopenia).
- Last, but not least, compared to the traditional posterior techniques, this approach is also advantageous in multiple-revision surgery cases as it allows us to reach and attempt fusion between vertebral bodies avoiding scar tissue, especially epidural fibrosis, from previous interventions.[14,15,20,21,22]

Expert Tip

LLIF has shown excellent results with regard to indirect decompression, fusion rates and subsidence avoidance, less paravertebral muscle damage, and avoidance of epidural scar tissue in revision cases.

18.3 Anesthesia

Our anesthesiology team, with large experience in obstetrics ("walking anesthesia"), postulated the following protocol:

- Epidural anesthesia is performed using an 18-gauge Tuohy needle (without catheter), inserted at the T10–T11 interspace. Ropivacaine 0.75 mg/ml was slowly injected, with 2 to 3 mg of morphine, according to the patient's weight.
- During epidural single-shot anesthesia, the lower motor function was maintained, allowing for continuous intraoperative monitoring of the lower extremity function (**Video 18.1**).
- Spinal anesthesia was performed using a dose of 2 to 3 mL of ropivacaine 0.5 mg/mL + morphine 150 µg, using a 25-gauge Whitacre needle, often in the L1–L2 interspace.
- In that case, intrathecal anesthesia causes complete motor block of lower extremities for 2 to 3 hours.

Expert Tip

Epidural anesthesia, even in single-shot scenario, permits intraoperative continuous control of lower extremities, obviating the necessity of other types of neuromonitoring during the procedure.

18.4 Surgical Technique

The surgical technique does not differ from that performed for LLIF under general anesthesia, as widely described in recent literature.

- The first anterior surgical time consists in the placement of the cage through an anterior, retroperitoneal, transpsoas approach.
- The patient is positioned in the strict lateral decubitus position, left or right depending on the chosen access side (▶ Fig. 18.1).
- To ensure patient/procedure safety and limit possible intraoperative nerve/vascular damage during cage placement, a standard fixed taping is performed.

Expert Tip

Patient positioning is paramount and should always be performed by the leading surgeon or an assistant surgeon experienced in the procedure. Maintaining of the correct position by adequate taping is equally important to avoid catastrophic vascular, bowel, or neurologic complications.

- Intraoperative neuromonitoring with triggered/multidirectional electromyogram (EMG) is not routinely utilized when epidural anesthesia is performed (**Video 18.2**).

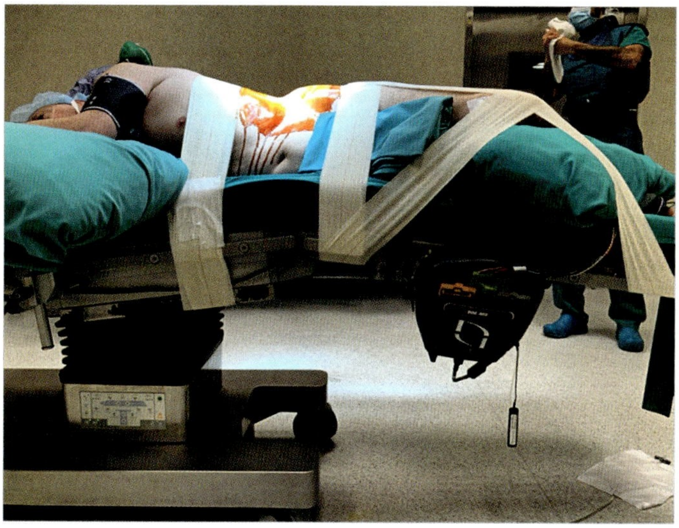

Fig. 18.1 Patient positioning in the strict lateral decubitus position. Minimal bending of the table should be done as seen; a standard fixed draping is performed.

- A standard transpsoas approach is performed, as described by Uribe and Deukmedjian,[23] with meticulous concern on standardization of the entire procedure, step by step, involving the entire surgical team.

Expert Tip

We highly advise a standardized blunt dissection through the muscle layers, keeping in mind the yellow/red/yellow/white rule (subcuticular fat/external oblique–internal oblique–transverse abdominal muscles/peritoneal fat/transverse abdominal fascia). Electrocautery use is not advised as multiple sensitive nerves can be damaged just performing the access (intercostal, iliohypogastric, ilioinguinal) and may cause pseudo-hernias of the abdominal wall.

- When epidural anesthesia is performed, real-time final motor neurologic monitoring can be performed after cage implant (**Video 18.3**).
- The "step-by-step" philosophy, in our experience, droughts down overall surgical time in a significant way (skin to skin in < 20 minutes regularly).
- In the second surgical time, pedicle screws are placed under direct 2D fluoroscopic guidance (in both the single lateral and standard prone position).

Expert Tip

Lateral decubitus pedicle screw placing can be demanding, so flipping the patient in a standard prone position is advised, at least at the early cases. Lateral positioning of the patient at the posterior edge of the table can help with lower screw insertion; navigation and robotics can be extremely helpful in this setting.

18.5 Postoperative Management

- *Immediate postoperative pain management:* Patients are managed with continuous intravenous analgesia (10 mg morphine, 90 mg ketorolac, and 30 mg metoclopramide in 50 ml saline solution, infused at 2 mL/hour) and intravenous paracetamol (3 × 1 g) for the first 24 hours.
- In case of persistent pain, sublingual morphine is administered if the visual analog scale (VAS) score is ≥ 4.
- Oral-only pain management is immediately started on the second postoperative day with pregabalin (2 × 50 mg, for 30 days), oxycodone/naloxone (2 × 5/2.5 mg for 15 days), and ibuprofen (3 × 600 mg for 15 days).

> **Expert Tip**
>
> *A standardized postoperative pain program is recommended, tailored to local site and geographical attitudes. Awake spine protocols have been shown to substantially reduce the need for opioid medications even in multilevel spine fusion procedures.*

- Additionally, enoxaparin (1 × 4,000 IU for 15 days) and lansoprazole (1 × 40 mg for 15 days) are administered starting on the second postoperative day.
- Patients are allowed to stand up as soon as they feel comfortable to do so.
- When epidural anesthesia is performed, patients can walk 3 to 4 hours after the surgical procedure.
- No brace or any other restrictions are ordered; standard "fast-track" physical therapy is started from the second postoperative day.
- Standing anteroposterior and lateral X-rays are taken on the second postoperative day.
- Discharge is allowed on the third postoperative day.

> **Expert Tip**
>
> *Early mobilization (3–4 hours after surgery) is possible, making a major reconstructive anterior/posterior surgery possible even in the context of ambulatory surgery center (ASC). A "fast-track" physical therapy protocol is highly recommended with no external brace restrictions necessary.*

18.6 Results

- A prospective, single-surgeon case series was conducted involving 145 consecutively operated patients who underwent ASF between September 2014 and December 2020, with a minimum follow-up of 2 years. The age of the patients was 24 to 82 years.
- *Diagnosis:* 72 lumbar stenosis (one to three levels), 30 degenerative spondylolisthesis, 30 discogenic instability, and 13 degenerative scoliosis.
- *Performed surgery:* 1 to 5 fused levels per patient, with direct decompression in 43 cases and with LLIF in 15 cases.
- The mean estimated blood loss was 6.2 mL/kg (range: 4.6–8.3 mL/kg); none of the patients required a postoperative blood transfusion.
- The mean surgical time was 40 minutes (range: 30–90 minutes) for the entire cohort.
- In the awake LLIF group (15 cases), the mean surgical time was 45 minutes (range: 40–70 minutes).
- The mean length of hospital stay was 2.8 days (range: 2–3 days).
- All the patients could stand and walk within 24 hours, within 3 to 4 hours for the last 45 patients.
- Five patients (2 in the LLIF group) required revision surgeries for adjacent segment disease (stenosis), at an average of 2 years after index surgery.
- In particular, in LLIF patients a re-instrumentation was performed for mechanical failure at 6 and 8 months after index surgery (screw loosening and proximal screw pullout).
- There was a significant improvement of the Oswestry Disability Index, which improved by 38 points at the last follow-up (range, 25–58).

> **Expert Tip**
>
> *According to our experience, the implementation of LLIF in a previously well-established posterior awake program has substantially reduced the operative surgical time of the lateral procedure, reducing the total OR occupation time, hospital stay, and overall costs. Cost-effectiveness of awake LLIF is still to be established and understood, but our preliminary results combining both lateral fusion and awake procedure benefits seem extremely promising.*

18.7 Case Example

A 53-year-old man presented with low back pain and left radicular pain with L4 distribution. The imaging showed L4/L5 instability with foraminal stenosis. He was not responding to 6 weeks of conservative treatment. An awake left side L4/L5 LLIF (lateral cage measuring 22 × 45 × 10) with

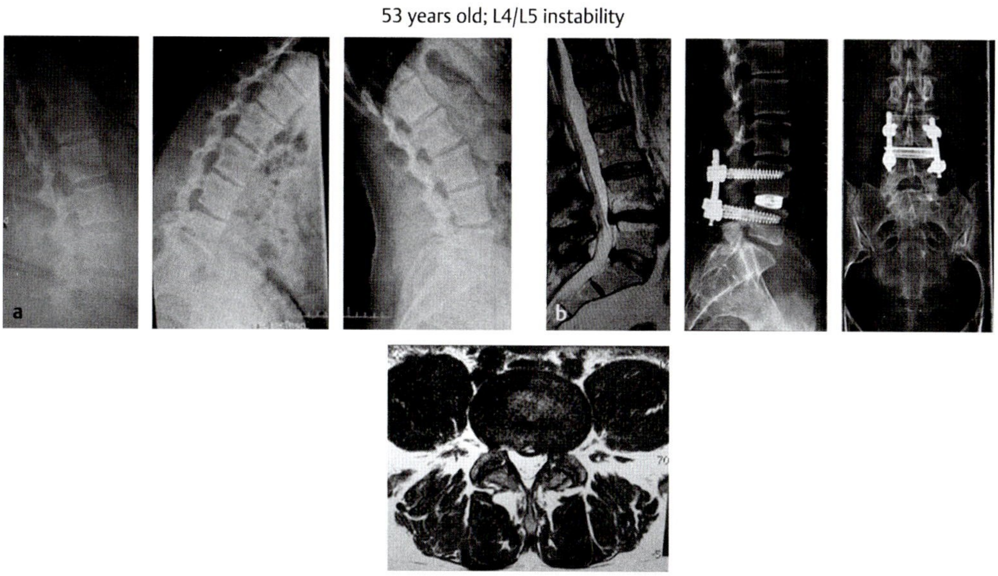

Fig. 18.2 (a) Lateral and flexion-estension X-rays of the presented patients, with preoperative RMN imaging. (b) Postoperative anteroposterior and lateral X-rays.

single lateral position posterior percutaneous L4/L5 screw placement was performed (total operative time of 60 minutes). Indirect decompression without laminectomy resulted in complete relief of symptoms, and he was able to walk 4 hours after the surgery.

Please notice the psoas and plexus anatomical distribution on axial magnetic resonance imaging (▶ Fig. 18.2).

18.8 Conclusion

ASF is safe and effective even when an LLIF is performed. In this particular scenario, when done under epidural, single-shot anesthesia, no standard neuromonitoring has been used in our series. A standardized surgical, step-by-step, procedure with engagement of the entire surgical team (circulating nurses/X-ray tech/anesthesiology) can guarantee significant improvement in the overall surgical time and significantly reduce intraoperative adverse events.

This setting permits lower overall surgery-related complications, diminished hospital stay, significant reduction of direct and indirect surgical costs, and eventually, but mostly importantly, significant improvement in surgery-related experience for the patient and his or her family.

References

[1] Breton JM, Ludwig CG, Yang MJ, et al. Spinal anesthesia in contemporary and complex lumbar spine surgery: experience with 343 cases. J Neurosurg Spine. 2021; 36(4):534–541

[2] Finsterwald M, Muster M, Farshad M, Saporito A, Brada M, Aguirre JA. Spinal versus general anesthesia for lumbar spine surgery in high risk patients: perioperative hemodynamic stability, complications and costs. J Clin Anesth. 2018; 46: 3–7

[3] Jadczak CN, Vanjani NN, Pawlowski H, et al. The current status of awake endoscopic surgery: a systematic review and meta-analysis. World Neurosurg. 2023; 180:e198–e209

[4] Perez-Roman RJ, Govindarajan V, Bryant J-P, Wang MY. Spinal anesthesia in awake surgical procedures of the lumbar spine: a systematic review and meta-analysis of 3709 patients. Neurosurg Focus. 2021; 51(6):E7

[5] Rajjoub R, Ghaith AK, El-Hajj VG, et al. Comparative outcomes of awake spine surgery under spinal versus general anesthesia: a comprehensive systematic review and meta-analysis. Eur Spine J. 2024; 33(3):985–1000

[6] Lu VM, Brusko GD, Urakov TM. Defining the time benefit of awake versus general anesthesia for single-level lumbar spine surgery. World Neurosurg. 2022; 158:e793–e798

[7] Shui M, Zhao D, Xue Z, Wu A. Impact of spinal/epidural anesthesia versus general anesthesia on perioperative outcomes in patients undergoing lumbar spine surgery: an updated

systematic review and meta-analysis. Clin Spine Surg. 2023; 36(6):227–236

[8] Sykes DAW, Tabarestani TQ, Chaudhry NS, et al. Awake spinal fusion is associated with reduced length of stay, opioid use, and time to ambulation compared to general anesthesia: a matched cohort study. World Neurosurg. 2023; 176:e91–e100

[9] De Biase G, Gruenbaum SE, Quiñones-Hinojosa A, Abode-Iyamah KO. Spine surgery under spinal vs general anesthesia: prospective analysis of quality of life, fatigue, and cognition. Neurosurgery. 2022; 90(2):186–191

[10] De Cassai A, Geraldini F, Boscolo A, et al. General anesthesia compared to spinal anesthesia for patients undergoing lumbar vertebral surgery: a meta-analysis of randomized controlled trials. J Clin Med. 2020; 10(1):102

[11] West JL, De Biase G, Bydon M, et al. What is the learning curve for lumbar spine surgery under spinal anesthesia? World Neurosurg. 2022; 158:e310–e316

[12] Ozgur BM, Aryan HE, Pimenta L, Taylor WR. Extreme lateral interbody fusion (XLIF): a novel surgical technique for anterior lumbar interbody fusion. Spine J. 2006; 6(4):435–443

[13] Domínguez I, Luque R, Noriega M, Rey J, Alia J, Marco-Martínez F. Extreme lateral lumbar interbody fusion. Surgical technique, outcomes and complications after a minimum of one year follow-up. Rev Esp Cir Ortop Traumatol. 2017; 61(1):8–18

[14] Tessitore E, Molliqaj G, Schaller K, Gautschi OP. Extreme lateral interbody fusion (XLIF): a single-center clinical and radiological follow-up study of 20 patients. J Clin Neurosci. 2017; 36:76–79

[15] Pereira EAC, Farwana M, Lam KS. Extreme lateral interbody fusion relieves symptoms of spinal stenosis and low-grade spondylolisthesis by indirect decompression in complex patients. J Clin Neurosci. 2017; 35:56–61

[16] Tohmeh AG, Khorsand D, Watson B, Zielinski X. Radiographical and clinical evaluation of extreme lateral interbody fusion: effects of cage size and instrumentation type with a minimum of 1-year follow-up. Spine. 2014; 39(26):E1582–E1591

[17] Castellvi AE, Nienke TW, Marulanda GA, Murtagh RD, Santoni BG. Indirect decompression of lumbar stenosis with transpsoas interbody cages and percutaneous posterior instrumentation. Clin Orthop Relat Res. 2014; 472(6):1784–1791

[18] Alimi M, Hofstetter CP, Tsiouris AJ, Elowitz E, Härtl R. Extreme lateral interbody fusion for unilateral symptomatic vertical foraminal stenosis. Eur Spine J. 2015; 24 Suppl 3: 346–352

[19] Berjano P, Balsano M, Buric J, Petruzzi M, Lamartina C. Direct lateral access lumbar and thoracolumbar fusion: preliminary results. Eur Spine J. 2012; 21 Suppl 1:S37–S42

[20] Berjano P, Langella F, Damilano M, et al. Fusion rate following extreme lateral lumbar interbody fusion. Eur Spine J. 2015; 24 Suppl 3:369–371

[21] Rodgers W, Cox C, Gerber E. Minimally invasive treatment (XLIF) of adjacent segment disease after prior lumbar fusions. Internet J Minim Invasive Spinal Technol. 2009; 4: 1–7

[22] Formica M, Berjano P, Cavagnaro L, Zanirato A, Piazzolla A, Formica C. Extreme lateral approach to the spine in degenerative and post traumatic lumbar diseases: selection process, results and complications. Eur Spine J. 2014; 23 Suppl 6: 684–692

[23] Uribe JS, Deukmedjian AR. Visceral, vascular, and wound complications following over 13,000 lateral interbody fusions: a survey study and literature review. Eur Spine J. 2015; 24 Suppl 3:386–396

Part III

Postoperative Considerations

III

19 Long-Acting Nerve Block Pumps for Postoperative Pain Management

Ernest E. Braxton Jr. and Andrew Lucic

Abstract

The trend toward minimally invasive surgical techniques and outpatient procedures has emphasized the need for effective postoperative analgesic plans, particularly amid rising opioid addiction rates. This chapter reviews the use of erector spinae blocks and paravertebral blocks as superior alternatives to epidural catheters for postoperative analgesia in outpatient spine surgery due to their lower risk profiles. Continuous infusion catheters are evaluated against single-shot nerve blocks, showing advantages in prolonged analgesia and reduced opioid consumption, despite potential risks such as catheter migration and infection. The chapter explores different catheter and pump types, with a focus on the benefits and drawbacks of electronic versus elastomeric pumps, and discusses various infusion strategies, including continuous infusion and high-pressure intermittent bolus modes. It also addresses postoperative management, stressing the importance of individualized pain management plans considering surgical approach, patient pain history, infection risk, and anticoagulation status. The chapter highlights the need for further research in continuous infusion techniques specific to spine surgery and emphasizes multidisciplinary consultation for optimal patient outcomes.

Keywords: ambulatory infusion pump, regional anesthesia, long-acting nerve pumps, erector spinae block, paravertebral block

Key Points

- Discuss nonopioid pain management strategies with ambulatory infusion pumps.
- Techniques and considerations for erector spinae blocks and paravertebral blocks.
- Compare and contrast electronic and elastomeric pumps for postoperative pain control.
- Explain the goals and rationale behind various infusion strategies.
- Develop strategies for patient education and troubleshooting problems with long-acting blocks.

19.1 Introduction

The current trend toward more minimally invasive surgical techniques and outpatient surgery can be enhanced with a strong postoperative analgesic plan. This is especially important in the current era of rising incidence of opioid addiction.[1] These trends have been commonplace in many hospitals and surgery centers with most types of orthopaedic surgery.[2,3] Over that last decade, the introduction of the erector spinae block has allowed for expansion of the nerve block as an excellent analgesic option for outpatient spine surgery.[4,5,6,7] Epidural catheters have been used in the past, but the technique comes with risks, limiting its use to the inpatient setting. These risks are motor block, sympathectomy, and risk of epidural hematoma. The erector spinae and paravertebral blocks theoretically carry these same risks but at a much lower incidence.[8] This allows them to be great options in a postoperative analgesic plan. This chapter will review the catheter types, continuous pump types, different infusion strategies, and patient education topics.

19.2 Continuous Infusion Catheters

Studies support the superiority of infusion catheters over single-shot blocks in various musculoskeletal surgeries (see ▶ Table 19.1).

- Continuous peripheral nerve blocks have shown the following[9,10]:
  - Better postoperative analgesia.
  - Increased patient satisfaction.
  - Improved surgical outcomes compared to single-shot nerve blocks in orthopaedic surgeries.
  - Prolonged pain relief.
  - Reduced opioid consumption.
  - Enhanced rehabilitation.

Table 19.1 Pros and cons of long-acting pain pumps

Pros	Cons
Improved analgesia	Burden of carrying extra equipment for patients
Reduced opioid requirements	Need for 24-h call service and development of an acute pain service
Improved patient satisfaction	Complications inherent to nerve block catheters: • Infection • Bleeding associated with anticoagulation • Block failures • Lock anesthesia toxicity
Increase sense of control for patients	
Improved reimbursement for anesthesia team	

- Meta-analysis findings of continuous catheter adductor canal blocks versus single-shot blocks in knee replacement surgery showed the following[11]:
  - Significant improvements in pain scores in knee replacement.
  - Reduced need for rescue analgesia with the continuous catheter approach.
  - Continuous femoral nerve blocks versus single-shot blocks demonstrated lower opioid requirements postoperatively for patients undergoing primary hip and knee arthroplasty.
- Mixed results for spine surgery, though current data appear favorable.[4]
- Advantages of continuous catheters:
  - Adjustable block density.
  - Prolonged block duration.
  - Lowered opioid consumption.
  - Patient control over analgesic plan.
- Negatives of continuous infusion catheters:
  - Risk of migration and block failure.
  - Potential leakage and infection.
  - Requirement to carry a pump and anesthetic reservoir.
- Alternative approach with liposomal formulations of local anesthetic: Currently FDA approved for limited nerve blocks (*not* including erector spinae, paravertebral, and other trunk blocks for spine surgery).[12]
- Downsides of liposomal formulations[13]:
  - Unpredictable release and analgesia.
  - Limited rescue options if the block fails, as no additional local anesthetic can be used for 96 hours due to toxicity concerns.

19.3 Blocks Amenable to Continuous Infusions

- **Epidural technique in postoperative analgesia**:
  - One of the oldest regional anesthesia techniques, dating back to 1900.
  - First injections by Jean Sicard and Fernand Cathelin in Paris, using cocaine injected into the sacral hiatus.[14]
  - Effective for pain management but has a high risk of motor block, increasing fall risk, impeding mobility, and prolonging hospital stays.[15]
  - Less ideal for patients requiring early mobilization postsurgery due to motor block risk.[16,17]
- **Challenges of epidural analgesia**:
  - High incidence of motor block requires careful patient monitoring.
  - Its use is limited in settings where continuous monitoring is not feasible.
  - Motor block can delay rehabilitation and extend hospital stays due to limited ambulation.[18,19]
- **Preferred blocks**:
  - Erector spinae and paravertebral blocks are preferred for certain spine surgeries.
  - Paravertebral catheters provide better lateral and anterior trunk coverage.
  - Paravertebral blocks may have a higher pneumothorax risk and require technical skill, making them less favored in some practices.[20]

Expert Tip

Consider placing "dry" erector spinae block/ paravertebral block catheters without a loading dose, to minimize the risk of local anesthetic toxicity. This strategy saves room for supplementary local anesthetics for your surgical block during surgery. To do this, have the acute pain team place the catheters using only saline. A small amount of lidocaine is permissible to reduce stimulation before placing the catheter. Have the acute pain service start dosing the nerve blocks 6 hours after surgical start to allow adequate time to metabolize the initial local given during surgery.

19.4 Catheter Types for Continuous Anesthesia Pumps

- **Catheter-through-needle systems** (▶ Fig. 19.1):
  - Suitable for epidural and paravertebral blocks, allowing greater catheter length positioning.
  - Require more skill, prone to leakage, and may increase infection risk.[16,18]
- **Catheter-over-needle systems** (▶ Fig. 19.2):
  - Easier to place; suitable for less experienced practitioners.
  - Reduced leakage at insertion but higher risk of dislodgment and less suitable for deeper blocks like paravertebral and epidural blocks.[17,18]

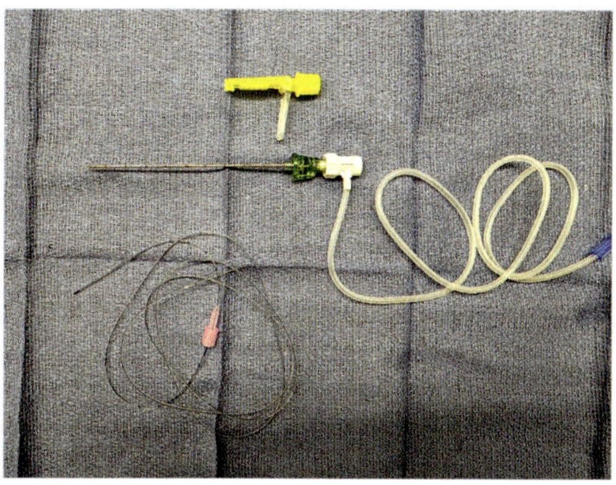

Fig. 19.1 Catheter-through-needle system. Shown here are a clamp-style catheter connector, an 18-gauge needle with a sideport valve assembly, and a polyamide catheter (Contiplex Continuous Nerve Block Set B, Braun, Bethlehem, PA).

19.5 Pump Types for Acute Pain Management

- **Electronic pumps** (▶ Fig. 19.3):
  - Precise dosage control, providing consistent analgesia and reducing opioid consumption.[21,22,23]

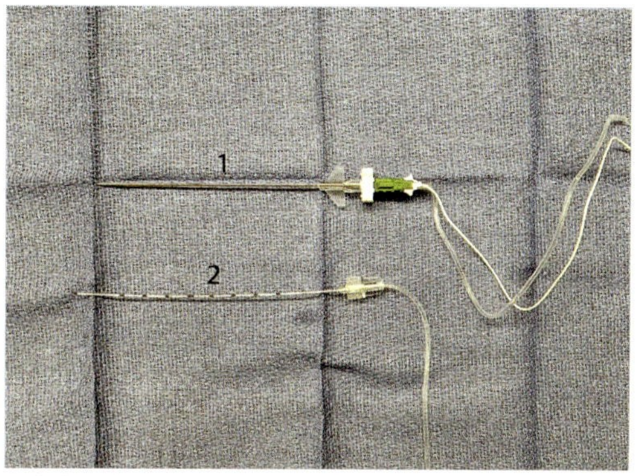

Fig. 19.2 Common pain catheters. Label 1 is the catheter over the needle system. Label 2 is the internal catheter (Pajunk Medical Systems, Alpharetta, GA).

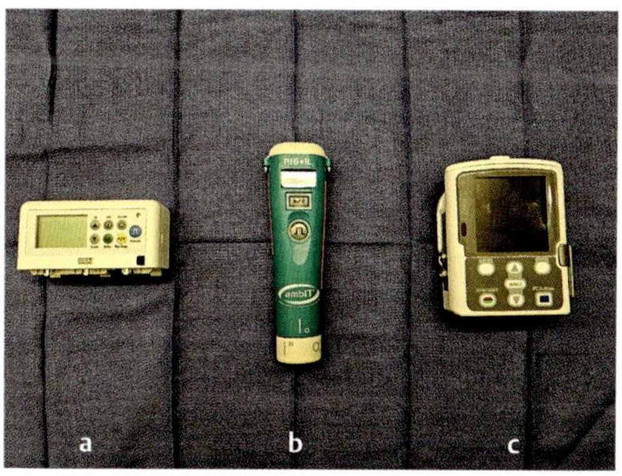

Fig. 19.3 Common electronic ambulatory infusion pumps. The pumps can administer a higher-pressure intermittent bolus (PIB) mode and have a patient control anesthesia function. **(a)** Nimbus II PainPro Ambulatory Infusion Pump (InfuTronix, Natick, MA). **(b)** Ambit pump (Avanos Medical Alpharetta, GA). **(c)** CADD-Solis VIP ambulatory Infusion pump (Smiths Medical, St. Paul, MN).

- Patient-controlled analgesia allows patients to control over their pain management.[24]
- *Drawback:* Complexity and training requirements for health care staff.[22]

- **Elastomeric pumps**:
  - Simple, battery free, and silent, offering comfort and reliability.[25]
  - Used in outpatient and home settings for pain management, infection treatment, and chemotherapy.[26]
  - *Drawback:* Fixed flow rate, potential flow restrictor variability, and no high-pressure intermittent bolus option.
- **Delivery Strategies for Local Anesthetic**:
  - *Continuous infusion:* Provides steady medication flow, ideal for nighttime pain control.
  - *Patient-controlled bolus:* Allows patients to self-administer within set limits, offering control over breakthrough pain.
  - *High-pressure intermittent bolus:* Effective for spreading anesthetic across multiple dermatomes, particularly useful in obstetric and certain thoracic surgeries.[27,28]
- **Postoperative management considerations**:
  - Individualize pain management plans based on pain history, surgical approach, infection risk, and anticoagulation status.
  - Continuous regional anesthesia may reduce opioid needs for patients with prior pain history.
  - *Paravertebral block:* Preferred for anterior/lateral surgical approaches for consistent analgesia.
  - *Erector spinae block:* Suitable for posterior approaches and patients requiring anticoagulants.
  - Limit infusions to 3 to 7 days to reduce infection risk.[29,30]

Expert Tip

- *In case of lateral spine surgeries, consider using a paravertebral catheter on the side of the lateral incision. While this may sacrifice some dermatomal coverage on the dorsal rami, a paravertebral will provide better lateral and anterior coverage. On the contralateral side, your acute pain team can place an erector spinal catheter for better dorsal coverage.*

- **Importance of patient education**:
  - It empowers patients for effective pain management and device operation postsurgery.
  - It reduces risk of adverse events and increases adherence to treatment.
  - Establishing a 24-hour support call service is crucial for addressing catheter-related issues (▶ Fig. 19.4).
  - Educate on pump use, wound care, signs of complications, and emergency procedures to improve patient outcomes.[17,26]

19.6 Conclusion

The use of long-acting nerve block pumps, specifically continuous infusion catheters, represents a significant advancement in postoperative pain management. Erector spinae and paravertebral blocks have emerged as superior alternatives to traditional epidural catheters due to their lower risk profiles and effectiveness in outpatient spine surgery. Continuous infusion techniques offer prolonged analgesia, reduced opioid consumption, and greater patient satisfaction, although they come with potential risks that must be carefully managed.

The choice between electronic and elastomeric pumps, as well as the selection of appropriate infusion strategies, should be tailored to individual patient needs and the specific clinical scenario. While electronic pumps provide precise control and flexibility, elastomeric pumps offer simplicity and reliability, making them suitable for various settings, including outpatient and home care. High-pressure intermittent bolus modes have shown promise in certain applications, though further research is needed to optimize their use in spine surgery.

Ultimately, effective postoperative pain management requires a multidisciplinary approach that includes anesthesiologists and spine surgeons. By considering factors such as patient history, surgical approach, and potential risks, health care providers can develop comprehensive pain management plans that enhance recovery, reduce complications, and improve overall patient outcomes. Continuous advancements in nerve block techniques and infusion pump technology will continue to play a crucial role in outpatient surgery by reducing pain and dependance on opioids.

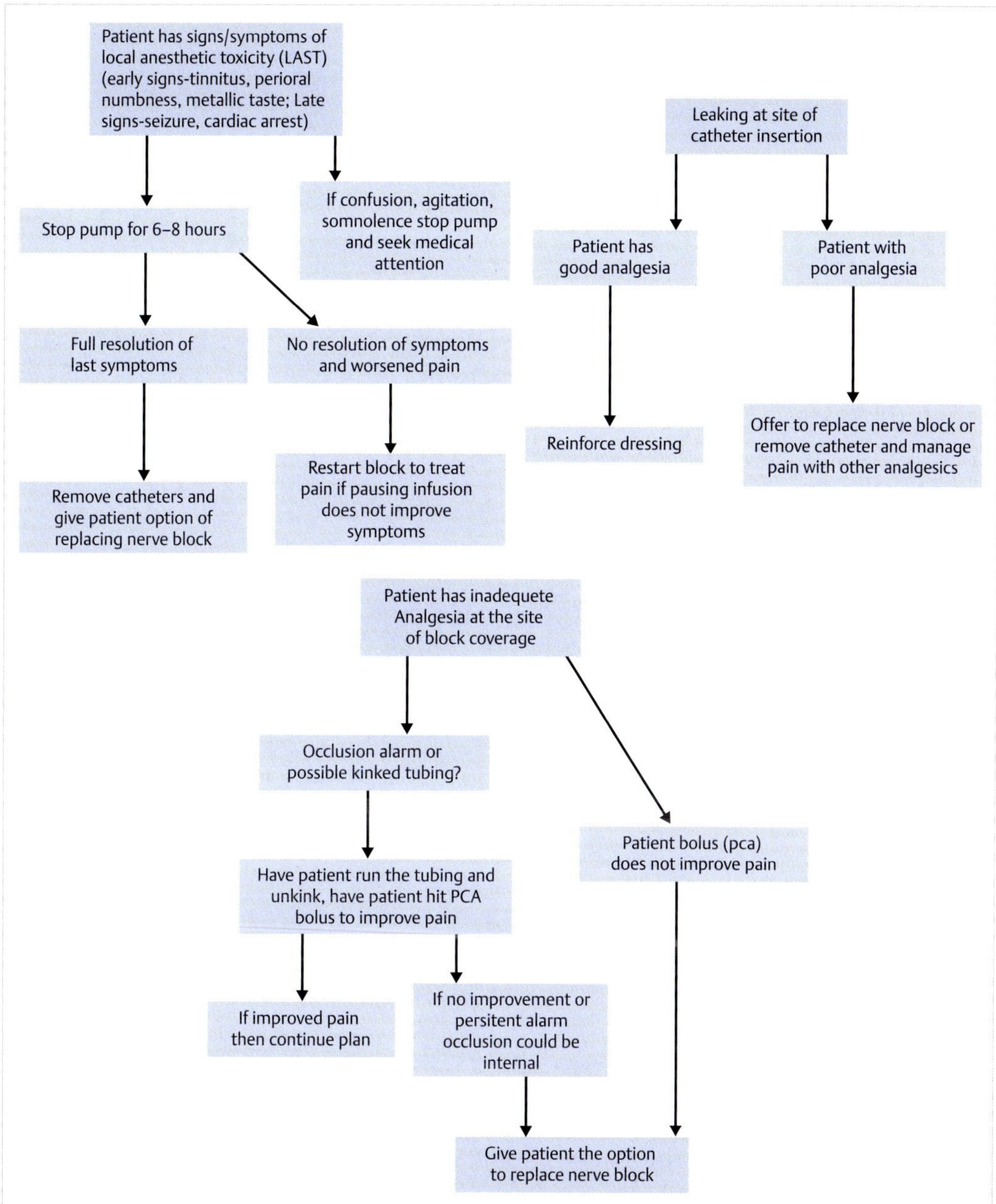

Fig. 19.4 Troubleshooting common patient questions in the outpatient setting.

References

[1] Makanji HS, Solomito MJ, Maffeo-Mitchell C, Esmende S, Finkel K. Utility of erector spinae plane blocks for postoperative pain management and opioid reduction following lumbar fusions. Clin Spine Surg. 2023; 36(4):E131–E134

[2] Memtsoudis SG, Cozowicz C, Bekeris J, et al. Peripheral nerve block anesthesia/analgesia for patients undergoing primary hip and knee arthroplasty: recommendations from the International Consensus on Anesthesia-Related Outcomes after Surgery (ICAROS) group based on a systematic review and meta-analysis of current literature. Reg Anesth Pain Med. 2021; 46(11):971–985

[3] Memtsoudis SG, Cozowicz C, Bekeris J, et al. Anaesthetic care of patients undergoing primary hip and knee arthroplasty: consensus recommendations from the International Consensus on Anaesthesia-Related Outcomes after Surgery group (ICAROS) based on a systematic review and meta-analysis. Br J Anaesth. 2019; 123(3):269–287

[4] Braxton EE, Brena KR, Spears H, Conrad E, Heinze JD. Ultrasound-guided bilateral erector spinae plane nerve blocks: a novel application for the management of acute postoperative pain in awake spine surgery. Illustrative case. J Neurosurg Case Lessons. 2022; 3(18):CASE21633

[5] Garg B, Ahuja K, Khanna P, Sharan AD. Regional anesthesia for spine surgery. Clin Spine Surg. 2021; 34(5):163–170

[6] Bellantonio D, Bolondi G, Cultrera F, et al. Erector spinae plane block for perioperative pain management in neurosurgical lower-thoracic and lumbar spinal fusion: a single-centre prospective randomised controlled trial. BMC Anesthesiol. 2023; 23(1):187

[7] Zhang A, Chen J, Zhang X, et al. Twelfth thoracic vertebra erector spinae plane block for postoperative analgesia and early recovery after lumbar spine surgery in elderly patients: a single-blind randomized controlled trial. BMC Anesthesiol. 2023; 23(1):402

[8] Sun Q, Zhang C, Liu S, et al. Efficacy of erector spinae plane block for postoperative analgesia lumbar surgery: a systematic review and meta-analysis. BMC Anesthesiol. 2023; 23 (1):54

[9] Ilfeld BM. Continuous peripheral nerve blocks: a review of the published evidence. Anesth Analg. 2011; 113(4):904–925

[10] Jensen AR, Sharma AK, Formanek B, et al. Continuous peripheral nerve blocks are associated with increased rates of emergency department visits after arthroscopic rotator cuff repair surgery. Orthopedics. 2020; 43(2):127–131

[11] Jabur A, Nam HJ, Dixon A, Cox T, Randall H, Sun J. The effects of continuous catheter adductor canal block for pain management in knee replacement therapy: a meta-analysis. Knee Surg Relat Res. 2023; 35(1):16

[12] Hamilton TW, Athanassoglou V, Trivella M, et al. Liposomal bupivacaine peripheral nerve block for the management of postoperative pain. Cochrane Database Syst Rev. 2016; 2016 (8):CD011476

[13] Surdam JW, Licini DJ, Baynes NT, Arce BR. The use of Exparel (liposomal bupivacaine) to manage postoperative pain in unilateral total knee arthroplasty patients. J Arthroplasty. 2015; 30(2):325–329

[14] Ter Meulen BC, Weinstein H, Ostelo R, Koehler PJ. The epidural treatment of sciatica: its origin and evolution. Eur Neurol. 2016; 75(1–2):58–64

[15] Patel N, Solovyova O, Matthews G, Arumugam S, Sinha SK, Lewis CG. Safety and efficacy of continuous femoral nerve catheter with single shot sciatic nerve block vs epidural catheter anesthesia for same-day bilateral total knee arthroplasty. J Arthroplasty. 2015; 30(2):330–334

[16] Loubert C, Fernando R. Falling after epidural analgesia: lessons from obstetric anesthesia. Can J Anaesth. 2016; 63 (5):519–523

[17] van Geffen G-J, Bruhn J. Continuous peripheral nerve blocks safe practice and management. In: Finucane BT, Tsui BCH, eds. Complications of Regional Anesthesia: Principles of Safe Practice in Local and Regional Anesthesia. Cham: Springer International Publishing; 2017:167–185

[18] Marya SKS, Arora D, Singh C, Kacker S, Desai R, Lodha V. A prospective comparative study of local infiltration versus adductor block versus combined use of the two techniques following knee arthroplasty. Arthroplasty. 2020; 2(1):15

[19] Buggy DJ, Hall NA, Shah J, Brown J, Williams J. Motor block during patient-controlled epidural analgesia with ropivacaine or ropivacaine/fentanyl after intrathecal bupivacaine for caesarean section. Br J Anaesth. 2000; 85(3):468–470

[20] Lönnqvist PA, MacKenzie J, Soni AK, Conacher ID. Paravertebral blockade. Failure rate and complications. Anaesthesia. 1995; 50(9):813–815

[21] Iyer SJ, Leo SA. Maintenance of neuraxial block in labor analgesia. Trends Anaesth Crit Care. 2012; 2(4):199–204

[22] Fernandes MTP, Hernandes FB, de Almeida TN, Sobottka VP, Poli-Frederico RC, Fernandes KBP. Patient-controlled analgesia (PCA) in acute pain: pharmacological and clinical aspects. In: Pain Relief-From Analgesics to Alternative Therapies. London: IntechOpen; 2017

[23] de Leon-Casasola O. A review of the literature on multiple factors involved in postoperative pain course and duration. Postgrad Med. 2014; 126(4):42–52

[24] Choi SH, Lee WK, Lee SJ, et al. Parent-controlled analgesia in children undergoing cleft palate repair. J Korean Med Sci. 2008; 23(1):122–125

[25] Kan K, Levine WC. Infusion pumps. In: Ehrenwerth J, Eisenkraft JB, Berry JM, eds. Anesthesia Equipment. St. Louis, MO: Elsevier; 2021:351–367

[26] Capdevila X, Pirat P, Bringuier S, et al. French Study Group on Continuous Peripheral Nerve Blocks. Continuous peripheral nerve blocks in hospital wards after orthopedic surgery: a multicenter prospective analysis of the quality of postoperative analgesia and complications in 1,416 patients. Anesthesiology. 2005; 103(5):1035–1045

[27] Finnerty DT, McMahon A, McNamara JR, Hartigan SD, Griffin M, Buggy DJ. Comparing erector spinae plane block with serratus anterior plane block for minimally invasive thoracic surgery: a randomised clinical trial. Br J Anaesth. 2020; 125 (5):802–810

[28] Altıparmak B, Korkmaz Toker M, Uysal Aİ, Turan M, Gümüş Demirbilek S. Comparison of the effects of modified pectoral nerve block and erector spinae plane block on postoperative opioid consumption and pain scores of patients after radical mastectomy surgery: a prospective, randomized, controlled trial. J Clin Anesth. 2019; 54:61–65

[29] Borghi B, D'Addabbo M, White PF, et al. The use of prolonged peripheral neural blockade after lower extremity amputation: the effect on symptoms associated with phantom limb syndrome. Anesth Analg. 2010; 111(5):1308–1315

[30] Stojadinovic A, Auton A, Peoples GE, et al. Responding to challenges in modern combat casualty care: innovative use of advanced regional anesthesia. Pain Med. 2006; 7(4):330–338

20 Postoperative Delirium and Awake Spine Surgery

Favour C. Ononogbu-Uche, Felix Toussaint, Taylor Wallace, Abdullah Wael Saleh, and Chakib Maurice Ayoub

Abstract

Postoperative delirium (POD), a common and often underappreciated complication in surgical patients, can have significant detrimental effects on patient outcomes, including increased mortality, prolonged hospital stays, and long-term cognitive impairment. Given the substantial burden of POD on health care systems and patients alike, it is imperative to explore innovative strategies to mitigate its incidence. Awake spine surgery, a relatively recent advancement in surgical technique, presents a promising approach to reducing POD risk. By leveraging the benefits of regional anesthesia and minimizing the neurochemical disturbances associated with general anesthesia, awake spine surgery can significantly reduce the likelihood of POD. This chapter delves into the mechanisms underlying this association, highlighting the neurophysiological factors at play. Additionally, we discuss the clinical evidence supporting the efficacy of awake spine surgery in POD prevention, including comparative studies and meta-analyses. Understanding the potential of awake spine surgery to reduce POD is crucial for optimizing patient care and improving postoperative outcomes. By adopting this approach in appropriate cases and implementing strategies to mitigate potential risks, we can contribute to a paradigm shift in POD prevention and enhance the overall surgical experience for our patients.

Keywords: postoperative delirium, awake spine surgery, regional anesthesia, general anesthesia, patient outcomes

Key Points

- Postoperative delirium (POD) is a common complication in surgical patients. It can have significant negative consequences, including increased mortality, prolonged hospital stays, and long-term cognitive impairment.
- Awake spine surgery is a surgical technique that allows for spinal procedures while the patient is awake. It uses regional anesthesia and mild sedation to ensure patient comfort and real-time neurological monitoring.
- Awake spine surgery has been shown to reduce the incidence of POD compared to traditional general anesthesia. This is likely due to the reduced neurochemical disturbances associated with general anesthesia.
- The mechanisms linking spine surgery and POD are complex and involve neurophysiological factors. These include the impact of anesthesia type on the brain, intraoperative stress response, and pain management strategies.
- Clinical studies and evidence support the use of awake spine surgery in POD prevention. Comparative studies and meta-analyses have demonstrated lower rates of POD in patients undergoing awake spine surgery compared to those receiving general anesthesia.
- Implementing awake spine surgery requires careful patient selection and a multidisciplinary approach. Preoperative assessment, intraoperative monitoring, and postoperative care are essential for optimizing patient outcomes.
- Future research is needed to further explore the benefits of awake spine surgery and to develop personalized approaches for POD prevention and management. This includes investigating new anesthetic techniques, monitoring technologies, and pharmacological interventions.
- By understanding the relationship between POD and awake spine surgery, health care providers can implement strategies to minimize the risk of POD and improve patient outcomes. This can lead to a paradigm shift in the management of POD.

20.1 Introduction

20.1.1 Definition of Postoperative Delirium

Postoperative delirium (POD) is a common complication in surgical patients, defined as an acute decline in cognitive function characterized by confusion, inattention, disorganized thinking, and an altered level of consciousness.[1] This condition typically occurs after surgery and anesthesia, presenting as a fluctuating course of symptoms that can persist for days to weeks, often until the point of hospital discharge.[2] POD is associated with an increased risk of long-term cognitive decline, extended hospital stays, higher mortality rates, and increased health care costs.[3] The profound effects of POD are often reflected in remarks from loved ones such as "he's never been the same since his operation," "he's become forgetful since," or "she's lost all interest in the family since."[4] Despite extensive research, the pathophysiology of POD remains unclear, underscoring the importance of early recognition and management to improve patient outcomes.

20.1.2 Overview of Awake Spine Surgery

Awake spine surgery is a technique that allows surgeons to perform spinal procedures while the patient is awake, using local anesthesia and mild sedation to ensure patient comfort.[5] This approach enables real-time neurological monitoring, which can be critical in avoiding nerve damage and ensuring optimal outcomes. Awake spine surgery has gained popularity due to its potential to reduce recovery time and the risks associated with general anesthesia, making it an attractive option for patients undergoing certain types of spinal procedures.[6]

20.1.3 Importance of Understanding the Relationship

The incidence of POD has been shown to be lower in patients undergoing awake spine surgery compared to those receiving general anesthesia.[7] Awake spine surgery offers several benefits, including a reduced risk of POD, shorter hospital stays, lower readmission rates, and decreased health care costs.[8] For patients at high risk of POD or those who cannot tolerate general anesthesia, awake spine surgery provides a safer alternative. Understanding the clinical features, epidemiology, and risk factors associated with POD, and the advantages of awake spine surgery, is essential for improving patient outcomes in spinal surgery. This chapter will explore the mechanisms, clinical studies, and management strategies related to POD and awake spine surgery.

20.2 Understanding Postoperative Delirium

20.2.1 Clinical Features

- POD is a multifaceted condition that profoundly affects cognitive and behavioral functions. Recognizing its diverse manifestations is crucial for timely diagnosis and effective management.[9]

Cognitive Disturbances

- **Memory impairment:** Patients may experience difficulties in recalling recent events or forming new memories. This impairment can hinder their ability to participate in postoperative recovery activities and follow-up care.[10]
- **Attention deficits:** There is often a significant reduction in the ability to focus or maintain attention. This can result in confusion and difficulty following instructions, complicating postoperative care.[10]
- **Disorientation:** Patients may become disoriented, struggling with a sense of time, place, or personal identity. This disorientation can be distressing and may exacerbate other symptoms (▶ Fig. 20.1).[11]

Behavioral Changes

- **Hyperactivity/agitation:** The patient experiencing POD may exhibit varying degrees of restlessness or aggression, ranging from mild irritability to severe agitation that requires intervention. Such behavior can disrupt the healing process and necessitate careful management.[11,12]
- **Hypoactivity:** The patient may present with lethargy and decreased motor activity, appearing withdrawn and inattentive, yet without the agitation common in other forms of POD. This subdued presentation can easily be overlooked, making diagnosis in the postoperative setting more challenging.[13]
- **Hallucinations:** Visual and auditory hallucinations are common, contributing to a heightened sense of fear and confusion. These symptoms often require prompt treatment to ensure patient safety.[14]

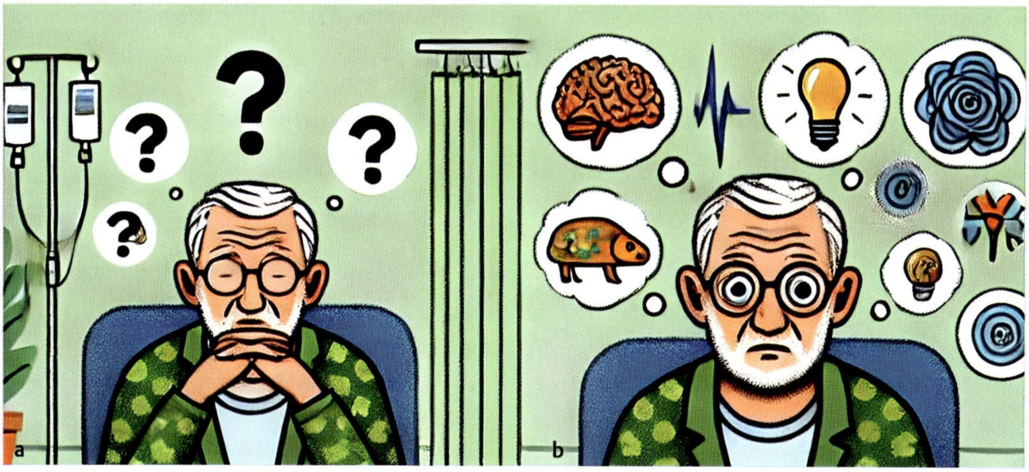

Fig. 20.1 (a) A cartoon depicting a patient experiencing cognitive disturbances such as memory impairment, attention deficits, and disorientation following surgery. (b) A patient experiencing behavioral changes such as hyperactivity/agitation, hallucinations, and emotional dysregulation/distress.

- **Emotional dysregulation and distress:** Rapid and unpredictable shifts in mood can occur, including episodes of anxiety, fear, or depression. Addressing these mood changes is vital for overall patient well-being (see ▸ Fig. 20.1).[15]

Importantly, patients may fluctuate through any of these discussed cognitive and behavioral states.

Onset and Duration

- POD typically emerges within the initial week following surgery, a critical period where patients are particularly vulnerable.[16]
- The duration of POD can range from a few hours to several weeks. Variability in duration depends on factors such as the patient's baseline cognitive status, the severity of the POD, and the effectiveness of the interventions implemented.[17]

20.2.2 Epidemiology and Incidence

Prevalence in Surgical Patients

- POD is prevalent in surgical settings, particularly among older adults. Studies indicate that 10 to over 50% of surgical patients may experience POD, with incidence rates varying based on patient demographics (age, commodities, etc.) and surgical complexity.[18,19]

Variation by Age and Surgery Type

- The risk of POD increases with age, particularly in individuals older than 65 years. This increased susceptibility is linked to age-related vulnerabilities in brain function.[20]
- Major surgeries, such as cardiac, vascular, orthopaedic, or mixed procedures, present higher risks due to the greater physiological and psychological stress involved.[21]

Expert Tip

Consider POD in patients older than 65 years, especially in those with preexisting neurodegenerative diseases such as Alzheimer's disease and Parkinson's disease.

20.2.3 Pathophysiology and Risk Factors

Neuroinflammatory Mechanisms

- Surgical procedures and postoperative infections can initiate systemic inflammatory responses. This inflammation can cross the blood–brain barrier, leading to neuroinflammation—a key contributor to the development of POD.[22]

Neurotransmitter Imbalances

- POD may be associated with disruptions in neurotransmitter systems, particularly acetylcholine, dopamine, and serotonin. Imbalances in these neurotransmitters may impair cognitive function and contribute to the onset of POD.[23]

Risk Factors

- **Age:** Older patients are at increased risk due to age-related changes in brain structure and function.[20]
- **Preexisting cognitive impairment:** Conditions such as dementia or mild cognitive impairment predispose individuals to POD.[24]
- **Comorbidities:** Chronic conditions like diabetes, cardiovascular disease, and renal impairment can exacerbate the risk of POD.[18]
- **Surgical factors:** The complexity and duration of surgery, along with intraoperative factors like blood loss and hypotension, significantly impact the likelihood of developing POD.[21]

20.2.4 Diagnosis and Assessment Tools

Montreal Cognitive Assessment

- This brief screening tool evaluates cognitive function and can help identify cognitive impairments related to POD. It is useful for assessing the severity and impact of POD on cognitive abilities.[25]

Confusion Assessment Method

- This is a widely used diagnostic tool that assesses POD based on key criteria: acute onset and fluctuating course, inattention, disorganized thinking, and altered level of consciousness. It is well suited to use in acute care and postprocedural settings.[26]

Delirium Rating Scale-Revised-9

- This scale measures the severity of POD and can track changes over time, aiding in the evaluation of treatment effectiveness. It is very comprehensive but also more time-consuming.[27]

4 A's Test

- This rapid screening tool assesses alertness, attention, acute change or fluctuating course, and disordered thinking, facilitating early detection of POD.[28]

Nurses' Delirium Screening Checklist

- This screening tool was developed for nursing staff to facilitate early detection and intervention in delirium. It is quick and easy to use and has shown high specificity when screening for POD.[29]

20.3 Awake Spine Surgery: An Overview

20.3.1 Definition and Techniques

- Awake spine surgery represents a significant advancement in spine surgery techniques. By utilizing regional anesthetic techniques and mild sedation, this approach allows for real-time neurological assessments and patient interaction during the procedure.[6]

Local Anesthesia and Sedation Protocols

- The surgery is performed under regional anesthetic techniques, including spinal or epidural anesthesia and muscle plane blocks, often combined with mild sedatives to ensure patient comfort while maintaining consciousness. This approach minimizes the risks associated with general anesthesia and allows for immediate feedback from the patient regarding neurological function.[6]

20.3.2 Indications and Contraindications

Suitable Conditions and Patient Profiles

- Awake spine surgery is particularly suited for procedures such as lumbar decompression and diskectomy. It is ideal for patients who require minimal surgical intervention (≤ 2 vertebrae levels) and neural feedback and those who may benefit from reduced exposure to general anesthesia such as aging populations.[5,6]
- Contraindications include patients with anxiety, bleeding disorders, multiple health comorbidities, or conditions requiring extensive surgical intervention that is not amenable to local anesthesia.[5,6]

Expert Tip

Avoid awake spine surgery in patients who are very anxious and in surgeries that will take longer than 3 hours.

20.3.3 Benefits and Challenges

Reduced Recovery Time

- One of the primary advantages of awake spine surgery is the expedited recovery process. Patients often experience a faster return to daily activities and a shorter hospital stay, which are beneficial for overall recovery and rehabilitation.[30]

Decreased Anesthesia-Related Complications

- By avoiding general anesthesia, the risk of complications such as postoperative nausea, cardiovascular issues, and respiratory issues is significantly reduced. This results in a smoother perioperative experience for the patient.[5]

Patient Selection and Intraoperative Cooperation

- Successful implementation of awake spine surgery depends on careful patient selection and ensuring that patients can remain still and cooperate throughout the procedure. Effective communication and patient education are essential to achieving positive outcomes.[31,32]

20.3.4 Comparison with Traditional Spine Surgery

Differences in Anesthesia, Recovery, and Outcomes

- While traditional spine surgery typically involves general anesthesia, which can have more significant physiological impacts and associated risks, awake spine surgery offers the advantage of reduced anesthesia-related complications and potentially faster recovery times.[6]

20.4 Mechanisms Linking Awake Spine Surgery and Postoperative Delirium

20.4.1 Neurophysiological Mechanisms

Impact of Anesthesia Types on the Brain

- The use of local anesthesia and mild sedation in awake spine surgery minimizes the neurochemical disturbances associated with general anesthesia. This may contribute to a lower incidence of postoperative POD by reducing the overall impact on brain function.[33]

Intraoperative Stress Response

- Managing intraoperative stress and anxiety is crucial. Strategies to minimize stress and ensure patient comfort can mitigate the neurophysiological impact of surgery and potentially reduce the risk of POD.[33]

20.4.2 Pain Management and Delirium

Nonopioid versus Opioid Analgesics

- The use of opioids is associated with an increased risk of delirium due to their effects on the central nervous system. Implementing nonopioid analgesics is preferred to minimize POD risk.[34]

Opioid-Sparing Approaches

- Strategies such as regional anesthesia and multimodal analgesia, which combine different pain relief modalities, can effectively manage pain while reducing the reliance on opioids. This approach may help in mitigating the risk of POD.[35]

20.4.3 Perioperative Factors

Intraoperative Monitoring

- Continuous monitoring of hemodynamic stability and neurological status during awake spine surgery is essential. This real-time assessment allows for immediate intervention if any signs of POD or other complications arise.[36]

Postoperative Care

- Early identification and management of POD are critical for improving patient outcomes. A multidisciplinary approach involving surgeons, anesthesiologists, nurses, and other health care professionals ensures comprehensive care and addresses any issues promptly.[37]
- Postoperative care should include regular cognitive assessments, effective pain management, and ensuring adequate hydration and nutrition to support recovery and reduce the risk of POD.[37,38]

By integrating these strategies and understanding the intricate relationship between awake spine surgery and postoperative POD, clinicians can enhance patient outcomes, minimize risks, and provide optimal care throughout the surgical journey.

20.5 Clinical Studies and Evidence

20.5.1 Review of Key Studies

Comparative Studies, Systematic Reviews, and Meta-Analyses on Delirium Incidence in Awake versus Traditional Spine Surgery

- Comparative studies indicate that awake spine surgery, performed under regional anesthetic techniques, offers advantages over traditional spine surgery conducted under general anesthesia.
- Demirel et al conducted a prospective randomized study comparing epidural versus general anesthesia for lumbar disk surgery, showing that regional anesthesia techniques like spinal or epidural anesthesia led to better postoperative cognitive outcomes than general anesthesia.[39]
- Perez-Roman et al conducted a systematic review and meta-analysis involving 3,709 patients, finding that awake spine surgery under spinal anesthesia offers benefits over general anesthesia, including reduced operating room time, lower postoperative pain scores, and earlier ambulation, which may lower the incidence of POD.[40]
- Breton et al reviewed 343 cases of complex lumbar spine surgery and highlighted that spinal anesthesia reduces adverse cognitive effects commonly associated with general anesthesia.[41]
- A systematic review and meta-analysis of 38 studies involving 7,820 patients found that awake lumbar spine surgeries with spinal anesthesia reduce operating room time, lower postoperative pain, and enable earlier ambulation compared to general anesthesia, contributing to a lower incidence of POD, especially in older patients.[42]
- Additionally, a Mayo Clinic study in 2021 reported that awake spine surgery reduces adverse effects like memory loss and cognitive dysfunction associated with general anesthesia, shortens hospital stays, and improves patient satisfaction.[43]
- These findings align with other research suggesting that spinal anesthesia can mitigate postoperative cognitive issues, including delirium.
- Overall, evidence suggests that awake spine surgery under regional anesthesia is a safer alternative to traditional spine surgery under general anesthesia, reducing the risk of delirium and enhancing recovery outcomes.
- Awake spine surgery opens the doors to patients who previously were considered to be “high risk” due to age, comorbidities, and risk of POD.[44]

20.5.2 Outcomes, Complications, and Best Practices

Short-Term Outcomes

- **Reduction in operating room time:** Awake spine surgery under spinal anesthesia significantly reduces total operating room time compared to general anesthesia, leading to better surgical resource utilization and shorter patient waiting times.[45] This is likely due to the knowledge that many regional anesthetic techniques, such as spinal anesthesia, only last for 2 to 3 hours, making the need for efficient surgery paramount.
- **Lower postoperative pain:** Patients undergoing awake spine surgery report lower immediate postoperative pain due to the effective localized pain relief provided by spinal anesthesia.[35]
- **Earlier ambulation:** Awake spine surgery facilitates earlier ambulation, often within hours postsurgery, benefiting recovery and reducing the risk of complications such as deep vein thrombosis.[46]
- **Shorter hospital stays:** Patients typically experience shorter hospital stays following awake spine surgery, attributed to quicker recovery and reduced need for intensive postoperative care.[46]

Long-Term Outcomes

- **Reduced risk of cognitive dysfunction:** Awake spine surgery under spinal anesthesia lowers the risk of long-term cognitive dysfunction, including POD, particularly in elderly patients.[47]
- **Patient satisfaction:** Long-term patient satisfaction is higher with awake spine surgery due to reduced adverse effects and quicker recovery.[48]
- **Long-term pain management:** Effective short-term pain management leads to better long-term pain outcomes, reducing the likelihood of chronic pain conditions.[46]
- **Lower incidence of postoperative complications:** Awake spine surgery is associated with a lower incidence of postoperative complications such as infections and pulmonary issues, benefiting long-term health.[40]

Comparative Summary

- General anesthesia in spine surgery is associated with higher risks of POD, longer operating room times, greater pain, delayed ambulation, and extended hospital stays. In contrast, spinal anesthesia used in awake spine surgery reduces delirium risk, operating room time, postoperative pain, and hospital stays. These benefits underscore the advantages of spinal anesthesia in improving recovery and reducing complications.[49]
- Overall, awake spine surgery under spinal anesthesia provides significant benefits over general anesthesia, including fewer cognitive issues and enhanced recovery.[47]

Impact on Hospital Stay

- **Spinal anesthesia (awake surgery):** Awake spine surgery under spinal anesthesia is linked to significantly shorter hospital stays, often 1 to 2 days after surgery, due to quicker recovery, earlier ambulation, and fewer complications.[30]
- **General anesthesia:** Traditional spine surgery under general anesthesia generally results in longer hospital stays, typically 3 to 5 days, due to slower recovery, increased postoperative pain, and a higher risk of complications such as nausea and cognitive impairment.[42]

20.5.3 Impact on Readmission Rates

- **Spinal anesthesia (awake surgery):** Awake spine surgery under spinal anesthesia is associated with lower readmission rates due to reduced postoperative pain, fewer complications, and higher patient satisfaction. Effective pain management and fewer cognitive issues lead to fewer readmissions.[47] Research from the Mayo Clinic and other studies confirm that spinal anesthesia results in shorter hospital stays and fewer readmissions.[46]
- **General anesthesia:** Spine surgeries under general anesthesia generally have higher readmission rates due to more frequent complications such as POD, infections, and pulmonary issues, which necessitate additional treatment.[42]

20.5.4 Best Practices

Patient Selection

- **Criteria:** Ideal candidates for awake spine surgery are those without severe obstructive sleep apnea, high obesity (BMI > 35), or significant anxiety about being awake during the procedure.
- **Preoperative assessment:** Conduct thorough physical and psychological evaluations to ensure patient suitability for spinal anesthesia.[42,46]

Multidisciplinary Approach

- **Team coordination:** Ensure close collaboration among neurosurgeons, anesthesiologists, and nursing staff for effective intraoperative communication and patient monitoring.
- **Training and protocols:** Implement standardized protocols and training to manage awake spine procedures efficiently.[46]

Intraoperative Management

- **Patient comfort:** Use noise-canceling headphones and music and maintain continuous communication to keep patients comfortable and informed.
- **Anesthesia techniques:** Administer spinal anesthesia with appropriate dosing to ensure effective analgesia while keeping patients responsive.[42,46]

Postoperative Care

- **Pain management:** Employ multimodal pain strategies to minimize opioid use and support recovery.
- **Early mobilization:** Promote early ambulation and physical therapy to accelerate recovery and prevent complications.[46]

Follow-Up and Monitoring

- **Regular check-ups:** Schedule follow-ups to monitor recovery, address complications early, and provide support.
- **Patient education:** Inform patients about postoperative expectations, signs of complications, and when to seek medical help to reduce readmission rates.[42]

Adhering to these practices enhances patient outcomes in awake spine surgery, improving recovery times, reducing complications, and increasing satisfaction.

20.6 Prevention and Management Strategies

20.6.1 Preoperative Assessment and Optimization

Screening for Risk Factors

Preoperative assessment and optimization are essential in spine surgery for reducing complications and improving outcomes. Screening for risk factors, such as comorbidities and nutritional issues, allows for targeted interventions to enhance surgical success.[50]

Preoperative Education

Providing patients with comprehensive education about the surgery and recovery process can reduce anxiety and improve postoperative outcomes, which may help in minimizing delirium risks.[51]

Intraoperative Techniques

- **Anesthetic considerations:** Using multimodal anesthesia and avoiding prolonged sedation can reduce the risk of POD. Regional anesthesia techniques, when appropriate, may also lower delirium incidence.[46,45]
- **Surgical techniques:** Minimally invasive surgical approaches can reduce operative stress and postoperative recovery time, potentially lowering the risk of delirium.[36]

Postoperative Care

- **Early mobilization:** Encouraging early mobilization and ambulation postsurgery is critical for reducing delirium risk and enhancing recovery.[46]
- **Multidisciplinary approach:** A team-based approach involving nurses, physical therapists, and geriatric specialists can improve overall patient outcomes and reduce delirium incidence.[46]

- **Delirium prevention protocols:** Implementing protocols to monitor and manage delirium, such as regular cognitive assessments and creating a supportive environment, is essential for preventing and addressing POD.[38]
- Together, these postoperative care strategies—early mobilization, a multidisciplinary approach, and adherence to delirium prevention protocols—form a robust framework for minimizing the risk of delirium in awake spine surgery patients, ultimately enhancing their recovery and overall well-being.

20.7 Future Directions and Research

20.7.1 Emerging Techniques in Awake Spine Surgery

- **Advances in surgical and anesthetic techniques:** The development of refined surgical methods and anesthetic techniques is expanding the feasibility and safety of awake spine surgery. Enhanced local and regional anesthesia, coupled with minimally invasive surgical approaches, allows for reduced operative times and quicker recoveries.[5]
- **Innovations in intraoperative monitoring:** Cutting-edge intraoperative monitoring technologies are improving the precision and safety of awake spine surgery. Real-time neurophysiological monitoring and advanced imaging techniques ensure better outcomes and lower the risk of complications[52]

20.7.2 Advances in Delirium Prevention and Management

- **New pharmacological agents:** Research into new pharmacological agents aims to prevent and manage POD more effectively. These drugs target specific pathways involved in delirium, offering more targeted prevention and treatment options.[53]
- **Enhanced recovery protocols:** Enhanced Recovery After Surgery (ERAS) protocols, which include multimodal pain management, early mobilization, and nutritional support, are being tailored to spine surgery to reduce delirium incidence and improve overall recovery.[38]

20.7.3 Ongoing Research and Clinical Trials

- **Potential for Personalized Medicine Approaches:** Personalized medicine is on the horizon, with ongoing research into genetic and biomarker-based strategies for tailored prevention and treatment of POD. Identifying individual risk profiles through genetic markers and biomarkers can lead to more precise and effective interventions.[54]
- **Genetic and biomarker research:** Studies are investigating specific genetic variants and biomarkers that could predict susceptibility to POD. This research aims to enable personalized risk assessment and the development of individualized preventive strategies.[55]

By focusing on these future directions, the field of spine surgery can continue to improve patient outcomes, reduce complications, and enhance the overall quality of care.

20.8 Clinical Example

20.8.1 Patient Background

- A 72-year-old man with severe central spinal canal stenosis at the L4–L5 vertebral level (▶ Fig. 20.2), complicated by Parkinson's disease, atrial fibrillation, obstructive sleep apnea, benign prostatic hyperplasia, and rapid eye movement behavioral disorder, presented for surgery. Despite having a previously implanted spinal cord stimulator, he had persistent low back and radicular pain, affecting his quality of life.

20.9 Preoperative Considerations

The patient's risk of POD necessitated careful preoperative planning.

- **Family presence:** His wife committed to staying with him during his hospital stay, and they received an informative handout on delirium.
- **Pain management:** The patient was advised to use up to 3,000 mg of Tylenol per day before and after surgery, with an emphasis on careful opioid use to minimize the risk of POD. The use

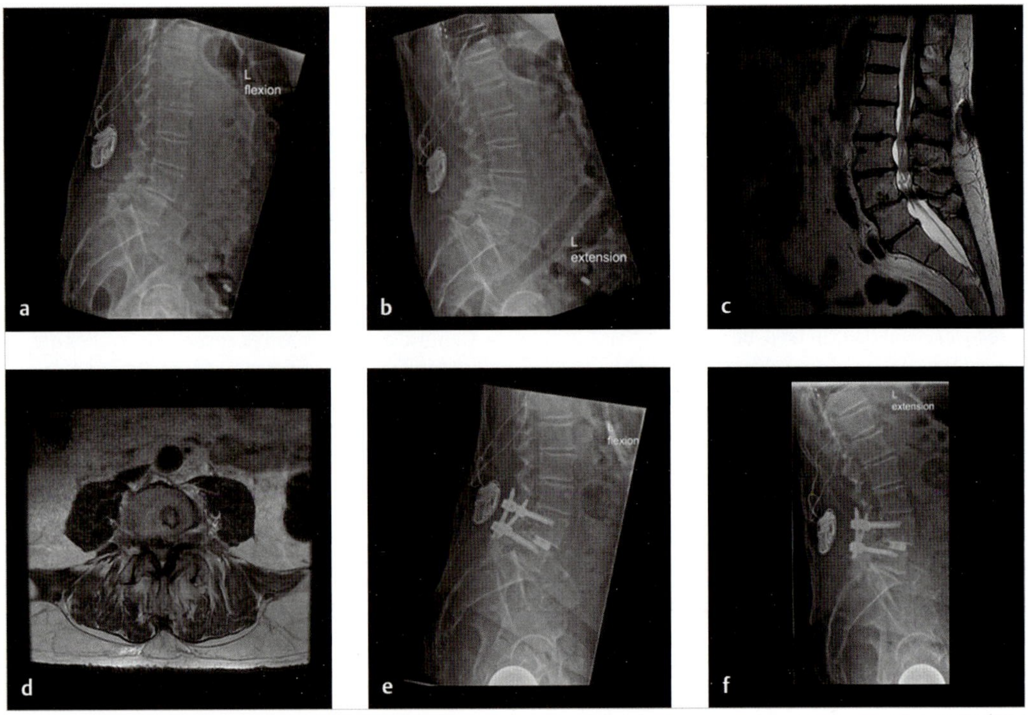

Fig. 20.2 **(a)** Preoperative flexion X-ray: grade 1 anterolisthesis of L4/L5 without dynamic instability. Multilevel degenerative disk disease and spinal cord stimulator leads terminating at T8–T9. **(b)** Preoperative extension X-ray: findings consistent with flexion view, with stable grade 1 anterolisthesis and no instability. **(c)** Sagittal T2-weighted magnetic resonance imaging (MRI): severe central stenosis at L4/L5 and moderate stenosis at L3/L4 and L1/L2, with slight progression at L1/L2. **(d)** Axial T2-weighted MRI at L4/L5: severe left foraminal stenosis with exiting L4 nerve root impingement. **(e)** Six-month postoperative flexion X-ray: stable fusion and adequate decompression at L4/L5 with intact interbody disk spacer and hardware. No evidence of instability. **(f)** Six-month postoperative extension X-ray: findings confirm adequate decompression, stable fusion, and intact hardware at L4/L5, with no instability or periprosthetic lucency.

of a regional anesthetic block was indicated to further minimize postoperative pain.

- **Hearing and vision:** The patient failed a hearing screen and required reading glasses. The team focused on clear communication and reducing background noise.
- **Early mobility and nutrition:** He was encouraged to stay active and maintain good nutrition and hydration before and after surgery.
- **Awake surgery:** Performing this procedure using a spinal anesthetic minimizes disruptions to the patient's Parkinson's oral medication regiment, resulting in better management of parkinsonian symptoms and reduced likelihood of POD.

20.10 Operative Course

- **Surgical plan:** The patient underwent an awake percutaneous lumbar interbody fusion (percLIF) at L4–L5 to reduce the risk of POD associated with general anesthesia.
- **Anesthetic technique:** A spinal block at L3–L4 with 0.75% bupivacaine was used as the primary anesthesia. To manage postoperative pain, an ultrasound-guided erector spinae plane (ESP) block was performed bilaterally at L3, using a mixture of 0.5% bupivacaine and 1.3% Exparel.
- **Surgical procedure:** In the operating room, the patient's identity and procedure were confirmed. He received spinal anesthesia, and a Foley catheter was placed. After positioning him

prone on a Jackson table, the team performed a timeout. A stab incision was made approximately 6 cm off midline, and the L4–L5 disk space was accessed through Kambin's triangle using instrument-tracking fluoroscopy (TrackX, Hillsborough, NC). Following the diskectomy, an expandable interbody fusion system was percutaneously hammered into the disk space. Next, the pedicles of L4 and L5 were cannulated bilaterally, and percutaneous screws were inserted. Correct placement was confirmed via a CT scan. A decompressive hemilaminectomy was then performed on the right L4 lamina, followed by bilateral rod placement. Posterolateral fusion was completed by drilling the facets bilaterally at L4 and L5, followed by placement of allograft and autograft. Following bacitracin irrigation, the fascia was closed.

Neuromonitoring confirmed quiet EMG signals throughout the procedure. Skin to skin time was 163 minutes and estimated blood loss during the procedure was less than 50 mL.

20.11 Postoperative Course

Postoperative care focused on preventing delirium and managing pain.

- **Family presence:** His wife provided emotional support and assisted with communication.
- **Pain management:** Scheduled Tylenol administration ensured pain control without deliriogenic medications such as opioids.
- **Early mobility:** Daily physical therapy sessions were prescribed postoperation to encourage walking with assistance soon after surgery to minimize POD risk.
- **Communication and sensory aids:** The team ensured his hearing and vision needs were met, and communication with the patient was clear and efficient.
- **Consistent delirium screening:** The patient was proactively screened for delirium twice daily during his admission using various screening tests including the Nursing Delirium Screening Scale (NuDESC). He consistently achieved a score of 0, indicative of the absence presence of delirium, on all assessment areas throughout his stay.
- **Nutrition and hydration:** His intake was monitored, supported by dietary counseling.

20.12 Outcome

- The surgery was successful with good correction of spondylolisthesis and decompression (► Fig. 20.2). The patient did not develop POD, demonstrating the effectiveness of the comprehensive perioperative strategies. He was discharged on postoperative day 5 to a skilled nursing facility with improved mobility plans and pain control, significantly enhancing his quality of life. Follow-up visits at 6 weeks and 3, 6, and 12 months confirmed no recurrence of symptoms and no continued need for the spinal cord stimulator.

20.13 Conclusion

20.13.1 Summary of Key Points

- POD is a cognitive decline often seen after surgery, with awake spine surgery offering a solution that minimizes its incidence. Utilizing local anesthesia and mild sedation rather than general anesthesia, awake spine surgery reduces risks such as longer hospital stays and increased postoperative pain, while facilitating quicker recovery and real-time neurological assessments.

20.13.2 Clinical Implications

- Awake spine surgery presents a significant advantage in reducing POD and associated complications compared to general anesthesia. It is particularly beneficial for high-risk patients and those unable to undergo general anesthesia. Proper patient selection and multidisciplinary care are essential for maximizing the benefits of this approach.

20.13.3 Call for Continued Research and Education

- Further research is needed to explore advanced anesthetic techniques, innovative monitoring technologies, and new pharmacological strategies to prevent POD. Continued education on the benefits of awake spine surgery and its implementation will help enhance patient outcomes and refine surgical practices.

References

[1] Pinho C, Cruz S, Santos A, Abelha FJ. Postoperative delirium: age and low functional reserve as independent risk factors. J Clin Anesth. 2016; 33:507–513

[2] Evered L, Silbert B, Knopman DS, et al. Nomenclature Consensus Working Group. Recommendations for the Nomenclature of Cognitive Change Associated with Anaesthesia and Surgery-20181. J Alzheimers Dis. 2018; 66(1):1–10

[3] Fineberg SJ, Nandyala SV, Marquez-Lara A, Oglesby M, Patel AA, Singh K. Incidence and risk factors for postoperative delirium after lumbar spine surgery. Spine. 2013; 38(20): 1790–1796

[4] Bedford PD. Adverse cerebral effects of anaesthesia on old people. Lancet. 1955; 269(6884):259–263

[5] Waguia R, Touko EK, Sykes DAW, et al. How to start an awake spine program: protocol and illustrative cases. IBRO Neurosci Rep. 2022; 13:69–77

[6] Fiani B, Reardon T, Selvage J, et al. Awake spine surgery: an eye-opening movement. Surg Neurol Int. 2021; 12:222

[7] Sieber FE, Zakriya KJ, Gottschalk A, et al. Sedation depth during spinal anesthesia and the development of postoperative delirium in elderly patients undergoing hip fracture repair. Mayo Clin Proc. 2010; 85(1):18–26

[8] Arizumi F, Maruo K, Kusuyama K, Kishima K, Tachibana T. Efficacy of intervention for prevention of postoperative delirium after spine surgery. Spine Surg Relat Res. 2020; 5(1): 16–21

[9] Whitlock EL, Vannucci A, Avidan MS. Postoperative delirium. Minerva Anestesiol. 2011; 77(4):448–456

[10] Vu T, Smith JA. An update on postoperative cognitive dysfunction following cardiac surgery. Front Psychiatry. 2022; 13:884907

[11] Vasilevskis EE, Han JH, Hughes CG, Ely EW. Epidemiology and risk factors for delirium across hospital settings. Best Pract Res Clin Anaesthesiol. 2012; 26(3):277–287

[12] Collet MO, Caballero J, Sonneville R, et al. AID-ICU cohort study co-authors. Prevalence and risk factors related to haloperidol use for delirium in adult intensive care patients: the multinational AID-ICU inception cohort study. Intensive Care Med. 2018; 44(7):1081–1089

[13] Mart MF, Williams Roberson S, Salas B, Pandharipande PP, Ely EW. Prevention and management of delirium in the intensive care unit. Semin Respir Crit Care Med. 2021; 42(1): 112–126

[14] Teller J, Gabriel MM, Schimmelpfennig SD, et al. Stroke, seizures, hallucinations and postoperative delirium as neurological complications after cardiac surgery and percutaneous valve replacement. J Cardiovasc Dev Dis. 2022; 9(11): 365

[15] Boehm LM, Jones AC, Selim AA, et al. Delirium-related distress in the ICU: A qualitative meta-synthesis of patient and family perspectives and experiences. Int J Nurs Stud. 2021; 122:104030

[16] Schaller SJ, Anstey M, Blobner M, et al. International Early SOMS-guided Mobilization Research Initiative. Early, goal-directed mobilisation in the surgical intensive care unit: a randomised controlled trial. Lancet. 2016; 388(10052): 1377–1388

[17] Wilson JE, Mart MF, Cunningham C, et al. Delirium. Nat Rev Dis Primers. 2020; 6(1):90

[18] Sadeghirad B, Dodsworth BT, Schmutz Gelsomino N, et al. Perioperative factors associated with postoperative delirium in patients undergoing noncardiac surgery: an individual patient data meta-analysis. JAMA Netw Open. 2023; 6(10): e2337239

[19] Deeken F, Sánchez A, Rapp MA, et al. PAWEL Study Group. Outcomes of a delirium prevention program in older persons after elective surgery: a stepped-wedge cluster randomized clinical trial. JAMA Surg. 2022; 157(2):e216370

[20] Schenning KJ, Deiner SG. Postoperative delirium in the geriatric patient. Anesthesiol Clin. 2015; 33(3):505–516

[21] Igwe EO, Nealon J, O'Shaughnessy P, et al. Incidence of postoperative delirium in older adults undergoing surgical procedures: a systematic literature review and meta-analysis. Worldviews Evid Based Nurs. 2023; 20(3):220–237

[22] Liu Y, Yang W, Xue J, et al. Neuroinflammation: the central enabler of postoperative cognitive dysfunction. Biomed Pharmacother. 2023; 167:115582

[23] Stollings JL, Kotfis K, Chanques G, Pun BT, Pandharipande PP, Ely EW. Delirium in critical illness: clinical manifestations, outcomes, and management. Intensive Care Med. 2021; 47 (10):1089–1103

[24] Deiner S, Silverstein JH. Postoperative delirium and cognitive dysfunction. Br J Anaesth. 2009; 103 Suppl 1:i41–i46

[25] Somnuke P, Srishewachart P, Jiraphorncharas C, et al. Early postoperative neurocognitive complications in elderly patients: comparing those with and without preexisting mild cognitive impairment: a prospective study. BMC Geriatr. 2024; 24(1):84

[26] Wei LA, Fearing MA, Sternberg EJ, Inouye SK. The confusion assessment method: a systematic review of current usage. J Am Geriatr Soc. 2008; 56(5):823–830

[27] Trzepacz PT, Mittal D, Torres R, Kanary K, Norton J, Jimerson N. Validation of the Delirium Rating Scale-revised-98: comparison with the delirium rating scale and the cognitive test for delirium. J Neuropsychiatry Clin Neurosci. 2001; 13(2): 229–242

[28] Saller T, MacLullich AMJ, Schäfer ST, et al. Screening for delirium after surgery: validation of the 4 A's test (4AT) in the post-anaesthesia care unit. Anaesthesia. 2019; 74(10):1260–1266

[29] Kim S, Choi E, Jung Y, Jang I. Postoperative delirium screening tools for post-anaesthetic adult patients in non-intensive care units: a systematic review and meta-analysis. J Clin Nurs. 2023; 32(9–10):1691–1704

[30] Wang MY, Grossman J. Endoscopic minimally invasive transforaminal interbody fusion without general anesthesia: initial clinical experience with 1-year follow-up. Neurosurg Focus. 2016; 40(2):E13

[31] Letchuman V, Agarwal N, Mummaneni VP, et al. Awake spinal surgery: simplifying the learning curve with a patient selection algorithm. Neurosurg Focus. 2021; 51(6):E2

[32] Hernandez NS, Begashaw B, Riesenburger RI, Kryzanski JT, Liu P. Spinal anesthesia in elective lumbar spinal surgery. Anesth Pain Med. 2023; 18(4):349–356

[33] Wu L, Zhao H, Weng H, Ma D. Lasting effects of general anesthetics on the brain in the young and elderly: "mixed picture" of neurotoxicity, neuroprotection and cognitive impairment. J Anesth. 2019; 33(2):321–335

[34] Yoo SH, Kang J, Kim HJ, et al. Opioid use and subsequent delirium risk in patients with advanced cancer in palliative care: a multicenter registry study. Sci Rep. 2024; 14(1):6004

[35] Sykes DAW, Tabarestani TQ, Chaudhry NS, et al. Awake spinal fusion is associated with reduced length of stay, opioid use, and time to ambulation compared to general anesthesia: a matched cohort study. World Neurosurg. 2023; 176: e91–e100

[36] Jung C, Hinken L, Fischer-Kumbruch M, et al. Intraoperative monitoring parameters and postoperative delirium: results of a prospective cross-sectional trial. Medicine (Baltimore). 2021; 100(1):e24160
[37] Epstein NE. Multidisciplinary in-hospital teams improve patient outcomes: a review. Surg Neurol Int. 2014; 5 Suppl 7: S295–S303
[38] Qureshi O, Arthur ME. Recent advances in predicting, preventing, and managing postoperative delirium. Fac Rev. 2023; 12:19
[39] Demirel CB, Kalayci M, Ozkocak I, Altunkaya H, Ozer Y, Acikgoz B. A prospective randomized study comparing perioperative outcome variables after epidural or general anesthesia for lumbar disc surgery. J Neurosurg Anesthesiol. 2003; 15 (3):185–192
[40] Perez-Roman RJ, Govindarajan V, Bryant JP, Wang MY. Spinal anesthesia in awake surgical procedures of the lumbar spine: a systematic review and meta-analysis of 3709 patients. Neurosurg Focus. 2021; 51(6):E7
[41] Breton JM, Ludwig CG, Yang MJ, et al. Spinal anesthesia in contemporary and complex lumbar spine surgery: experience with 343 cases. J Neurosurg Spine. 2021; 36(4):534–541
[42] Rajjoub R, Ghaith AK, El-Hajj VG, et al. Comparative outcomes of awake spine surgery under spinal versus general anesthesia: a comprehensive systematic review and meta-analysis. Eur Spine J. 2024; 33(3):985–1000
[43] Schulte PJ, Roberts RO, Knopman DS, et al. Association between exposure to anaesthesia and surgery and long-term cognitive trajectories in older adults: report from the Mayo Clinic Study of Aging. Br J Anaesth. 2018; 121(2):398–405
[44] Sykes DAW, Tabarestani TQ, Salven DS, et al. Awake spinal anesthesia facilitates spine surgery in poor surgical candidates: a case series. Neurochirurgie. 2023; 69(3):101444
[45] McLain RF, Kalfas I, Bell GR, Tetzlaff JE, Yoon HJ, Rana M. Comparison of spinal and general anesthesia in lumbar laminectomy surgery: a case-controlled analysis of 400 patients. J Neurosurg Spine. 2005; 2(1):17–22
[46] De Biase G, Gruenbaum SE, West JL, et al. Spinal versus general anesthesia for minimally invasive transforaminal lumbar interbody fusion: implications on operating room time, pain, and ambulation. Neurosurg Focus. 2021; 51(6):E3
[47] De Biase G, Gruenbaum SE, Quiñones-Hinojosa A, Abode-Iyamah KO. Spine surgery under spinal vs general anesthesia: prospective analysis of quality of life, fatigue, and cognition. Neurosurgery. 2022; 90(2):186–191
[48] Goth A, Karim HMR, Yunus M, Chakraborty R, Dey S, Bhattacharyya P. Effect of postoperative anesthesiologists' single visit on patient satisfaction: a hospital-based non-randomized study. Cureus. 2023; 15(2):e34518
[49] Morino T, Hino M, Yamaoka S, et al. Risk factors for delirium after spine surgery: an age-matched analysis. Asian Spine J. 2018; 12(4):703–709
[50] Wang TY, Price M, Mehta VA, et al. Preoperative optimization for patients undergoing elective spine surgery. Clin Neurol Neurosurg. 2021; 202:106445
[51] Raats JW, Steunenberg SL, de Lange DC, van der Laan L. Risk factors of post-operative delirium after elective vascular surgery in the elderly: a systematic review. Int J Surg. 2016; 35: 1–6
[52] De Jesus Encarnacion Ramirez M, Chmutin G, Nurmukhametov R, et al. Integrating augmented reality in spine surgery: redefining precision with new technologies. Brain Sci. 2024; 14(7):645
[53] Vlisides P, Avidan M. Recent advances in preventing and managing postoperative delirium. F1000 Res. 2019; 8:F1000 Faculty Rev-607
[54] Inouye SK, Westendorp RGJ, Saczynski JS. Delirium in elderly people. Lancet. 2014; 383(9920):911–922
[55] Ayob F, Lam E, Ho G, Chung F, El-Beheiry H, Wong J. Preoperative biomarkers and imaging tests as predictors of post-operative delirium in non-cardiac surgical patients: a systematic review. BMC Anesthesiol. 2019; 19(1):25

21 Evidence for Awake Spine Surgery

Shaun E. Gruenbaum and Kingsley Abode-Iyamah

Abstract

Awake spine surgery is currently a growing field in advancement of anesthetics for spinal surgery. Historic data have shown the safety of regional anesthesia for spinal pathology, and there is increasing evidence showing the benefits of awake spinal over general anesthesia for spine surgery. These benefits include intraoperative benefits such as decreased operating time but also extends to other benefits such as decreased fatigue. Many of the benefits of awake spinal surgery may result in the patient's ability to mobilize earlier than those undergoing general anesthesia as a result of better pain control from this cohort. As this field continues to grow with many more centers adopting the technique, ensuring a robust protocol especially for emergent airway management will be paramount for success.

Keywords: awake spine surgery, spinal anesthesia, regional anesthesia, general anesthesia, airway management

Key Points

- Spinal techniques used in awake spinal surgery have been well established to be safe for surgery.
- There are many benefits of awake spinal surgery, including decreased fatigue, improved hemodynamic control, better postoperative pain management, shorter length of procedure and length of stay, decreased postoperative nausea and vomiting, improved patient and surgeon satisfaction, faster time to ambulation, and lower risk of urinary retention.
- Patient selection and a standardized protocol are critical aspects of developing an awake program.
- Recognizing potential airway risk and having an established emergency airway management are critical to complication avoidance in awake spine surgery.

21.1 Introduction

Low back pain is a leading cause of disability worldwide, with a high global point prevalence of 7.5%.[1] The total number of patients living with low back pain has risen considerably in recent years from under 400 million in 1990 to more than 600 million by 2017, with the highest prevalence observed in Southern Latin America and the lowest in East Asia. Compared with nonoperative treatment, spine surgery offers significant advantages of reducing symptoms and disability, with self-rated improvements noted at 2 and 4 years after initiation of therapy.[2] The number of elective spine surgeries performed annually has therefore exponentially increased in recent years, and spine surgery has emerged as one of the most rapidly growing categories of surgical procedures.[3]

Owing to significant advancements in surgical techniques and an aging demographic, the eligibility for spine surgery has considerably broadened in recent years. However, despite the reported advantages of spine surgery over nonoperative treatment approaches, many patients report poorer physical and mental functioning postsurgery. Nearly half of operated patients continue to report persistent pain, disability, and a poor quality of life, and many of these patients require reoperations for persistent back pain. This phenomenon, coupled with the increased susceptibility of older patients to postoperative cognitive decline, has propelled a growing interest among patients in exploring alternative anesthetic options to general anesthesia. The reasons are multifaceted, encompassing concerns over the side effects of general anesthesia, the desire for quicker recovery times, and the wish to avoid cognitive impairments.

Patients undergoing surgical treatment for spine surgery have two anesthetic options, each offering its potential advantages and disadvantages (▸ Fig. 21.1). The first option, general anesthesia, has historically been the most common approach due to its high level of patient acceptance and awareness (i.e., most patients presenting for spine surgery expect that they will receive general anesthesia), its ability to facilitate the surgeons extending the duration of surgery, and

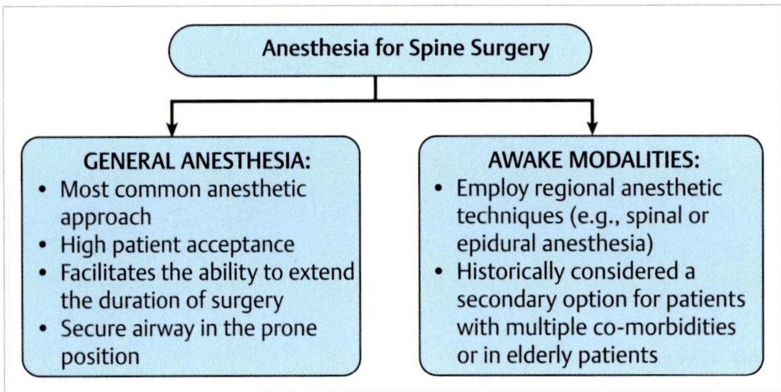

Fig. 21.1 Anesthetic options for spine surgery patients include general anesthesia and awake modalities that employ regional (i.e., neuraxial) anesthetic techniques.

because it allows for the placement of a secure airway device while the patient is positioned prone. Alternatively, awake spine surgery modalities employ regional anesthetic techniques (e.g., spinal or epidural anesthesia) and have historically been considered a secondary option for patients with multiple comorbidities or in elderly patients.

In this chapter, we will explore the nuances of awake spine surgery as an alternative to general anesthesia. Specifically, we will discuss the historical context of spinal anesthesia for spine surgery, how awake spine surgery is performed, clinical outcomes that compare awake spine surgery with general anesthesia, potential drawbacks of awake spine surgery, and emergency management approaches. Finally, we will discuss the logistics of starting an awake spine surgery program, including establishing an awake spine anesthetic protocol.

21.2 Historical Context

- The origins of local anesthetics can be traced to the mid-19th century with the isolation of cocaine, the first effective local anesthetic.
- German chemist Friedrich Gaedcke (1928–1890) was the first to isolate cocaine, the active ingredient in coca leaves, in 1855.
- Austrian ophthalmologist Karl Koller (1857–1944) is credited with the clinical introduction of cocaine as a local anesthetic in 1884, in which he used cocaine for eye surgery. He highlighted cocaine's efficacy in numbing the eye without affecting the patient's consciousness.
- American neurologist James Leonard Corning (1855–1923) is credited with performing the first spinal anesthetic. He injected cocaine between the vertebrae of a dog to produce temporary paralysis, and later, he applied this technique to a human patient to relieve pain from spinal neurosis.
- German surgeon August Bier (1861–1949) is recognized for successfully performing the first documented clinical application of spinal anesthesia in 1898. He described a technique in which he administered cocaine intrathecally to a 34-year-old patient with tuberculosis undergoing an ankle resection.[4]
- By the early 1950s, spinal anesthesia had considerably evolved and was commonly performed for various surgical procedures, including lumbar spine surgery.
- The earliest descriptions of spinal anesthesia for spine surgery in 1952 reported successful lumbar spine surgeries performed after a single spinal injection of tetracaine.[5,6]
- In 1959, American anesthesiologist John Ditzler published a landmark paper that detailed the use of hyperbaric spinal anesthesia in surgery for a herniated intervertebral disk, in which he retrospectively compared the outcomes of 766 patients undergoing spinal anesthesia with 333 general anesthetics administered over a 20-year span.[7]
- Epidural anesthesia has been investigated in limited situations due to its ability to provide continuous pain relief in the perioperative period and the capacity for careful dose adjustment.[8]
- Despite these potential advantages, the adoption of epidural anesthesia in spine surgery has been significantly limited by concerns for increased infection risk, risk of epidural bleeding at the operative site, and difficulty assessing the patient's neurological status after surgery.[9]

- For select surgical procedures, such as endoscopic lumbar decompression surgery, alternative awake spine surgery techniques, such as combining conscious sedation and local anesthesia (without neuraxial blockade), have also been recently described.[10]
- The period from 1950s to the early 2000s reflects broader shifts in anesthetic practices, surgical techniques, and patient care paradigms and marks a transition from the use of spinal anesthesia without any sedation to a more sophisticated, multimodal approach that incorporates preemptive analgesia and moderate sedation alongside spinal anesthesia.
- Early descriptive studies focused primarily on spinal technique, postoperative recovery times, and avoiding complications related to general anesthesia.[11,12,13,14,15,16,17,18]
- Awake spine surgery modalities were generally reserved for patients deemed high risk for general anesthesia due to coexisting medical conditions.
- By the late 1990s, however, studies began to emerge demonstrating some potential benefits of awake spine surgery under spinal anesthesia compared with general anesthesia.[19]
- Studies have demonstrated that awake surgery with spinal anesthesia results in better hemodynamic stability, less mortality, less intraoperative blood loss due to sympathetic blockade and lower intrathoracic pressures, reduced risk of venous thrombosis, lower rates of postoperative renal failure, and improved postoperative cognition.[20,21,22]
- Spinal anesthesia is currently a commonly used technique for a wide range of surgical procedures, particularly those below the umbilicus, including many orthopaedic procedures, vascular and endovascular surgery, urological surgery, gynecological surgeries including cesarean sections, pain management during vaginal birth and delivery, and lower abdominal procedures including hernia surgeries (▶ Table 21.1). A recent compilation of nine Cochrane systemic reviews concluded that awake surgery with neuraxial anesthesia offers significant advantages over general anesthesia, including potentially reducing 30-day mortality rates.[21]
- The evolution and expansion of spinal anesthesia across various surgical domains have recently sparked increasing interest. The recent COVID-19 pandemic further underscored the value and interest of spinal anesthesia in spine surgery, in which critical resources such as ventilators and hospital beds were limited.[23,24]
- Moreover, in response to the current opioid crisis, several states have implemented stricter legislation governing the prescription of narcotics. In recent years, surgeons have been more inclined to consider minimally invasive surgical approaches combined with multimodal analgesic strategies, including the adoption of awake spine surgery techniques, such as a comprehensive approach to these legislative changes.[25]

Table 21.1 Modern uses of spinal anesthesia

Modern uses of spinal anesthesia
• Orthopaedic surgery
• Vascular and endovascular surgery
• Urological surgery
• Cesarean sections
• Pain management during vaginal birth and delivery
• Examinations under anesthesia
• Hernia surgery

Note: Spinal anesthesia is a versatile and widely used technique in regional anesthesia that has been applied to a broad spectrum of surgical procedures, typically below the umbilicus. Some of the procedures that can benefit from spinal anesthesia are listed in the table.

21.3 Benefits of Awake Spine Surgery

The literature on awake spine surgery has significantly evolved marking a shift from initial demonstrations of safety, leading some experts to question whether awake anesthetic modalities should become the standard of care in the future for selected spine surgeries.[26,27] To date, several outcome variables have been examined, with significant insights gained about their potential advantages and limitations. A summary of the potential benefits of awake spine surgery is presented in ▶ Table 21.2.

Table 21.2 Potential benefits of awake spine surgery under spinal anesthesia compared to general anesthesia

Perioperative metric	Conclusions of systematic reviews
Benefits of awake spine surgery	
Safety profiles	Fewer postoperative complications associated with awake spine surgery under spinal anesthesia compared with general anesthesia (OR: 0.29; 95% CI: 0.16–0.53; $p < 0.00001$)[49]
Postoperative pain	Reduced pain scores in awake spine surgery with spinal anesthesia compared to spine surgery done under general anesthesia (MD: −2.80; 95% CI: −4.55 to −1.06; $p = 0.002$)[49]
Postoperative analgesic requirements	Reduced analgesic requirements in awake spine surgery with spinal anesthesia compared to spine done surgery under general anesthesia (OR: 0.06; 95% CI: 0.02–0.25; $p > 0.00001$)[49]
Costs	Reduced costs in awake spine surgery with spinal anesthesia compared to spine surgery done under general anesthesia (MD: −226.14; 95% CI: −0324.73 to −127.55; $p < 0.00001$)[49]
Postoperative nausea and vomiting (PONV)	Reduced PONV in awake spine surgery with spinal anesthesia compared to spine surgery done under general anesthesia (RR: 0.60; 95% CI: 0.39–0.90)[67]
Anesthesia times	Reduced anesthesia times for awake spine surgery with spinal anesthesia compared to spine surgery done under general anesthesia for lumbar laminectomies (MD: −26.53; 95% CI: −38.16 to −14.49; $p = 000001$) and lumbar laminectomies (MD: −11.21; 95% CI: −19.66 to −2.75; $p = 0.009$)[49]
Operative times	Shorter operative times for awake spine surgery with spinal anesthesia compared to spine surgery done under general anesthesia (MD: −14.94; 95% CI: −20.43 to −9.45; $p < 0.00001$)[49]
Blood loss	Reduced blood loss in awake spine surgery with spinal anesthesia compared to spine surgery done under general anesthesia (MD: −52.36; 95% CI: −81.55 to −23.17; $p = 0.00004$)[49]
Hospital length of stay	Reduced hospital length of stay in awake spine surgery with spinal anesthesia compared to spine surgery done under general anesthesia (MD: 0.61; 95% CI: −0.29 to −0.03; $p = 0.02$)[49]
Urinary retention	Reduced postoperative urinary retention in awake spine surgery with spinal anesthesia compared to spine surgery done under general anesthesia (RR: 0.61; 95% CI: 0.37–0.99)[67]
Mixed results	
Surgeon satisfaction	Mixed results
Postanesthesia care unit recovery times	Mixed results
Hemodynamic effects	Mixed results
Limited data	
Patient satisfaction	Limited data suggest higher patient satisfaction in awake spine surgery with spinal anesthesia compared to spine surgery done under spinal anesthesia
Deep vein thrombosis (DVT)	Limited data suggest a lower risk of DVT in awake spine surgery with spinal anesthesia compared to spine surgery done under spinal anesthesia

(Continued)

Table 21.2 *(Continued)* Potential benefits of awake spine surgery under spinal anesthesia compared to general anesthesia

Perioperative metric	Conclusions of systematic reviews
Carbon footprint	Limited data suggest a lower carbon footprint in awake spine surgery with spinal anesthesia than in spine surgery done under spinal anesthesia
Time to mobilization	Limited data suggest potential faster mobilization or no differences in awake spine surgery with spinal anesthesia compared to surgery done under general anesthesia
Fatigue and quality of life	Limited data suggest a potential reduction in postoperative fatigue in awake spine surgery with spinal anesthesia compared to surgery done under general anesthesia
Cognition	Limited data suggest no differences in cognition in awake spine surgery with spinal anesthesia compared to surgery done under general anesthesia

Abbreviations: CI, confidence interval; MD, mean difference; OR, odds ratio; RR, relative risk.

21.3.1 Safety of Awake Spine Surgery

- The earliest foundational studies demonstrated safety, reliability, and effectiveness without significantly increasing complication rates in herniated disk surgeries, establishing awake spine surgery as a viable alternative to general anesthesia.[7,17]
- Retrospective studies and prospective randomized controlled trials have consistently demonstrated that awake spine surgery has similar complication rates to those under general anesthesia across various procedures, including spondylosis, endoscopic lumbar fusion, transforaminal lumbar interbody fusion (TLIF), diskectomy and microdiskectomy, and spinal tumor resection.[28,29,30,31,32,33,34,35,36,37,38]
- Similar complication rates for awake spine surgery and spine surgery under general anesthesia have been demonstrated in elderly patients[39,40,41] and those with multiple comorbidities, including obesity, anxiety, and obstructive sleep apnea (OSA).[42,43]
- The safety and reliability of awake spine surgery were demonstrated in high-risk patients (American Society of Anesthesiologists [ASA] class III or IV), with a high rate of patient and surgeon satisfaction.[44] Single case reports have further demonstrated the safety and efficacy of awake spine surgery for select, very high-risk patients, including a patient with severe cardiac disease[34] and in a 4-week pregnant patient.[45]
- Awake spine surgery techniques have recently been successfully applied in more complex scenarios, including reoperations and multilevel operations, further evidenced by similar complications and revision rates.[30,46]
- Reflecting on the unique challenges posed by the recent COVID-19 pandemic, recent retrospective studies have highlighted the benefits of spinal anesthesia in awake lumbar spine surgeries, such as shorter hospital stays, no readmissions, high patient satisfaction, and effective pain management.[47,48]
- A recent systematic review and meta-analysis reported that awake spine surgery with spinal anesthesia was associated with fewer postoperative complications compared to spine surgery done under general anesthesia, with an odds ratio of 0.29 and 95% confidence interval of 0.16 to 0.53 ($p < 0.00001$).[49] These findings underscore the broader applicability and benefits of awake spine surgery, supporting its role as a feasible alternative to general anesthesia for various surgeries and patient populations.

21.3.2 Hemodynamic Effects

- The assessment of hemodynamic effects during awake spine surgery under spinal anesthesia versus general anesthesia has yielded mixed outcomes.
- Several studies have demonstrated better hemodynamic stability in awake spine surgery patients compared to general anesthesia across a broad spectrum of lumbar spine surgeries, with fewer observed intraoperative hypotensive episodes, intraoperative blood pressure and

heart rate changes, and vasopressor and fluid requirements.[46,50,51,52,53]

- Other studies demonstrated similar intraoperative hemodynamics or less hemodynamic stability in patients undergoing awake spine surgery under spinal anesthesia, with lower heart rates and mean arterial pressures observed in awake spine patients in the immediate postoperative period.[32,35,54]

21.3.3 Postoperative Pain and Analgesic Requirements

- The localized nature of spinal anesthesia, which might reduce the physiological stress response and inflammation associated with surgery, has led many experts to hypothesize that awake spine surgery under spinal anesthesia results in better pain control and reduced analgesic requirements, especially in the immediate postoperative period.
- Moreover, a reduction in the use of systemic opioids and other analgesics might lead to fewer side effects such as nausea, vomiting, and sedation, potentially facilitating a faster recovery.
- Better pain control in the early postoperative period might also contribute to higher patient satisfaction rates and earlier mobilization.
- Several studies have shown that patients undergoing awake spine surgery under spinal anesthesia have lower pain scores in the immediate postoperative period. For example, patients undergoing lumbar laminectomy showed lower peak pain scores in the postanesthesia care unit (PACU) in patients who underwent awake spine surgery with spinal anesthesia compared with general anesthesia.[54] Similar trends were demonstrated with patients undergoing lumbar disk surgery and fusions.[31,32,50,53]
- Several studies have also demonstrated a reduction in analgesic requirements in patients who underwent awake spine surgery with spinal anesthesia compared with patients who had general anesthesia.[50,54,55,56,57,58]
- Although no significant differences were observed in postoperative analgesic requirements or pain between patients undergoing spinal anesthesia for lumbar disk surgery and those under general anesthesia,[35] there was reduced need for an additional dose of intraoperative fentanyl in patients undergoing awake spine surgery.
- The reduction in pain and postoperative analgesic requirements might be short-lived and typically does not persist beyond the immediate postoperative period.[30,46,54]
- A systematic review and meta-analysis reported that awake spine surgery with spinal anesthesia was associated with an overall reduction in pain scores compared to spine surgery done under general anesthesia with a mean difference of –2.80 and 95% confidence interval of –4.55 to –1.06 ($p = 0.002$).[49]
- The same systematic review and meta-analysis further demonstrated that awake spine surgery with spinal anesthesia was associated with reduced analgesic requirements compared with traditional spine surgery under general anesthesia, with an odds ratio of 0.06 and 95% confidence interval of 0.02 to 0.25 ($p > 0.00001$).
- Although differences in pain management and analgesic requirements are unlikely to persist beyond the immediate postoperative period, these differences are still clinically relevant for several reasons. First, the early postoperative period is critical for patient recovery, and effective pain management during this phase can significantly influence the overall recovery trajectory. Moreover, reduced pain and lower analgesic needs can facilitate earlier mobilization, which is vital for preventing deep vein thrombosis (DVT) and pulmonary complications. Better pain control and fewer analgesic requirements can also result in fewer opioid-related side effects, improved patient satisfaction, and faster recovery times.

21.3.4 Surgeon Satisfaction

Surgeon satisfaction with awake spine surgery under spinal anesthesia versus general anesthesia is an important consideration that can significantly influence the choice of anesthetic technique.

- Retrospective studies and randomized controlled trials have both demonstrated variability in surgeon preferences, with some studies reporting higher surgeon satisfaction with awake spine surgery under spinal anesthesia[50,57] and other studies demonstrating a preference for spine surgery under general anesthesia.[32,55,59]

- The varying preferences of surgeons are likely dependent on multiple factors. For example, surgeons more experienced with awake spine surgery techniques might be more comfortable managing the intraoperative dynamics of an awake patient.
- Their satisfaction could stem from positive outcomes and patient feedback they have encountered. By contrast, surgeons less familiar with or trained in managing awake procedures might lean more toward general anesthesia, where the controlled environment of an unconscious patient reduces the variables they must manage during the surgery, such as patient movement and anxiety.
- The availability of a skilled anesthesiology team experienced in managing spinal anesthesia can also influence a surgeon's preference. Surgeons might be more satisfied with awake spine surgery if they trust their anesthesia colleagues to manage patient comfort effectively during the operation.
- Institutional protocols and the availability of necessary staff and equipment to support awake patients can also play an important role, and surgeons with well-equipped settings are more likely to report satisfaction with awake procedures.

21.3.5 Patient Satisfaction

- Although limited studies have focused specifically on patient preference in this context, patient satisfaction is high for awake spine surgery under spinal anesthesia.[57]
- A single randomized controlled trial demonstrated that patient satisfaction was higher for those who underwent awake lumbar disk surgery with spinal anesthesia compared to those who received general anesthesia.[35] Although these studies provide valuable insights into patient perspectives, it is essential to note that these preferences might be subject to various biases,[60] including influences from surgeon preference and the underlying reasons for avoiding general anesthesia.

21.3.6 Costs and Carbon Footprint

The rising costs of health care and increasing environmental concerns have prompted a reassessment of current medical practices, including surgical interventions. Many experts have called for efforts to cut down costs, environmental waste, and the overall carbon footprint.[61]

- Reduction in costs associated with awake spine surgery compared to general anesthesia can be attributed to several factors, including reduced hospital stay and resource utilization, increased operating room efficiency, and turnover.
- General anesthesia typically requires a combination of drugs that include anesthetics, muscle relaxants, and opioids, which are most expensive compared to spinal anesthesia.
- Several studies have demonstrated a reduction in anesthetic, and total costs were lower in patients undergoing spinal anesthesia for spine surgery compared to those who received general anesthesia.[32,35,37,46,55,62] This cost reduction associated with awake spine surgery was demonstrated for direct and indirect health care costs.
- A systematic review and meta-analysis reported that awake spine surgery with spinal anesthesia was associated with an overall reduction in costs compared to spine surgery done under general anesthesia, with a mean difference of −226.14 and 95% confidence interval of −0324.73 to −127.55 ($p < 0.00001$).[49]
- Concerning the environmental impact, general anesthesia typically requires more disposable items, including breathing circuits, carbon dioxide absorbers, and various single-use instruments, all contributing to medical waste.
- By contrast, spinal anesthesia simplifies the setup, markedly reducing the quantity of waste generated during each surgery.
- Moreover, anesthetic gases like desflurane and nitrous oxide have global warming potential, and reducing their use not only diminishes direct emissions but also aligns with broader goals to cut health care–related contributions to climate change.[63]
- A recent study has confirmed a marked reduction in the environmental carbon footprint associated with awake spine surgery under spinal anesthesia compared to general anesthesia.[64,65]

21.3.7 Postoperative Nausea and Vomiting

Reducing postoperative nausea and vomiting (PONV) is a significant benefit, as it enhances patient comfort and satisfaction and expedites recovery and discharge processes. Moreover, a reduction in PONV results in a decreased need for antiemetic medications, which avoids the side effects of these drugs, including drowsiness and further gastrointestinal disturbances. Several contributing factors are thought to contribute to the reduced PONV observed in awake spine surgery patients, including avoidance of volatile anesthetic agents and reduction of opioids, both of which are associated with PONV, more stable hemodynamics, and reduced stress response to surgery.

- Awake spine surgery has been shown to reduce the incidence of severe nausea compared with general anesthesia,[19,46] especially in the first 24 hours after surgery.[54]
- Awake spine surgery patients had fewer antiemetic requirements than those under general anesthesia.[57,66]
- A single retrospective case series demonstrated no differences in nausea rates between awake lumbar spine surgery under spinal anesthesia and that under general anesthesia.[53]
- The most recent systematic review and meta-analysis to date reported that awake spine surgery with spinal anesthesia was associated with an overall reduction in PONV compared to spine surgery done under general anesthesia, with a relative risk of 0.60 and 95% confidence interval of 0.39 to 0.90.[67]

21.3.8 Anesthesia, Surgical, and Operating Room Times

In evaluating the impact of anesthetic technique on anesthesia, surgical, and operating times for spine surgery, evidence from multiple studies present a somewhat mixed but favorable view toward awake spine surgery, particularly noting its potential for reducing various time metrics compared to general anesthesia.

- Several studies have reported shorter anesthesia and surgical times for patients undergoing awake spine surgery with spinal anesthesia.[31,32,46,54,56,57,62,66,68]
- These trends were further highlighted in elderly patients who underwent spinal anesthesia for lumbar decompression compared with general anesthesia.[39]
- Other studies found no differences in operative times between awake lumbar spine surgery with spinal anesthesia compared with that under general anesthesia,[30,32,53,58] although shorter anesthesia times between groups were observed in some of these studies.[55]
- A recent systematic review and meta-analysis reported that awake spine surgery with spinal anesthesia was associated with an overall reduction in total anesthesia time for both lumbar discectomies (mean difference of −26.53 and 95% confidence interval of −38.16 to −14.49; $p = 000001$) and lumbar laminectomies (mean difference of −11.21 and 95% confidence interval of −19.66 to −2.75; $p = 0.009$), as well as shorter operative times (mean difference of −14.94 and 95% confidence interval of −20.43 to −9.45; $p < 0.00001$).[49]
- The reduction in perioperative time metrics could be due to several factors. First, spinal anesthesia typically requires less time for induction, and it can similarly allow patients to recover much faster at the end of the surgery, facilitating earlier transfer from the operating room.
- Spinal anesthesia can contribute to the efficiency of the surgery itself due to time constraints associated with the duration of local anesthetic action. Shorter anesthesia times can also lead to quicker turnover between surgeries, enhancing operating room efficiency.
- These findings suggest that awake spine surgery with spinal anesthesia enhances the patient's immediate recovery experience and contributes to broader operational efficiencies within surgical practices.

21.3.9 Deep Vein Thrombosis

The potential reduction in the risk of DVT in patients undergoing awake spine surgery versus those receiving general anesthesia is another important metric of interest in surgical medicine.

- A recent large retrospective study demonstrated significantly less incidence of DVT in patients who underwent spine surgery under spinal anesthesia compared those who received general anesthesia.[19]
- While data on DVT risk are limited, the theoretical advantages of spinal anesthesia in reducing DVT risk can be substantial, based on known physiological response and patient recovery profiles, including earlier mobilization, more stable hemodynamics and avoidance of the activation of the coagulation system that is associated with general anesthesia and surgery.

21.3.10 Blood Loss

Blood loss during spine surgery is a significant concern that can impact postoperative recovery, the need for blood transfusions, and overall patient outcomes.

- Most studies to date have demonstrated that awake spine surgery under spinal anesthesia results in less blood loss compared with spine surgery performed under general anesthesia,[32,39,50,62,69] with a reduced need for blood transfusions and volume supplementation.[46,53]
- Possible mechanisms for reduced blood loss in awake spine surgery under spinal anesthesia include the sympathetic blockade associated with spinal anesthesia, which can decrease the force of blood flow, reduce surgical bleeding, and reduce venous pressure at the surgical site.
- Other studies failed to demonstrate any differences between the two anesthetic techniques.[30,55] These conflicting findings might be due to differences in surgical technique and experience among surgeons in different study groups, individual patient factors, and the type of surgical procedure, potentially impacting surgical blood loss.
- When combining all the studies that have been performed to date, a recent systematic review and meta-analysis reported that awake spine surgery with spinal anesthesia was associated with an overall reduction in blood loss compared to spine surgery done under general anesthesia, with a mean difference of −52.36 and 95% confidence interval of −81.55 to −23.17 ($p = 0.00004$).[49]

21.3.11 Hospital Length of Stay

The hospital length of stay (LOS) following spine surgery is a critical metric influencing health care costs, patient satisfaction, and resource allocation.

- Several studies have demonstrated that awake spine surgery under spinal anesthesia can significantly reduce the LOS compared to traditional spine surgery under general anesthesia.[28,58,62,68,69]
- This trend was also demonstrated in elderly patients who underwent awake spine surgery under spinal anesthesia versus general anesthesia for lumbar decompression.[39] Factors associated with a reduced hospital LOS associated with awake spine surgery include faster recovery from anesthesia, reduced incidence of PONV and other complications associated with general anesthesia, and enhanced pain management.
- Some studies report no differences in hospital LOS between spinal anesthesia and general anesthesia for spine surgery,[36,53,54,55] which can be attributed to institutional protocols and discharge criteria, patient demographics and health status differences between different study populations, and the nature and duration of the surgery studied.
- A recent systematic review and meta-analysis reported that awake spine surgery with spinal anesthesia was associated with an overall reduction in hospital LOS compared to spine surgery done under general anesthesia, with a mean difference of −0.61 and 95% confidence interval of −0.29 to −0.03 ($p = 0.02$).[49]

21.3.12 Postanesthesia Care Unit Admission Times

The PACU admission time is a critical phase in the recovery process, reflecting how quickly patients recover from anesthesia and are ready to move on to the next stage of care.

- A limited number of studies have shown that patients undergoing awake spine surgery under spinal anesthesia experience shorter PACU times than those receiving general anesthesia.[46,53,55] These studies highlight the benefit of spinal anesthesia in facilitating quicker recovery from anesthesia, allowing patients to meet discharge criteria from the PACU sooner.
- A few studies have indicated no differences in PACU admission times between awake spine surgery patients and those who underwent general anesthesia or longer PACU admission times associated with awake spine surgery under spinal anesthesia.[32,57]
- The individual variability in findings across studies underscores the influence of other variables such as surgical technique, patient demographics and health between study populations, and differences in PACU discharge protocols.
- Most evidence suggests that awake spine surgery with spinal anesthesia tends to result in shorter PACU times. This reduction might be due to the nature of spinal anesthesia, which

can facilitate faster recovery compared with general anesthesia, reduced incidence of early postoperative complications, PONV, and more effective pain management with earlier mobilization after surgery.

21.3.13 Urinary Retention

- Postoperative urinary retention (PUR) is a common and significant concern after elective spine surgery. PUR can significantly impact patient comfort and overall recovery, including prolonged hospital admission times.
- Spinal anesthesia can potentially reduce the risk of PUR by several mechanisms, including less autonomic nervous system interference with spinal anesthetics compared to general anesthetics, faster mobility, and a reduction in the duration of surgery.
- Some studies have reported significantly lower rates of urinary retention in patients undergoing decompressive lumbar spine surgery and lumbar microdiskectomy under spinal anesthesia compared to those who received general anesthesia.[56,57]
- A prospective, nonrandomized study in patients undergoing elective spine surgery demonstrated that awake surgery with spinal anesthesia was independently associated with a lower incidence of PUR than surgery under general anesthesia, even after adjusting for potential confounding risk factors.[70]
- Some studies have found no differences in the incidence of urinary retention between spinal and general anesthesia in patients undergoing lumbar laminectomy and lumbar disk surgery,[35,54] suggesting that other perioperative factors may play a more critical role in developing PUR after spine surgery.
- A recent systematic review and meta-analysis reported that awake spine surgery with spinal anesthesia was associated with an overall reduction in urinary retention compared to spine surgery done under general anesthesia, with a relative risk of 0.61 and 95% confidence interval of 0.37 to 0.99.[67]

21.3.14 Time to Mobilization

The time to mobilization after spine surgery is a critical factor in patient recovery, influencing outcomes such as the risk of complications, overall patient satisfaction, and length of hospital stay.

- Faster mobilization was demonstrated for awake spine surgery patients undergoing spinal fusions.[31,58]
- However, one randomized controlled trial observed no differences in the time to mobilization between patients undergoing spinal anesthesia for lumbar disk surgery and those under general anesthesia.[35]
- While evidence suggests that spinal anesthesia might facilitate faster mobilization after certain types of spine surgeries, such as lumbar spine fusion, the overall impact of anesthetic technique on mobilization times can vary and should be further examined in future studies.

21.3.15 Fatigue and Quality of Life

- Postoperative fatigue is a common and significant concern after lumbar spine surgery, as it can significantly affect a patient's overall recovery trajectory and quality of life after surgery.[59]
- A single prospective, nonrandomized study demonstrated that patients who underwent spinal anesthesia for awake lumbar spine surgery had less fatigue and increased quality of life 1 month after surgery compared to patients who underwent general anesthesia.[71]
- Although the data on quality of life are limited, awake spine surgery with spinal anesthesia might reduce the intensity and duration of postoperative fatigue, thereby supporting a better overall recovery and enhanced quality of life.

21.3.16 Cognition

- Cognition after spine surgery is a significant concern, and cognitive function can be impacted by various factors related to the surgical and anesthetic techniques used.
- De Biase et al demonstrated that patients who underwent spinal anesthesia for awake lumbar spine surgery had similar cognitive function 1 month after surgery compared to patients who underwent general anesthesia.[71]

21.4 Practical Considerations and Perioperative Approach

Although the literature provides limited guidance on when regional anesthesia might be preferable over general anesthesia, successfully awake spine surgery hinges on careful patient selection. Moreover, specific clinical scenarios might favor awake spine surgery, especially for patients at higher risk of general anesthesia complications or for whom a faster postoperative recovery associated with awake spine surgery is desirable. In addition to choosing the appropriate patient, awake spine surgery requires a highly skilled surgical team and proficient anesthesia team, with each component playing a critical role in the safe and effective execution of awake spine surgery.

21.4.1 Patient Selection

- Patients with significant comorbidities, such as respiratory or cardiovascular conditions, may benefit from awake spine surgery because it avoids potential complications related to general anesthesia, including hemodynamic instability and postoperative cognitive dysfunction.
- Some patients have a strong preference to avoid general anesthesia, making awake spine surgery an attractive alternative anesthetic approach.
- Patient refusal is the only absolute contraindication for awake spine surgery with spinal anesthesia, while several relative contraindications should be considered when planning an awake spine procedure (▶ Table 21.3).
- An anticipated easy spinal insertion increases the likelihood of successful awake spine surgery without converting to general anesthesia. For example, a history of previous spine surgeries is not considered a contraindication to awake spine surgery but can have important implications for planning the anesthetic approach.[72] Anatomical landmarks for placing spinal anesthesia can be altered, making it more challenging to accurately and safely insert the spinal needle. Moreover, scar tissue can form externally around the vertebrae and muscles and internally within the dural sac.[73]
- Some studies have reported a 100% success rate in patients with a history of lumbar spine surgery undergoing awake spine surgery under spinal anesthesia,[74] leading to the conclusion that prior spine surgery should not be viewed as a contraindication to awake spine surgery.

Table 21.3 Absolute and relative contraindications to awake spine surgery under spinal anesthesia

Absolute contraindications	Relative contraindication
Patient refusal	Anxiety or severe claustrophobia
	High risk of airway compromise
	Coagulopathy
	Preload-dependent states
	Undetermined neurological disease

21.4.2 Surgical Indications

- The types of surgeries described for awake spine surgery have evolved with time, with the earliest applications of awake spine surgery primarily limited to herniated disk surgery and lumbar laminectomies.[7,14]
- As the benefits of awake spine surgery became more apparent and anesthesiologists and surgeons have grown more comfortable with awake anesthetic approaches, the range of spine surgeries performed under these conditions has expanded (▶ Table 21.4). Extension of awake anesthesia techniques to minimally invasive spine surgery such as TLIF combines the advantages of awake surgery with the many benefits demonstrated by minimally invasive surgical approaches, including less disruption of the musculoskeletal structures surrounding the

Table 21.4 Surgical indications for awake spine surgery

Surgical indications for awake spine surgery
• Diskectomy and microdiscectomy
• Lumbar decompression • Laminectomy
• Fusion surgery, including minimally invasive transforaminal lumbar interbody fusion (TLIF)
• Percutaneous vertebroplasty
• Spinal tumor surgery

Note: Awake spine surgery has been applied to various spine surgical procedures, demonstrating its versatility and adaptability. It is typically reserved for shorter lumbar spine surgeries that are associated with a low expected risk of blood loss. Some of the spine surgical procedures are listed in the table.

spine, smaller incisions, less postoperative pain, and less blood loss.[75]

- Awake spine surgery has also been described for spine tumor resection[34,76] and percutaneous vertebroplasty,[77] and has even been successfully described in a first-term pregnant patient undergoing lumbar microdiskectomy.[45]
- Some experts have extended awake spine surgery to include the lower thoracic region, demonstrating favorable outcomes.[78]
- Although the time constraints of spinal anesthesia have historically limited awake spine surgery to one or two vertebral levels, successful awake spine fusion surgery has been demonstrated to include up to five vertebral levels.[79]

21.4.3 Spinal Technique

- Spinal anesthesia is a regional anesthetic method that involves injecting a local anesthetic into the cerebrospinal fluid (CSF) in the subarachnoid space, resulting in a reversible block of central nerve impulses.
- Positioning for the spinal procedure should be done with the patient's comfort in mind while maintaining optimal spine curvature to facilitate needle placement.
- Plain isobaric bupivacaine effectively creates a robust surgical block, making it a popular local anesthetic choice for awake spine surgery.[16,18,80]
- Mepivacaine produces a surgical block that is equal to bupivacaine in quality but has a much shorter duration of action. Mepivacaine is, therefore, often reserved for shorter (< 2 hours) awake spine surgeries.
- Some protocols have advocated for adding fentanyl to the block to increase the duration of the spinal's analgesic effects, but this can be associated with pruritus, and we typically avoid it in our practice.
- Achieving adequate pain control extends beyond the surgical procedure itself and involves a carefully coordinated regiment of additional analgesics to manage the discomfort that the spinal block alone might not fully address (► Fig. 21.2).

21.4.4 Preemptive Analgesia

- Effective perioperative pain control is essential for patients undergoing awake spine surgery due to the inherently painful nature of these procedures.
- Inadequate pain control after spine surgery has profound negative implications on the patient's recovery process and has been associated with increased urinary retention[81] and a poor quality of life.[82]
- Given that the analgesic effects of spinal medications are limited in duration, effective pain management strategies must anticipate the emergence of pain as the spinal blockade recedes. This approach not only enhances patient comfort but also contributes to better overall outcomes by mitigating the physiological and psychological impacts of pain.

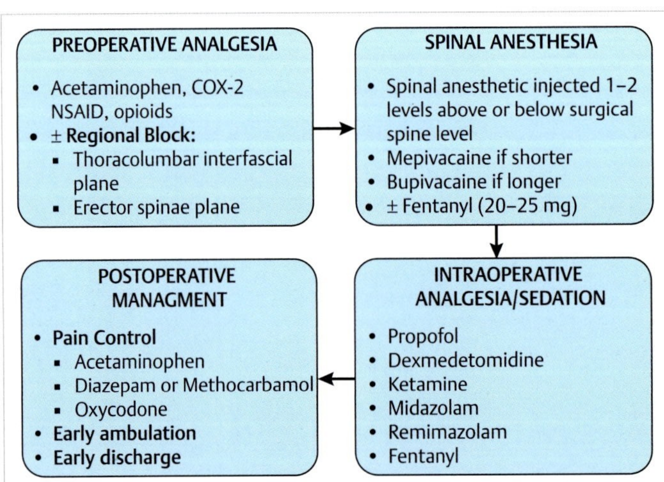

Fig. 21.2 Overview of perioperative considerations and technical approach for awake spine surgery. Successful awake spine surgery requires a comprehensive anesthetic protocol, including pharmacological approaches across different perioperative stages.

- Several pharmacologic approaches targeting different pain pathways have been described with variable effects on recovery after spine surgery. Preemptive treatment with opioids or nonsteroidal anti-inflammatory drugs (NSAIDs) can provide some pain relief in the early postoperative period, but their effects are often short-lived.[83]
- Alternatively, preoperative pregabalin is less sedating and has been associated with reduced early postsurgical pain at rest and with movement, less opioid consumption, and improvements in overall quality of life after spine surgery.[84,85]
- The erector spinae plane (ESP) block is a recent regional anesthesia technique targeting erector spinae muscles and the associated vertebral spaces. This technique involves the injection of local anesthetic into the plane deep into the erector spinae muscle group, which lies close to the transverse processes of the vertebrae. By blocking these nerves, the ESP block can provide extensive analgesia for the lumbar spine region.[86,87,88]
- The use of ESP block for patients undergoing spine surgery has been shown in extensive, prospective studies and meta-analyses to significantly reduce pain scores and opioid requirements in the early postoperative period.[89,90,91,92,93] The ESP block was also associated with a shortened hospital stay in spine surgery patients.[94]
- The broad analgesic coverage and low complication risk associated with ESP blocks have made it an attractive modality for preemptive analgesia in patients undergoing awake spine surgery with spinal anesthesia.[95,96]
- The ESP block with supplemental sedation has also been described as a viable anesthetic option for lumbar decompression surgery, even in the absence of neuraxial blockade.[97]
- An ultrasound-guided thoracolumbar interfascial plane (TLIP) block is another novel regional block technique that might be beneficial for patients undergoing awake spine surgery. A recent prospective, randomized controlled trial demonstrated that bilateral TLIP blocks in patients undergoing lumbar spine surgery resulted in a significant reduction in perioperative opioid and anesthetic consumption and shortened hospital LOS without an increase in complication rates.[98]
- A recent systematic review and meta-analysis[99] concluded that there is moderate-quality evidence that TLIP blocks effectively reduce pain scores at rest and with movement for up to 24 hours after lumbar surgery and reduce the incidence of PONV.

21.4.5 Perioperative Sedation

- Sedation should be minimal to maintain patient cooperation, reduce unintentional movements during surgery, and maintain a patent airway with adequate respirations.[14] ► Table 21.5 summarizes the levels of sedation and perioperative sedation goals for awake spine surgery.
- Preoperative anxiety is common before spine surgery and can be attributed to concerns about the procedure's outcome, potential complications, the prospect of pain, or concerns related to the anesthesia itself.[100]
- Compared with general anesthesia, patients awaiting laminectomy or diskectomy feared spinal surgery more than general anesthesia.[100]
- Recognizing and addressing this anxiety preemptively is vital, regardless of the type of anesthesia chosen for spine surgery. Studies have shown that the perioperative medical staff can play an essential role in reduce patient anxiety levels during the perioperative period.[100]

21.5 Challenges and Additional Considerations

21.5.1 Challenging Spinal Insertion

- Traditional methods of spinal anesthesia rely on palpation and anatomical landmarks to guide needle insertion, which can be particularly challenging in patients with atypical anatomy due to obesity, spinal deformities (e.g., scoliosis), previous spine surgery, or degenerative changes.[73,101,102]
- In patients with scoliosis, a thoracolumbar curve of greater than 50% has been associated with reduced spread of local anesthetic, resulting in a higher likelihood of a unilateral, inadequate, or patchy block.[101]
- Using ultrasound to visualize the spinal structures can significantly enhance the ease

Table 21.5 Levels of sedation and sedation goals during awake spine surgery

Levels of sedation	Responsiveness	Cardiovascular/respiratory function
Minimal sedation	• Normal response to verbal commands	• Cognitive function and coordination might be mildly impaired • Airway reflexes, ventilation, and cardiovascular functions are unaffected
Moderate (i.e., conscious) sedation[a]	• Responds purposefully to verbal commands	• Spontaneous ventilation is adequate • Cardiovascular function is maintained
Deep sedation	• The patient may not respond to verbal commands but might respond purposefully to repeated or painful stimulation	• Spontaneous ventilatory function might be impaired • Assistance might be required to maintain a patent airway • Cardiovascular function is typically maintained
General anesthesia	• The patient is not arousable, even with painful stimulation	• Assistance is often required to maintain a patent airway • Positive pressure ventilation may be required because of depressed spontaneous ventilation or drug-induced depression of neuromuscular function • Cardiovascular function may be impaired

Note: The American Society of Anesthesiologists defines four levels of sedation, each with its distinct characteristics.
[a]The goal of awake spine surgery should be to provide moderate sedation (i.e., conscious sedation) to relieve anxiety while maintaining a patent airway and responsive patient.

and safety of spinal anesthesia,[103] even in patients with poorly palpable surface landmarks or abnormal spinal anatomy.[104] Some studies have also suggested that the use of ultrasound can also be a useful preoperative tool for assessing the feasibility of neuraxial anesthesia when it is expected to be technically challenging.[105,106] Some experts have even suggested that ultrasound use be made mandatory for spinal placement due to its accessibility and ease of use.[107] In contrast, others suggest that it is a valuable technique but not indicated for routine use.[108]

21.5.2 Complications of Spinal Anesthesia

- Postdural puncture headache (PDPH) is the most common complication after spinal anesthesia, resulting from CSF leakage through a puncture hole in the dura mater.
- The incidence of PDPH can vary considerably depending on the relative ease of insertion and the type and diameter of the spinal needle used.[109]
- Rarer complications of spinal anesthesia that have been described in the context of awake spine surgery include pneumocephalus[110] and vasovagal events.[111]

21.5.3 Potential Drawbacks of Awake Spine Surgery

- Trend analyses from the early 2000s to the present day have indicated an increase in the utilization of awake spine surgery, reflecting improvements in surgical outcomes and patient satisfaction.[112]
- Despite these positive trends, the overall proportion of spine surgeries performed using awake techniques remains relatively small. This phenomenon can be attributed to several barriers, including patient perceptions and concerns within the medical community. Understanding these obstacles is critical for addressing them and further increasing the adoption of awake spine surgery practices (▶ Table 21.6).
- One potential drawback of awake spine surgery is the lack of patient awareness and the

Table 21.6 Potential drawbacks to the widespread adoption of awake spine surgery

Potential drawbacks to the widespread adoption of awake spine surgery
• Lack of patient awareness of spinal anesthesia as an anesthetic option
• Less surgeon satisfaction compared to general anesthesia
• Lack of ability to extend the surgery if needed
• Anesthesiologist preference toward general anesthesia due to an established airway in the prone position
• Concerns regarding patient movement and anxiety
• Concerns regarding the length and surgery and the need for redosing spinal medication
• Concerns for possible intraoperative complications and management in an awake patient in the prone position
• Concerns over the logistics of starting an awake spine program
• Concerns over the perceived risks and benefits of awake spine surgery
• Concerns over the learning curve associated with awake spine surgery

Note: Despite more than 70 years of literature encompassing numerous studies and meta-analyses demonstrating its safety and effectiveness, several factors have contributed to the slow integration of awake spine surgery into mainstream practice.

availability of spinal anesthesia as an anesthetic option for spine surgery. A recent study demonstrated that only 16% of patients eligible for awake lumbar spine surgery were aware of the possibility of spinal anesthesia as an anesthetic option until the surgeon discussed this with the patient.[113]

- In addition to a lack of widespread patient knowledge, surgeons' preference for general anesthesia over awake spine surgery has also been shown to impact patient choices. The strong preference of many surgeons for general anesthesia is in part thought to be driven by the lack of randomized control trials and skepticism over the benefits of awake spine surgery compared to general anesthesia.[114]
- Anesthesiologists have expressed similar concerns over the perceived risks of awake spine surgery and the lack of randomized controlled trials, despite numerous moderate-quality evidence that demonstrates outcomes and benefits of an awake spine over general anesthesia approaches.[115] Moreover, managing the airway in a patient under conscious sedation in the prone position can be particularly challenging and complex, whereas general anesthesia offers the advantage of having a controlled airway while in the prone position.
- There is considerable debate over the perceived risks and benefits of awake spine surgery compared with spine surgery under general anesthesia. Although several retrospective studies have demonstrated some advantages of awake spine surgery over general anesthesia, some experts have cautioned against drawing definitive conclusions due to the inherent methodological limitations of these studies, particularly selection bias.[116]
- Moreover, surgical approaches to lumbar spine surgery, especially those involving advanced and minimally invasive techniques, are recognized for their significant learning curves. Owing to the limited duration of analgesia provided by spinal anesthetics, there are concerns about balancing the time necessary to perform these procedures with the effective duration of spinal anesthesia. However, studies have demonstrated a lack of learning curve when spinal anesthesia is adopted for lumbar spine surgery, particularly for experienced surgical and anesthetic teams that are already familiar with managing spinal anesthetic techniques for other procedures.[117]

21.6 Emergency Airway Management

21.6.1 Risks of Airway Compromise

- Emergency airway management in prone spine surgery presents unique challenges,[118] and airway compromise can have significant consequences. Several potential risk factors are associated with airway compromise in awake spine procedures, and each factor should be considered when planning emergency airway management strategies (▸ Fig. 21.3).
- The patient's medical history plays a crucial role in evaluating the risk of airway compromise during awake spine surgery. Patients with a history of anxiety or panic disorders may have heightened sensitivity to the stressors associated with surgery, which can exacerbate their risk of hyperventilation or breath-holding during the procedures, and anxiety can also lead to increased airway reactivity, causing bronchospasm.
- Patients with a history of OSA have a higher risk of airway collapse during sedation due to the relaxation of the pharyngeal muscles. Similarly, congenital or anatomical variations in the airway structure, such as a deviated septum, enlarged tonsils, or previous surgeries, may complicate airway management and should be considered.
- Patients with a history of respiratory conditions such as chronic obstructive pulmonary disease (COPD), asthma, or restrictive lung disease are at increased risk of bronchospasm and hypoventilation, especially when sedatives are used. The importance of close monitoring of breathing patterns and maintaining adequate ventilation without oversedation cannot be overstated.
- Even in the absence of OSA or respiratory conditions, oversedation can decrease the patient's ability to maintain their airway, resulting in potential airway obstruction, hypoventilation, or apnea. It is essential to titrate the sedatives judiciously to a level that reduces anxiety and provides comfort but still allows the patient to maintain airway reflexes and adequate spontaneous breathing.
- Allergic reactions to medications can also lead to airway compromise through mechanisms such as angioedema or anaphylaxis, which can rapidly progress to airway obstruction. The anesthesia team must be prepared to recognize and promptly manage allergic reactions aggressively with medications such as antihistamines, corticosteroids, and epinephrine.

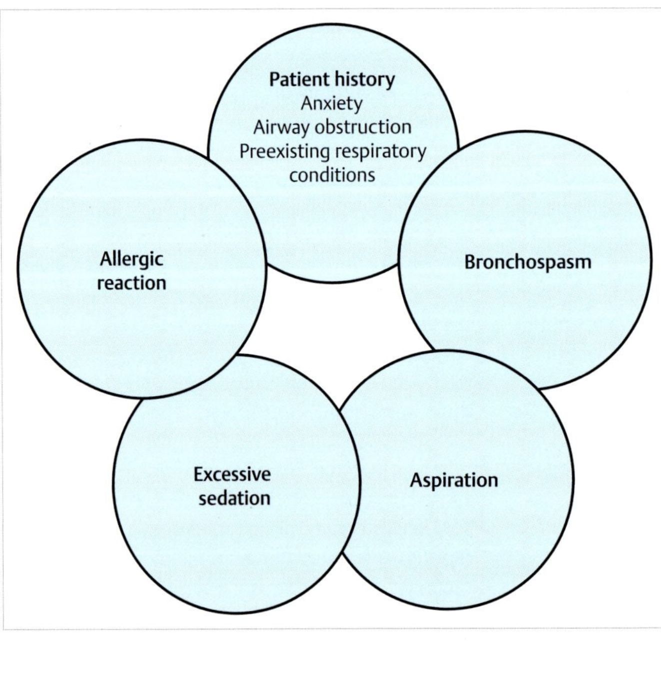

Fig. 21.3 Risk factors associated with airway compromise during awake spine surgery.

- Bronchospasm can result from airway irritation caused by sections, aspiration, or allergic reactions, leading to significant airflow resistance, hypoxia, and hypercapnia. Management includes the administration of bronchodilators, and if severe, advanced airway management techniques may be required.
- Aspiration of gastric contents can also occur during awake spine surgery, particularly if a patient has not fasted appropriately or has gastroesophageal reflux disease (GERD). Aspiration can cause chemical pneumonitis and mechanical obstruction of the airway. Preventive measures include following fasting guidelines and using medications to reduce gastric acidity.

21.6.2 Airway Management

- A comprehensive emergency airway management plan is an integral component of awake spine surgery and requires the coordinated effects of the entire operating room team and thorough preparation to address airway emergencies rapidly and effectively. During an airway emergency, each team member should understand their respective roles (▶ Table 21.7).

Table 21.7 Personnel and their respective roles during an intraoperative airway emergency

Operating room team member	Role in emergency airway management
Surgery team	
Surgeon	• Stop the surgery, remove surgical instruments and pack the wound • Place a sterile dressing over the surgical site
Surgeon assistant	• Aid the surgeon to prepare the patient for supine positioning
Surgical scrub technician	• Assist with removing surgical instruments and provide sterile dressing
Anesthesia team	
Anesthesiologist	• Assess the patient • Notify the surgical team of the airway emergency • Hold the head while the horseshoe or head pillow is removed • Attempt mask ventilation with 100% oxygen • Consider supraglottic airway insertion while waiting for the stretcher • If unsuccessful, all staff should assist in turning the patient supine • Once the patient is turned supine, the anesthesia team should secure the airway
In-room anesthesia provider	• At first signs of airway compromise, stimulate the patient • Increase oxygen flows • Stop all sedation • Call the anesthesiologist for help
Anesthesia technician	• Bring in difficult airway equipment • Prepare airway equipment and have a supraglottic airway ready
Nursing team	
Circulator nurse 1	• Call for additional help, including activating the overhead emergency response system • Bring the stretcher into the room
Circulator nurse 2	• Move equipment out of the way to make room for the incoming stretcher • Aid in removing the arm board • Cut the safety straps off the patient

Note: A comprehensive airway management plan requires the coordinated efforts of the entire operating team, with each team member having a clearly defined role and responsibilities.

- When an airway emergency occurs, all efforts are directed at safely repositioning the patient from the prone or sitting position to supine as quickly as possible, which requires bringing a stretcher into the operating room in a quick and efficient manner.
- The anesthesia team may need to use a laryngeal mask airway (LMA) or another airway device to assist ventilation while waiting for the patient to be moved or as a bridge to a more definitive airway device (i.e., endotracheal tube). Simultaneously, the surgical team must take swift action to cover and protect the port sites or surgical field to maintain sterility while the patient is being repositioned and airway management is conducted.

21.7 Establishing an Awake Spine Program

21.7.1 Establishing an Anesthetic Protocol

- Although no specific comprehensive guidelines have been proposed, some experts have published algorithms[119] and videos[75] that can be especially useful for reducing the learning curve associated with starting an awake spine surgery program.
- These algorithms and protocols were developed through rigorous research and clinical experience, providing a comprehensive framework addressing the technical, clinical, and logistical aspects of awake spine surgery.[24]
- These protocols offer a standardized approach to awake spine surgery, ensuring patients receive care based on best practices and evidence-based medicine. This consistency is vital for maintaining high-quality care across different surgeons and anesthesiologists.

21.8 Conclusions

Awake spine surgery represents a significant advancement in the field of spine surgery, offering a viable alternative to general anesthesia. This technique has demonstrated considerable benefits in terms of safety, efficacy, and feasibility, particularly for patient populations such as the elderly and those with multiple comorbidities. The evolution of awake spine surgery from the early 1950s to the present day highlights its potential to reduce the incidence of perioperative complications, lower health care costs, improve hemodynamic stability, and enhance patient satisfaction. The choice between awake spine surgery under spinal anesthesia and under general anesthesia should ultimately be tailored to the individual patient's needs, surgical requirements, and the expertise of the surgeon and anesthesiologist. Future research and clinical trials will be essential in further delineating the benefits and broadening the applicability of this technique, ensuring that patients receive the most appropriate, safe, and effective care.

References

[1] Wu A, March L, Zheng X, et al. Global low back pain prevalence and years lived with disability from 1990 to 2017: estimates from the Global Burden of Disease Study 2017. Ann Transl Med. 2020; 8(6):299

[2] Weinstein JN, Tosteson TD, Lurie JD, et al. Surgical vs nonoperative treatment for lumbar disk herniation: the Spine Patient Outcomes Research Trial (SPORT)—a randomized trial. JAMA. 2006; 296(20):2441–2450

[3] Kobayashi K, Sato K, Kato F, et al. Trends in the numbers of spine surgeries and spine surgeons over the past 15 years. Nagoya J Med Sci. 2022; 84(1):155–162

[4] Bier A. Versuche über Cocainisirung des Rückenmarkes. Deutsche Zeitschrift für Chirurgie. 1899; 51:361–369

[5] Cole F. Spinal anesthesia for spinal operations. Am J Surg. 1952; 84(3):326–327

[6] Siris JH, Miller ML. Spinal anesthesia in lumbar disk surgery. Curr Res Anest Anal. 1952; 31(3):208–210

[7] Ditzler JW, Dumke PR, Harrington JJ, Fox JD. Should spinal anesthesia be used in surgery for herniated intervertebral disk. Anesth Analg. 1959; 38(2):118–124

[8] Matheson D. Epidural anaesthesia for lumbar laminectomy and spinal fusion. Can Anaesth Soc J. 1960; 7:149–157

[9] Yoshimoto H, Nagashima K, Sato S, Hyakumachi T, Yanagibashi Y, Masuda T. A prospective evaluation of anesthesia for posterior lumbar spine fusion: the effectiveness of preoperative epidural anesthesia with morphine. Spine. 2005; 30(8):863–869

[10] Wu T, Liu D, Meng F, Lu JH, Chen YF, Fan Z. Awake unilateral biportal endoscopic decompression under local anesthesia for degenerative lumbar spinal stenosis in the elderly: a feasibility study with technique note. Clin Interv Aging. 2024; 19:41–50

[11] Faluhelyi A, Varga E, Koczor J. Spinal anesthesia in operations on the lumbosacral region of the spine. Magy Traumatol Orthop Helyreallito Seb. 1987; 30(2):137–140

[12] Horton JM. Anesthesia for surgery of the spine and spinal cord. Int Anesthesiol Clin. 1977; 15(3):253–263

[13] Khvisiuk NI, Kuznetsova NL. Anesthesiologic safety provision in surgical interventions on the spine. Ortop Travmatol Protez. 1971; 32(10):8–12

[14] Pitkänen M. Regional anaesthesia for low back operations. Anaesthesia. 1998; 53 Suppl 2:21–22

[15] Reynolds AF, Dautenhahn DL, Pollay M, Fagraeus L. Safety and efficacy of epidural analgesia in spine surgery. Ann Surg. 1986; 203(2):225–227

[16] Rung GW, Williams D, Gelb DE, Grubb M. Isobaric spinal anesthesia for lumbar disk surgery. Anesth Analg. 1997; 84 (5):1165–1166

[17] Silver DJ, Dunsmore RH, Dickson CM. Spinal anesthesia for lumbar disc surgery: review of 576 operations. Anesth Analg. 1976; 55(4):550–554

[18] Tetzlaff JE, Baird BA, Yoon HJ. Spinal anesthesia with plain bupivicaine for lumbar spine surgery. Can J Anaesth. 1990; 37(4, Pt 2):S61

[19] Tetzlaff JE, Dilger JA, Kodsy M, al-Bataineh J, Yoon HJ, Bell GR. Spinal anesthesia for elective lumbar spine surgery. J Clin Anesth. 1998; 10(8):666–669

[20] Amirfarzan H, Romagnoli S, Schumann R. Spinal vs. general anesthesia for hip-fracture surgery. N Engl J Med. 2022; 386(8):802

[21] Guay J, Choi P, Suresh S, Albert N, Kopp S, Pace NL. Neuraxial blockade for the prevention of postoperative mortality and major morbidity: an overview of Cochrane systematic reviews. Cochrane Database Syst Rev. 2014; 2014(1): CD010108

[22] Uzoigwe C, Symes T. Spinal vs. general anesthesia for hip-fracture surgery. N Engl J Med. 2022; 386(8):801

[23] Barry TWL, Jeanette TSLJ, Ashokka B, Lopez KG, Thambiah J, Kumar N. In the extraordinary times of coronavirus disease 2019: clinical strategies for performing spinal surgery. Asian Spine J. 2020; 14(5):721–729

[24] Letchuman V, Agarwal N, Mummaneni VP, et al. Pearls and pitfalls of awake spine surgery: a simplified patient-selection algorithm. World Neurosurg. 2022; 161:154–155

[25] Basil GW, Wang MY. Trends in outpatient minimally invasive spine surgery. J Spine Surg. 2019; 5 Suppl 1:S108–S114

[26] Fiani B, Reardon T, Selvage J, et al. Awake spine surgery: an eye-opening movement. Surg Neurol Int. 2021; 12:222

[27] Lee JK, Park JH, Hyun SJ, Hodel D, Hausmann ON. Regional anesthesia for lumbar spine surgery: can it be a standard in the future? Neurospine. 2021; 18(4):733–740

[28] Abode-Iyamah K, Ghaith AK, Bhandarkar AR, et al. Single-level awake transforaminal lumbar interbody fusion: a Mayo Clinic institutional experience and national analysis. Neurosurg Focus. 2021; 51(6):E4

[29] Breton JM, Ludwig CG, Yang MJ, et al. Spinal anesthesia in contemporary and complex lumbar spine surgery: experience with 343 cases. J Neurosurg Spine. 2021; 36(4): 534–541

[30] Dashtbani M, Dori MM, Hassani M, Omidi-Kashani F. A survey on the short-term outcome of microlumbar discectomy with general versus spinal anesthesia. Clin Orthop Surg. 2019; 11(4):422–426

[31] De Biase G, Gruenbaum SE, West JL, et al. Spinal versus general anesthesia for minimally invasive transforaminal lumbar interbody fusion: implications on operating room time, pain, and ambulation. Neurosurg Focus. 2021; 51(6): E3

[32] Kahveci K, Doger C, Ornek D, Gokcinar D, Aydemir S, Ozay R. Perioperative outcome and cost-effectiveness of spinal versus general anesthesia for lumbar spine surgery. Neurol Neurochir Pol. 2014; 48(3):167–173

[33] Liu G, Zhao J, Yuan L, Shi F, Zhang L. Spinal anesthesia for L5-S1 interlaminar endoscopic lumbar discectomy: a retrospective study. BMC Musculoskelet Disord. 2023; 24(1):818

[34] Öğrenci A, Akar E, Koban O, et al. Spinal anesthesia in surgical treatment of lumbar spine tumors. Clin Neurol Neurosurg. 2020; 196:106023

[35] Vural C, Yorukoglu D. Comparison of patient satisfaction and cost in spinal and general anesthesia for lumbar disc surgery. Turk Neurosurg. 2014; 24(3):380–384

[36] Wahood W, Yolcu Y, Alvi MA, Goyal A, Long TR, Bydon M. Assessing the differences in outcomes between general and non-general anesthesia in spine surgery: results from a national registry. Clin Neurol Neurosurg. 2019; 180:79–86

[37] Walcott BP, Khanna A, Yanamadala V, Coumans JV, Peterfreund RA. Cost analysis of spinal and general anesthesia for the surgical treatment of lumbar spondylosis. J Clin Neurosci. 2015; 22(3):539–543

[38] Wang MY, Grossman J. Endoscopic minimally invasive transforaminal interbody fusion without general anesthesia: initial clinical experience with 1-year follow-up. Neurosurg Focus. 2016; 40(2):E13

[39] Kindris F, Zegarek G, Krappel FA, Perrig WN, Schmid SL. Spinal versus general anesthesia for lumbar decompression or sequestrectomy in patients over 75 years. Clin Spine Surg. 2023; 36(7):E329–E331

[40] Lessing NL, Edwards CC , II, Brown CH , IV, et al. Spinal anesthesia in elderly patients undergoing lumbar spine surgery. Orthopedics. 2017; 40(2):e317–e322

[41] Wang AY, Olmos M, Ahsan T, et al. Safety and feasibility of spinal anesthesia during simple and complex lumbar spine surgery in the extreme elderly (≥ 80 years of age). Clin Neurol Neurosurg. 2022; 219:107316

[42] Ahsan T, Wang AY, Karimi H, et al. Assessing the safety and efficacy of spinal anesthesia in patients with significant comorbidities. World Neurosurg. 2023; 177:e110–e117

[43] Sykes DAW, Tabarestani TQ, Salven DS, et al. Awake spinal anesthesia facilitates spine surgery in poor surgical candidates: a case series. Neurochirurgie. 2023; 69(3):101444

[44] Patil H, Garg N, Navakar D, Banabokade L. Lumbar spine surgeries under spinal anesthesia in high-risk patients: a retrospective analysis. World Neurosurg. 2019; 124:e779–e782

[45] Babici D, Johansen PM, Newman SL, O'Connor TE, Miller TD. Microdiscectomy under local anesthesia and spinal block in a pregnant female. Cureus. 2021; 13(12):e20241

[46] Finsterwald M, Muster M, Farshad M, Saporito A, Brada M, Aguirre JA. Spinal versus general anesthesia for lumbar spine surgery in high risk patients: Perioperative hemodynamic stability, complications and costs. J Clin Anesth. 2018; 46:3–7

[47] Daneshi SA, Nabiuni M, Taheri M, Pour Roustaei Ardekani R. Spinal versus general anesthesia for spine surgery during the COVID-19 pandemic: a case series. Anesth Pain Med. 2023; 13(2):e134783

[48] Khattab MFM, Sykes DAW, Abd-El-Barr MM, et al. Spine surgery under awake spinal anesthesia: an Egyptian experience during the COVID-19 pandemic. Neurosurg Focus. 2021; 51(6):E6

[49] Perez-Roman RJ, Govindarajan V, Bryant JP, Wang MY. Spinal anesthesia in awake surgical procedures of the lumbar spine: a systematic review and meta-analysis of 3709 patients. Neurosurg Focus. 2021; 51(6):E7

[50] Attari MA, Mirhosseini SA, Honarmand A, Safavi MR. Spinal anesthesia versus general anesthesia for elective lumbar spine surgery: a randomized clinical trial. J Res Med Sci. 2011; 16(4):524–529

[51] Becq MC, Verdin M, Riegel B, et al. Hemodynamic effects of genu-pectoral position during the surgery of lumbar disk herniation: spinal anesthesia versus general anesthesia. Agressologie. 1994; 34(Spec No 1):49–50

[52] Deng H, Coumans JV, Anderson R, Houle TT, Peterfreund RA. Spinal anesthesia for lumbar spine surgery correlates with fewer total medications and less frequent use of vasoactive agents: a single center experience. PLoS One. 2019; 14(6):e0217939

[53] Lessing NL, Edwards CC , II, Dean CL, et al. Spinal anesthesia for geriatric lumbar spine surgery: a comparative case series. Int J Spine Surg. 2020; 14(5):713–721

[54] Jellish WS, Thalji Z, Stevenson K, Shea J. A prospective randomized study comparing short- and intermediate-term perioperative outcome variables after spinal or general anesthesia for lumbar disk and laminectomy surgery. Anesth Analg. 1996; 83(3):559–564

[55] Ahmed Jonayed S, Alam MS, Al Mamun Choudhury A, Akter S, Chakraborty S. Efficacy, safety, and reliability of surgery on the lumbar spine under general versus spinal anesthesia- an analysis of 64 cases. J Clin Orthop Trauma. 2021; 16: 176–181

[56] McLain RF, Kalfas I, Bell GR, Tetzlaff JE, Yoon HJ, Rana M. Comparison of spinal and general anesthesia in lumbar laminectomy surgery: a case-controlled analysis of 400 patients. J Neurosurg Spine. 2005; 2(1):17–22

[57] McLain RF, Tetzlaff JE, Bell GR, Uwe-Lewandrowski K, Yoon HJ, Rana M. Microdiscectomy: spinal anesthesia offers optimal results in general patient population. J Surg Orthop Adv. 2007; 16(1):5–11

[58] Sykes DAW, Tabarestani TQ, Chaudhry NS, et al. Awake spinal fusion is associated with reduced length of stay, opioid use, and time to ambulation compared to general anesthesia: a matched cohort study. World Neurosurg. 2023; 176: e91–e100

[59] De Biase G, Otamendi-Lopez A, Chen S, et al. Impact of postoperative fatigue following minimally-invasive lumbar spine surgery. J Clin Neurosci. 2023; 112:64–67

[60] Kundu M, Abdulla E, Rahman MM. Letter: spine surgery under spinal vs general anesthesia—prospective analysis of quality of life, fatigue, and cognition. Neurosurgery. 2023; 92(1):e9

[61] Alsoof D, Kasthuri V, McDonald C, et al. How much are patients willing to pay for spine surgery? An evaluation of attitudes toward out-of-pocket expenses and cost-reducing measures. Spine J. 2023; 23(12):1886–1893

[62] Agarwal P, Pierce J, Welch WC. Cost analysis of spinal versus general anesthesia for lumbar diskectomy and laminectomy spine surgery. World Neurosurg. 2016; 89:266–271

[63] Romanello M, Napoli CD, Green C, et al. The 2023 report of the Lancet Countdown on health and climate change: the imperative for a health-centred response in a world facing irreversible harms. Lancet. 2023; 402(10419):2346–2394

[64] Wang AY, Ahsan T, Kosarchuk JJ, Liu P, Riesenburger RI, Kryzanski J. Assessing the environmental carbon footprint of spinal versus general anesthesia in single-level transforaminal lumbar interbody fusions. World Neurosurg. 2022a; 163:e199–e206

[65] Wang AY, Ahsan T, Kosarchuk JJ, Liu P, Riesenburger RI, Kryzanski J. Dataset for carbon footprints of transforaminal lumbar interbody fusions performed under spinal or general anesthesia. Data Brief. 2022b; 42:108218

[66] McLain RF, Bell GR, Kalfas I, Tetzlaff JE, Yoon HJ. Complications associated with lumbar laminectomy: a comparison of spinal versus general anesthesia. Spine. 2004; 29(22): 2542–2547

[67] Rajjoub R, Ghaith AK, El-Hajj VG, et al. Comparative outcomes of awake spine surgery under spinal versus general anesthesia: a comprehensive systematic review and meta-analysis. Eur Spine J. 2024; 33(3):985–1000

[68] Ghaith AK, Akinduro OO, El-Hajj VG, et al. General versus nongeneral anesthesia for spinal surgery: a comparative national analysis of reimbursement trends over 10 years. Neurosurgery. 2024; 94(2):413–422

[69] Amoroso K, Okano I, Sarin M, et al. Comparative effectiveness of anesthetic technique on outcomes after lumbar spine surgery: a retrospective propensity score-matched analysis of the National Surgical Quality Improvement Program, 2009–2019. Reg Anesth Pain Med. 2023; 48(7): 343–348

[70] Hernandez NS, Wang AY, Kanter M, et al. Assessing the impact of spinal versus general anesthesia on postoperative urinary retention in elective spinal surgery patients. Clin Neurol Neurosurg. 2022; 222:107454

[71] De Biase G, Gruenbaum SE, Quiñones-Hinojosa A, Abode-Iyamah KO. Spine surgery under spinal vs general anesthesia: prospective analysis of quality of life, fatigue, and cognition. Neurosurgery. 2022; 90(2):186–191

[72] Kim SH, Jeon DH, Chang CH, Lee SJ, Shin YS. Spinal anesthesia with isobaric tetracaine in patients with previous lumbar spinal surgery. Yonsei Med J. 2009; 50(2):252–256

[73] Sun KO. Spinal anaesthesia following previous spinal surgery. Eur J Anaesthesiol. 1994; 11(4):321–323

[74] Jost U, Wolter E, Böhrer H. Spinal anaesthesia in 50 patients with previous lumbar spinal surgery. Anasthesiol Intensivmed Notfallmed Schmerzther. 2004; 39(2):78–80

[75] De Biase G, Chen S, Akinduro O, Quinones-Hinojosa A, Abode-Iyamah K. Awake robotic minimally invasive L4–5 transforaminal lumbar interbody fusion. World Neurosurg. 2021; 148:93

[76] Shtaya A, Luong CB, Pereira E. Awake intradural spinal tumor resection; case report and literature review. World Neurosurg. 2018; 114:344–347

[77] Balkarlı H, Kılıç M, Öztürk İ. Neuraxial anesthesia after local anesthesia for management of percutaneous vertebroplasty complication during vertebroplasty. Rev Bras Anestesiol. 2017; 67(2):205–209

[78] Wang AY, Liu P, Balonov K, Riesenburger R, Kryzanski J. Use of spinal anesthesia in lower thoracic spine surgery: a case series. Oper Neurosurg (Hagerstown). 2022; 23(4):298–303

[79] Lessing NL, Edwards CC , II, Lin C, Brown CH , IV. Complex lumbar spine fusion for an elderly patient under spinal anesthesia. Orthopedics. 2017; 40(5):e915–e917

[80] Tetzlaff JE, O'Hara J, Bell G, Grimm K, Yoon HJ. Influence of baricity on the outcome of spinal anesthesia with bupivacaine for lumbar spine surgery. Reg Anesth. 1995; 20(6): 533–537

[81] Aiyer SN, Kumar A, Shetty AP, Kanna RM, Rajasekaran S. Factors influencing postoperative urinary retention following elective posterior lumbar spine surgery: a prospective study. Asian Spine J. 2018; 12(6):1100–1105

[82] Leslie K, Troedel S, Irwin K, et al. Quality of recovery from anesthesia in neurosurgical patients. Anesthesiology. 2003; 99(5):1158–1165

[83] Yukawa Y, Kato F, Ito K, Terashima T, Horie Y. A prospective randomized study of preemptive analgesia for postoperative pain in the patients undergoing posterior lumbar interbody fusion: continuous subcutaneous morphine,

continuous epidural morphine, and diclofenac sodium. Spine. 2005; 30(21):2357–2361
[84] Gianesello L, Pavoni V, Barboni E, Galeotti I, Nella A. Perioperative pregabalin for postoperative pain control and quality of life after major spinal surgery. J Neurosurg Anesthesiol. 2012; 24(2):121–126
[85] Khurana G, Jindal P, Sharma JP, Bansal KK. Postoperative pain and long-term functional outcome after administration of gabapentin and pregabalin in patients undergoing spinal surgery. Spine. 2014; 39(6):E363–E368
[86] Gille O, Jolivet E, Dousset V, et al. Erector spinae muscle changes on magnetic resonance imaging following lumbar surgery through a posterior approach. Spine. 2007; 32(11): 1236–1241
[87] Harbell MW, Seamans DP, Koyyalamudi V, Kraus MB, Craner RC, Langley NR. Evaluating the extent of lumbar erector spinae plane block: an anatomical study. Reg Anesth Pain Med. 2020; 45(8):640–644
[88] Zhang JF, Zhang WW, Wang J, Guo H, Wang T. Distribution of the T12 erector spinal muscle plane block in the dorsal region guided by ultrasound. J Orthop Surg Res. 2021; 16 (1):48
[89] Akyuz ME, Firidin MN. Bilateral ultrasound-guided erector spinae plane block for postoperative persistent low back pain in lumbar disc surgery. Eur Spine J. 2022; 31(7):1873–1878
[90] Bellantonio D, Bolondi G, Cultrera F, et al. Erector spinae plane block for perioperative pain management in neurosurgical lower-thoracic and lumbar spinal fusion: a single-centre prospective randomised controlled trial. BMC Anesthesiol. 2023; 23(1):187
[91] Breebaart MB, Van Aken D, De Fré O, et al. A prospective randomized double-blind trial of the efficacy of a bilateral lumbar erector spinae block on the 24h morphine consumption after posterior lumbar inter-body fusion surgery. Trials. 2019; 20(1):441
[92] Chin KJ, Lewis S. Opioid-free analgesia for posterior spinal fusion surgery using erector spinae plane (ESP) blocks in a multimodal anesthetic regimen. Spine. 2019; 44(6):E379–E383
[93] Makanji HS, Solomito MJ, Maffeo-Mitchell C, Esmende S, Finkel K. Utility of erector spinae plane blocks for postoperative pain management and opioid reduction following lumbar fusions. Clin Spine Surg. 2023; 36(4):E131–E134
[94] van den Broek RJC, van de Geer R, Schepel NC, Liu WY, Bouwman RA, Versyck B. Evaluation of adding the erector spinae plane block to standard anesthetic care in patients undergoing posterior lumbar interbody fusion surgery. Sci Rep. 2021; 11(1):7631
[95] Braxton EE, Brena KR, Spears H, Conrad E, Heinze JD. Ultrasound-guided bilateral erector spinae plane nerve blocks: a novel application for the management of acute postoperative pain in awake spine surgery. Illustrative case. J Neurosurg Case Lessons. 2022; 3(18):CASE21633
[96] Xiao X, Zhu T, Wang L, Zhou H, Zhang Y. Efficacy of postoperative analgesia by erector spinal plane block after lumbar surgery: a systematic review and meta-analysis of randomized controlled trials. Comput Math Methods Med. 2022; 2022:3264142
[97] Kang TH, Kim WJ, Lee JH. Efficacy of the erector spinae plane block with sedation for unilateral biportal endoscopic spine surgery and comparison with other anesthetic methods. Acta Neurochir (Wien). 2023; 165(9):2651–2663
[98] Chen K, Wang L, Ning M, Dou L, Li W, Li Y. Evaluation of ultrasound-guided lateral thoracolumbar interfascial plane block for postoperative analgesia in lumbar spine fusion surgery: a prospective, randomized, and controlled clinical trial. PeerJ. 2019; 7:e7967
[99] Long G, Liu C, Liang T, Zhan X. The efficacy of thoracolumbar interfascial plane block for lumbar spinal surgeries: a systematic review and meta-analysis. J Orthop Surg Res. 2023; 18(1):318
[100] Lee JS, Park YM, Ha KY, Cho SW, Bak GH, Kim KW. Preoperative anxiety about spinal surgery under general anesthesia. Eur Spine J. 2016; 25(3):698–707
[101] Ballarapu GK, Nallam SR, Samantaray A, Kumar VAK, Reddy AP. Thoracolumbar curve and Cobb angle in determining spread of spinal anesthesia in scoliosis. An observational prospective pilot study. Indian J Anaesth. 2020; 64(7):594–598
[102] Berkowitz S, Gold MI. Spinal anesthesia for surgery in patients with previous lumbar laminectomy. Anesth Analg. 1980; 59(11):881–882
[103] Oh TT, Ikhsan M, Tan KK, et al. A novel approach to neuraxial anesthesia: application of an automated ultrasound spinal landmark identification. BMC Anesthesiol. 2019; 19(1):57
[104] Chin KJ, Chan VW, Ramlogan R, Perlas A. Real-time ultrasound-guided spinal anesthesia in patients with a challenging spinal anatomy: two case reports. Acta Anaesthesiol Scand. 2010; 54(2):252–255
[105] Chin KJ, Chan V. Ultrasonography as a preoperative assessment tool: predicting the feasibility of central neuraxial blockade. Anesth Analg. 2010; 110(1):252–253
[106] Chin KJ, Ramlogan R, Arzola C, Singh M, Chan V. The utility of ultrasound imaging in predicting ease of performance of spinal anesthesia in an orthopedic patient population. Reg Anesth Pain Med. 2013; 38(1):34–38
[107] Longbottom J, Clegg I, Bhatia K. Should ultrasound of the spine be mandatory before performing a lumbar central neuraxial block? Br J Hosp Med (Lond). 2014; 75(3):178
[108] Chin KJ. Recent developments in ultrasound imaging for neuraxial blockade. Curr Opin Anaesthesiol. 2018; 31(5): 608–613
[109] Zhang D, Chen L, Chen X, et al. Lower incidence of postdural puncture headache using whitacre spinal needles after spinal anesthesia: a meta-analysis. Headache. 2016; 56(3): 501–510
[110] Badiger SV, Desai SN, Dasar S. Pneumocephalus following spinal anaesthesia for spine surgery. Indian J Anaesth. 2016; 60(5):361–362
[111] Keenan C, Wang AY, Balonov K, Kryzanski J. Postoperative vasovagal cardiac arrest after spinal anesthesia for lumbar spine surgery. Surg Neurol Int. 2022; 13:42
[112] Azad TD, Alomari S, Khalifeh JM, et al. Adoption of awake spine surgery: trends from a national registry over 14 years. Spine J. 2022; 22(10):1601–1609
[113] De Biase G, Chen S, Ziu E, et al. Assessment of patients' willingness to participate in a randomized trial of spinal versus general anesthesia for lumbar spine surgery. World Neurosurg. 2022; 161:e635–e641
[114] De Biase G, Carter RE, Otamendi-Lopez A, et al. Assessment of surgeons' attitude towards awake spine surgery under spinal anesthesia. J Clin Neurosci. 2023; 107:48–53
[115] Amoroso K, Hughes AP, Soffin EM. Spine surgery under neuraxial vs. general anesthesia: the current state of

comparative outcomes research. Curr Opin Anaesthesiol. 2023; 36(5):516–524

[116] Abbatematteo JM, Snyder LA. Commentary: spine surgery under spinal vs general anesthesia: prospective analysis of quality of life, fatigue, and cognition. Neurosurgery. 2022; 90(6):e174–e175

[117] West JL, De Biase G, Bydon M, et al. What is the learning curve for lumbar spine surgery under spinal anesthesia? World Neurosurg. 2022; 158:e310–e316

[118] Aziz MF, Dillman D, Fu R, Brambrink AM. Comparative effectiveness of the C-MAC video laryngoscope versus direct laryngoscopy in the setting of the predicted difficult airway. Anesthesiology. 2012; 116(3): 629–636

[119] Letchuman V, Agarwal N, Mummaneni VP, et al. Awake spinal surgery: simplifying the learning curve with a patient selection algorithm. Neurosurg Focus. 2021; 51 (6):E2

22 Beyond General Anesthesia: The Protocols Powering Awake Spine Surgery

Shahenda Khedr, Kingsley Abode-Iyamah, Benjamin Frederick Gruenbaum, and Marie De Ruyter

Abstract

Awake spine surgery has seen increased adoption, but successful outcomes depend on proper patient selection and a multifaceted approach to patient management. This chapter discusses and defines a protocol selection, preoperative and intraoperative surgical preparation, anesthesia management, planned and emergency airway management, and postoperative care in details that are essential in ensuring the procedure's success and patient safety.

Keywords: patient selection criteria, surgical positioning, contraindications for awake spine surgery, anesthesia protocol, planned and emergent airway management, perioperative management, intraoperative management, postoperative management

Key Points

- Awake spine surgery is a minimally invasive approach that reduces recovery time and enhances patient safety by using local anesthetic and allowing for real-time neural feedback during procedures such as lumbar fusions, laminectomies/diskectomies, anterior cervical diskectomy and fusions, and dorsal column simulator placements.
- Systematic reviews and meta-analyses show that awake spine surgery significantly reduces operative time, anesthesia duration, postoperative complications, and hospital length of stay while improving postoperative pain management and decreasing the need for analgesics.
- Successful outcomes depend on careful patient selection, considering medical conditions including comorbidities, mental health, and surgical history. Suitable candidates typically include those needing procedures on a maximum of two vertebrae levels and those who can tolerate a prone position throughout surgery.
- The anesthesia protocol involves preoperative pain management, intraoperative administration of isobaric bupivacaine and flexible sedative regimens, and postoperative pain control using oral narcotics, muscle relaxants, acetaminophen, nonsteroidal anti-inflammatory drugs, and other medications.
- Effective airway management during surgery ensures spontaneous breathing and readiness for emergencies, with protocols for maintaining oxygenation and handling potential complications.
- Postoperative care focuses on pain control, muscle relaxation, early ambulation, comprehensive neurological assessments, and thorough patient education to ensure a smooth recovery.

22.1 Introduction

Awake spine surgery stands as an innovative procedure that represents a significant advancement in the field of spinal surgery, offering a minimally invasive approach that reduces recovery time and prioritizes patient safety using local anesthetic. Procedures suitable for this approach include lumbar fusions, laminectomies/diskectomies, anterior cervical diskectomy and fusions, and dorsal column simulator placement.[1] Awake spine surgery is also advantageous because it allows for real-time neural feedback from patients.[1] Numerous research articles support the advantages of awake spine surgery across various procedures:

- A systematic review and meta-analysis of 3,079 patients who underwent a spinal procedure highlight the benefits of awake spine surgery compared to general anesthesia (GA), demonstrating the following[2]:
  - Significant reductions in operative time.
  - Reduced anesthesia time.
  - Fewer postoperative complications.
  - Shorter hospital length.
  - Improvement in postoperative pain levels.
  - Decreased need for postoperative analgesia.

- Retrospective reviews on patients undergoing spinal anesthesia (SA) for lumbar decompression, foraminotomy, or microdiskectomy showed that compared to patients who underwent GA, SA resulted in the following[3,4,5]:
  - Significantly fewer drugs administered during the procedure.
  - Less frequent use of vasoactive agents.
  - Reduced time in the operating room.
  - Shorter duration in the postanesthesia care unit (PACU).
  - Lower postoperative pain levels.
  - Fewer complications.
  - Lower costs overall compared with patients who underwent GA.
- A randomized controlled trial for patients who underwent a diskectomy, laminectomy, foraminotomy, or cord tumor resection found that SA offered the following benefits[6]:
  - Lower postoperative analgesia needs.
  - Decreased blood loss.
  - Maintained better perioperative hemodynamic stability.
  - No increase in adverse side effects compared to the GA approach.
- Numerous studies found that awake minimally invasive surgery transforaminal lumbar interbody fusion (MIS-TLIF) to be beneficial, as demonstrated by the following findings[7,8,9,10]:
  - It is a safe and effective technique.
  - It demonstrates easier access and reduced damage to soft tissue during operation.
  - It allows for faster postoperative mobilization.
  - It reduces the use of opioids and time to ambulation.
  - It shortens hospital length of stay, operating room time, and postoperative pain.

Over the years, awake spine surgery has been gradually adopted, with non-GA operations rising from nearly 0% in 2005 to 2.1% in 2019.[11] This trend is associated with lower complication rates, shorter hospital stays, and reduced readmission rates, indicating growing acceptance and recognition of the benefits of this procedure.[11] However, the success of awake spine surgery is contingent on patient selection, as not everyone is a suitable candidate for awake procedures due to factors such as an inability to tolerate a prone position because of preexisting medical conditions, mental health disorders, or past medical/surgical history.

The protocol below outlines a framework for awake spine surgery by establishing criteria for patient selection and providing detailed guidelines for positioning during surgery, nonemergent and emergent airway management, anesthesia administration, surgical selection, and postoperative care to ensure optimal outcomes and patient safety.

22.2 Patient Selection

When considering patient selection for awake spine surgery, it is important to weigh both the indications and contraindications for performing this procedure to ensure optimal outcomes. Studies by Fiani et al, Waguia et al, De Biase et al, and Letchuman et al have published the following indications and contraindications for awake spinal surgeries [1,2,3,4,5,6,7,12,13,14,15]:

- Indications for SA:
  - Surgeries involving a maximum of two vertebrae levels.
  - Minimally invasive surgeries or those utilizing endoscopic techniques.
  - Surgeries requiring neural feedback.
  - Particularly suited for aging populations.
  - Ideal for patients seeking to avoid GA.

Expert Tip

The most definitive contraindication is the patient's unwillingness to undergo awake spine surgery.

- Preferred use of GA:
  - Patients under the age of 15 years.
  - Individuals prone to restlessness and agitation over a longer procedure.
- Contraindications to awake spine surgery:
  - Procedures with a longer duration, such as those with degenerative pathologies or involving more than two vertebrae (though the time frame is restricted to each case, and there is no absolute contraindication).

Expert Tip

The majority of these are relative contraindications and may vary depending on the surgeon's and anesthesiologist's level of comfort and clinical judgment.

- Patients with respiratory compromise, poorly controlled pulmonary disease (baseline room air oxygen saturation < 95%).
- Patients with poorly controlled cardiac disease or those at high risk of aspiration.
- Patients with a high body mass index (BMI; ≥ 37 kg/m²).
- Patients diagnosed with obstructive sleep apnea:
  - Not good candidates for local anesthesia because intubation will be significantly challenging if needed.
  - These patients are also at a higher risk of CO_2 accumulation during surgery due to limited chest wall expansion while in the prone position.
- Patients with mental health issues such as anxiety, depression, or claustrophobia.
- Patients with bleeding disorders or those diagnosed with intracranial hypertension.
- Patients who smoke.
- Patients who have had previous unsuccessful back surgery.
- Those who have prior history of lumbar spinal surgery at the level of the spinal anesthetic (due to potential problems with administration).
- Patients with radiologically evident arachnoiditis or severe spinal stenosis.
- Spinal pathology above the level of the conus medullaris.

Expert Tip

If there is no severe spinal stenosis, a standard intrathecal block should typically achieve a level of anesthesia up to T4.

- Special considerations:
  - The decision to operate is relative to the patient's case and the discussion between the surgeon and anesthesiologist.
  - The time frame of surgery can be extended through the administration of injections such as additional doses of local anesthetics, sedatives, analgesics, and nerve blocks.

A patient who is a candidate for SA should not only meet the indication criteria but also be able to tolerate lying in the prone position for the entire duration of the surgery without presenting challenges to airway management, which could arise due to anatomical or psychological considerations. Taking all the above indications for surgery into account, as well as assessing a patient's ability to maintain the prone position and ensuring a secure airway throughout the procedures, is imperative for achieving favorable outcomes and a successful awake spine surgery.

Expert Tip

It is crucial to establish guidelines in collaboration with anesthesiology and any dedicated teams until protocols for awake spine surgery are thoroughly established and standardized.

22.3 Surgical Selection

Regarding patient selection, an algorithm was curated by Letchuman et al[13] through a collaborative effort involving neurosurgeons, anesthesiologists, nurses, and physical therapists at the University of California, San Francisco. A retrospective review of patients who underwent awake lumbar spinal surgery was conducted to verify the algorithm's effectiveness and to establish a selection criterion.

22.3.1 Patient Selection Criteria for Spinal Procedures

For all patients undergoing spinal decompression or spinal fusion, the following stepwise approach for selection is recommended (▶ Fig. 22.1). Start by evaluating patient factors that could impact their ability to tolerate awake surgery, such as history of anxiety, BMI over 37 kg/m²,[1] and a history of sleep apnea or compromised airway. If any of those factors are present, GA is recommended.

Expert Tip

The BMI cutoff is determined based on the guidelines established by the surgeon and the anesthesiology team. It is important to note that some sources have published a BMI cutoff of less than 30 kg/m².

[1] Letchuman et al[13] suggest a BMI cutoff over 30 kg/m². However, we suggest that patients with a BMI of less than 37 kg/m² can be suitable candidates for awake spine surgery and should be considered for this approach.

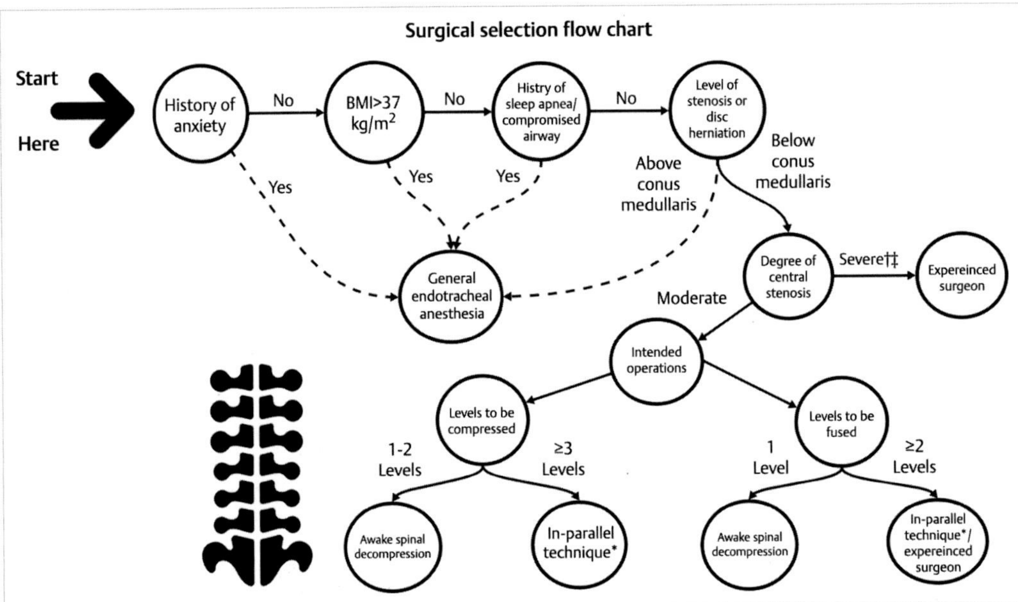

Fig. 22.1 Patient selection flowchart for awake lumbar spinal surgery: individuals with no history of anxiety, BMI ≤ 37, no history of sleep apnea, no airway compromise, pathology below the conus medullaris, and maximal moderate central stenosis are ideal candidates for awake intervention. *For three or more levels to be compressed or fused, the in-parallel technique is recommended. †Adequate space for the spinal anesthetic to enter the intradural compartment must be available—hence the need for an experienced surgeon. ‡Requires an experienced surgeon due to increased risk of CSF leak. (Based on Letchuman V, Agarwal N, Mummaneni VP, et al. Awake spinal surgery: simplifying the learning curve with a patient selection algorithm. Neurosurg Focus. 2021;51(6):E2.)

- If the patient does not present these risk factors, the evaluation continues with the level of stenosis or disk herniation, particularly whether it is above or below the conus medullaris, which further informs the decision for GA.
- For patients with stenosis below the conus medullaris, the degree of central stenosis is assessed—severe cases warranting an experienced surgeon.
- Letchuman et al recommend opting for GA in the presence of facet cysts.[13] However, we suggest that local anesthesia can still be a viable approach, provided the procedure is performed by an experienced surgeon.
- Finally, when considering the surgical operation, either decompression or fusion is considered. The number of levels to be compressed or fused dictates the surgical approach. Letchuman et al recommend that for spinal levels involving three or more segments, either an experienced surgeon or GA should be utilized.[13] However, based on the successful implementation of a the "in-parallel" technique,[2] we propose the following:
  - For spinal decompression, one to two levels can be managed with local anesthesia, while procedures involving three or more levels should utilize the "in-parallel" technique.
  - For spinal fusion, one level can be managed with local anesthesia, while two levels should be managed by an experienced surgeon. Similar to spinal decompression, procedures involving three or more levels should utilize the "in-parallel" technique.

[2] The "in-parallel" technique is a novel awake technique designed for performing simultaneous lumbar spinal surgery on three-segment pathology.[16] This technique is reliant on two independent surgeons to synchronously perform extensive operations under the time constraints of regional anesthesia and can be utilized for spinal decompression or fusion of three or more levels.

Expert Tip

When the "in-parallel" technique is not feasible, it is essential to have an experienced surgeon who can complete the surgery within the required time constraints. Alternatively, if the patient can tolerate an extended duration, additional intraoperative injections may be administered to prolong surgical time.

The following questionnaire serves as a supplemental tool for assessing patient selection:

Multilevel awake MIS-TLIF screening questionnaire

Screening questions	Yes	No
1. History of anxiety		
2. BMI ≥ 37 kg/m^2		
3. History of sleep apnea or compromised airway		
4. Previous history of CSF leak		
If all the above are marked as "No," you can continue with the questionnaire **If any of the above is marked as "Yes," you should proceed under General endotracheal anesthesia**		
5. Is it a revision surgery?		
If the answer to question 5 is "No," move to question 6 **If the answer to question 5 is "Yes," move the question 5.1**		
5.1. Need to drill bone?		
If the answer to question 5.1 is "No," move to question 6 **If the answer to question 5.1 is "Yes," you should proceed under General endotracheal anesthesia**		
6. Two levels		
If the answer to question 6 is "No." move to question 7 **If the answer to question 6 is "Yes," you can proceed under Spinal anesthesia**		
7. Three levels		
7.1. One to two levels of canal stenosis		
7.2. More than two levels of canal stenosis		
If the answer to question 7.1 is "Yes," you can proceed under Spinal anesthesia **If the answer to question 7.2 is "Yes," you should proceed under General endotracheal anesthesia**		

22.4 Preoperative Course

The approach to preoperative care in terms of the nurse's role remains consistent for both patients undergoing awake spine surgery and those receiving GA.[12] The nursing role involves conducting and documenting a thorough neurological assessment, which will be utilized to track the patient's progress postoperatively. Furthermore, the nurse reinforces the information given to the patient by the provider using the teach-back technique to ensure that the patient has adequate comprehension of the treatment plan, the postoperative expectations, and the educational objectives.

22.4.1 Positioning

Proper patient positioning during awake spine surgery is crucial to ensure optimal patient comfort and readiness for the surgical procedure. The following recommendations have been outlined:

- Both De Biase et al, and Waguia et al[12] recommend placing the patient in the supine position following the injection of SA to ensure comfort and stability before the anesthesia takes full effect.
- After stabilization, both guidelines advocate transitioning the patient into a prone position to prepare for the surgical procedure.
- The use of a horseshoe headrest with face foam is recommended, allowing patients to adjust until they are comfortable before the surgical site is prepared.
- Prone positioning is particularly important for laminectomy and MIS-TLIF procedures, as outlined by De Biase et al, with both procedures performed on a Wilson radiolucent frame atop a Jackson table.[7,9]
- Both studies also highlight the use of active noise canceling headphones and patient-preferred music to enhance the surgical experience and comfort. This patient-centered approach acknowledges the potential stressors of surgery and the benefits of creating a more relaxed environment.[17]
- The primary difference in the two sets of guidelines is in Waguia et al's mention of the placement of urinary catheters and neuromonitoring leads after the patient is placed in the supine position, adding a more comprehensive approach to presurgical patient setup.[12]

It is important to discuss the different types of tables available because each table has its own set of advantages and is chosen based on the specific requirements of the surgery, including the surgical approach, the area of the spine being operated on, and the patient's physical condition. The choice of table significantly contributes to the success of surgery by providing optimal exposure to the surgical site, minimizing patient movement, and reducing the risk of complications. Below are several types of tables and frames commonly used during spine surgeries:

- **Jackson table:** It is a table designed for versatile positioning during spine surgery, including prone, supine, and lateral positions. The Jackson table has a unique design that enables the surgeon to safely perform a 360-degree rotation of the patient without removing the patient from the table, providing C-arm and O-arm access, thereby facilitating anterior and posterior positioning during a single operating room visit. It includes the 360-degree patient rotation when used in conjunction with the radiolucent imaging top, in addition to a lateral tilt (25 degrees) in both directions. Additional features include a hand pendant of the advanced control base, which controls the height, lateral tilt, and Trendelenburg/reverse Trendelenburg as well as customized support pads to enhance the positioning of patients with varying body types. It is designed for many common spine surgeries including laminectomies, decompression, osteotomies, anterior/posterior fusions, surgical correction of deformities, anterior/posterior cervical procedures, kyphoplasties, vertebroplasties, and intradiscal electrothermal therapy surgeries.[18] This table is known for its ability to provide excellent abdominal decompression, which is beneficial during lengthy spine procedures.[19]

Expert Tip

Additional pillows may be necessary to provide the patient with extra comfort.

- **Mizuho OSI Modular Table System:** Originally known as the Jackson table, this table offers a versatile system of spine, imaging, and orthopaedic trauma procedure. This system consists of the Jackson table and the advanced control base. This multifunctional base can hold multiple different types of tops for different procedures, including a spinal surgery top with an open frame design for posterior spinal surgery and a radiolucent imaging top for supine and lateral positioning. Common procedures performed using this system include those performed on the Jackson table.[18]

- **Wilson frame:** This is a frame designed to support patients in a flexed position during lumbar procedures including laminectomy, decompression, disk surgery, and microdiskectomy procedures. This frame provides unrestricted (360-degree) radiolucency at the operating site, allowing for clear and unobstructed imaging using either a C-arm or X-ray. It is an attachment that can be placed on a regular operating table to create a convex platform, supporting the patient in a prone position. It allows for flexion of the spine, facilitating access to the posterior spine. Additionally, the Wilson frame is equipped with lordosis control, a mechanism that allows the pads to flexibly adjust to modify spinal lordosis, which enhances surgical site accessibility. The frame also incorporates two full-length gel pads that offer optimal comfort and are capable of lateral adjustments up to 10 inches, which improves ventilation and alleviates pressure on the abdomen. Furthermore, the frame features an easy-to-use and safe crank system that allows for easy removal and adjustments.[20] Benefits of utilizing the Wilson frame include minimizing intra-abdominal pressure and blood loss during the operative course.[21]
- **Andrews table:** The Andrews table or Andrews Spinal Surgery Table, like the Wilson frame, is specifically designed to support patients in a prone position, enhancing surgical access to lumbar and thoracic regions of the spine. Patients are positioned in a modified knee-chest position with adjustable tibial support that can produce a hip flexion with a range from 90 to 60 degrees, to be tailored to the operation performed. This table also allows for C-arm integration to support lateral intraoperative and anteroposterior views.[22] In comparison to the Wilson frame, the positioning that the Andrews table also provides is known to minimize intra-abdominal pressure and blood loss.[21]

22.4.2 Anesthesia Protocol: Preoperative

Below we outline a protocol for preventive pain management and localized anesthesia, both crucial for awake spine surgery.[7,12,13]

- Preemptive anesthesia:
  - *Acetaminophen:* 1,000 mg orally or intravenously (IV) is commonly agreed upon in the current literatures.
    - Additional medications:
      - *Gabapentin:* 600 mg orally for patients younger than 70 years and those without chronic kidney disease (glomerular filtration rate > 60) as recommend by Letchuman et al.[13]
      - *Midazolam:* 0.01 to 0.02 mg IV for anxiety, as recommended by De Biase et al,
      - *Fentanyl:* 1 to 2 μg/kg IV for pain (De Biase et al),
      - *Dexamethasone:* 8 mg IV.[12]
      - COX-2 selective nonsteroidal anti-inflammatory drug (NSAID).[12]
- Erector spinae plane (ESP) block:
  - It is recommended that the ESP block is administered by the anesthesia team in the preoperative holding area using light sedation.[12]
  - This allows the block to function at maximum capacity when the incision is made, improving efficiency in the operating room.
    - Procedure for ESP block[12]:
      - The patient is positioned sitting, in either a lateral or a prone position based on the surgeon's preference.
      - Skin over the lumbar spine should be prepped with chlorhexidine.
      - Low-frequency curvilinear ultrasound probe should be placed in the parasagittal orientation.
      - The transverse process of either the L2 or the L3 vertebra, whichever is more visible, is located.
      - A 21-gauge, 100-mm nerve block needle is precisely guided in a plane through the erector spinae muscle group until it touches the transverse process's dorsal aspect.
      - After ensuring no blood return with a negative aspiration, 2 to 3 mL of saline is injected to verify placement within the correct submuscular layer.
      - This is followed by the injection of 30 mL of a solution comprising 133 mg liposomal bupivacaine (10 mL) and 50 mg bupivacaine 0.25% (20 mL).

- The needle is then withdrawn, and the same steps are applied to the opposite side.

22.5 Intraoperative Course

22.5.1 Anesthesia Protocol: Intraoperative

In the intraoperative management of awake spine surgery, protocols exhibit both convergence and divergence in their approaches to SA and sedation, emphasizing the nuanced application of dosages and medication tailored to enhance patient comfort and surgical efficacy:

- De Biase et al[7]:
  - They recommend 12.5 to 15 mg of isobaric intrathecal bupivacaine, with or without the addition of intrathecal narcotics (fentanyl or hydromorphone).

> **Expert Tip**
>
> *For fusion procedures, a dose of 15 mg is more effective, while a lower dose is typically used for decompression. Additionally, the anesthesiologist may consider using mepivacaine for shorter cases.*

  - Administered one level above planned surgical intervention using a landmark technique to remain below L2–L3, which is important in cases of significant canal stenosis.
  - The spinal block is typically performed with the patient in a sitting position on the transport stretcher, monitored with electrocardiogram (ECG), noninvasive blood pressure, and pulse oximetry.
  - Premedication should be given with up to 100 µg of fentanyl and/or 2 mg of midazolam prior to anesthesia.
  - After the initial withdrawal of the cerebrospinal fluid (CSF), have the dosage of the bupivacaine is injected. To ensure that the dosage is delivered intrathecally, CSF is drawn again midway through, and the rest of the dosage is then delivered.
  - There is a possibility for the occurrence of pruritus due to intrathecal narcotic; intraoperative sedatives such as dexmedetomidine (0.1–0.2 µg/kg/h IV infusion) or propofol (10–25 µg/kg/min IV infusion) for sedation are recommended to alleviate patient discomfort.
- Waguia et al[12]:
  - Similarly emphasized the use of bupivacaine for SA, paired with IV propofol for sedation.
  - Conversely, the authors respecify spinal anesthetic application at the L3–L4 or L4–L5 levels with 12.5 to 15 mg of isobaric bupivacaine to ensure a dense block of the lower thoracic and the entire lumbar region for over 4 hours.
  - Sedation is managed through titrated IV propofol infusion, intentionally avoiding long-term benzodiazepines or opioids to facilitate quick patient recovery, illustrating a precise and controlled approach to sedation and anesthesia placement.
- Letchuman et al[13]:
  - They outline a regimen starting with procedural IV sedation using less than 2 mg of midazolam and less than 100 µg of fentanyl.
  - This is followed by lumbar SA with 15 mg of isobaric bupivacaine and 10 to 25 µg of fentanyl, administered near the operative level (one space above or below).
  - This approach requires patients to self-position on a Jackson table.
  - General sedation is maintained at a Ramsay Sedation Scale of 2 to 3, using 25 to 50 µg/kg/min of propofol and 2 µg/kg/min of ketamine with alternatives to intravenous sedation such as dexmedetomidine or a combination of fentanyl and midazolam.
  - Each incision or percutaneous screw tract in the surgical site should be infiltrated with 10 mL (20 mL or 1.3% liposomal bupivacaine diluted with 20 mL of normal saline to a total volume of 40 mL) of liposomal bupivacaine.
  - Reinjection of 1 mL of 0.5% of bupivacaine is recommended for extended analgesia.
  - During the operation, blood pressure and prophylaxis nausea should be managed as follows:
    - Blood pressure should be maintained via fluid boluses, phenylephrine guttae, or ephedrine should be administered to maintain a minimum of 65 mm Hg or 80% of the patient's baseline mean arterial pressure.
    - Nausea should also be managed using intravenous dexamethasone and Zofran

(4 mg), with dexamethasone being held for diabetic patients.

- Commonalties and differences across the mentioned protocols:
  - Isobaric bupivacaine is consistently used for SA in all protocols.
  - Protocol diverges in the adjunct use of narcotics, the selection and dosages of sedatives, and the strategies employed to ensure patient comfort and operative efficiency.

22.5.2 Airway Management

In the guidelines for airway management during awake spine surgery, both De Biase et al, and Waguia et al[12] emphasize the importance of maintaining spontaneous breathing in the prone position with the assistance of light to moderate sedation. Both studies recommend the use of a nasal cannula for oxygen delivery to the patient. An important aspect is the prevention of carbon dioxide accumulation. De Biase et al, suggest the use of an open horseshoe with open face foam for this purpose (▶ Fig. 22.2).

Approaches regarding sedation vary slightly. De Biase et al, outline a versatile flexible approach that allows for titration using dexmedetomidine, propofol infusion, midazolam, or fentanyl, depending on patient and anesthesiologist preference. In contrast, Waguia et al recommend propofol infusion for inducing mild sedation, as per the anesthesiologist's preference, without mentioning the use of other sedatives.[12]

Both guidelines agree on the necessity of having emergency airway management equipment readily available. Both recommend the availability of a laryngeal mask airway (LMA) and video laryngoscopy equipment to address the potential need for transitioning to GA or handling emergent airway management situations.

In the event of an airway emergency during surgery, when a patient experiences difficulty breathing, the anesthesiologist should declare an "airway emergency" to alert the team. This announcement mobilizes the team, with each member quickly assuming their predefined roles. It is our recommendation that the following roles and steps are promptly executed:

- A circulator is designated to press an orange button for airway emergencies, turn on the X-ray light, and obtain a stretcher from the hallway.
- Another circulator clears the area by moving equipment such as the C-arm or X-ray machine, cutting patient straps, and removing the arm board.
- The surgeon stops the procedure, removes surgical instruments, and covers the wound with a transparent dressing provided by a scrub tech. The surgeon's assistant and the scrub tech help in these tasks.
- An anesthesia tech responds with a GlideScope equipped with fiberoptic technology, prepares an LMA, brings in a difficult airway cart that includes a bronchoscope, and hands induction drugs to the anesthesiologist or anesthesia provider.
- Either a CRNA (Certified Registered Nurse Anesthetist) or a resident takes steps to improve the patient's oxygenation by stimulating the patient, increasing oxygen flow, stopping sedation, and attaching a mask to the breathing circuit while holding the patient's head.
- The anesthesiologist directs the care and assists in positioning the patient properly.
- The entire team works together to bring a stretcher in, aiming to quickly turn the patient from a prone to a supine position to better secure the airway.
- While waiting for the stretcher and the difficult intubation cart, the team attempts to oxygenate the patient with 100% oxygen, with or without using an oral or nasal airway.
- If the patient is unconscious and unresponsive, they consider inserting an LMA, which could be challenging in obese patients due to restricted head and neck movement.
- If LMA placement is successful and provides adequate ventilation and oxygenation, the team might decide to continue with the surgery using the LMA or proceed to intubate through it if necessary.
- Once the patient is positioned supine, mask ventilation begins with 100% oxygen, followed by a transition to GA, muscle relaxation is induced, and intubation with the GlideScope is attempted.
- Confirmation of tube placement is ensured with end-tidal CO_2 monitoring and listening for breath sounds bilaterally.

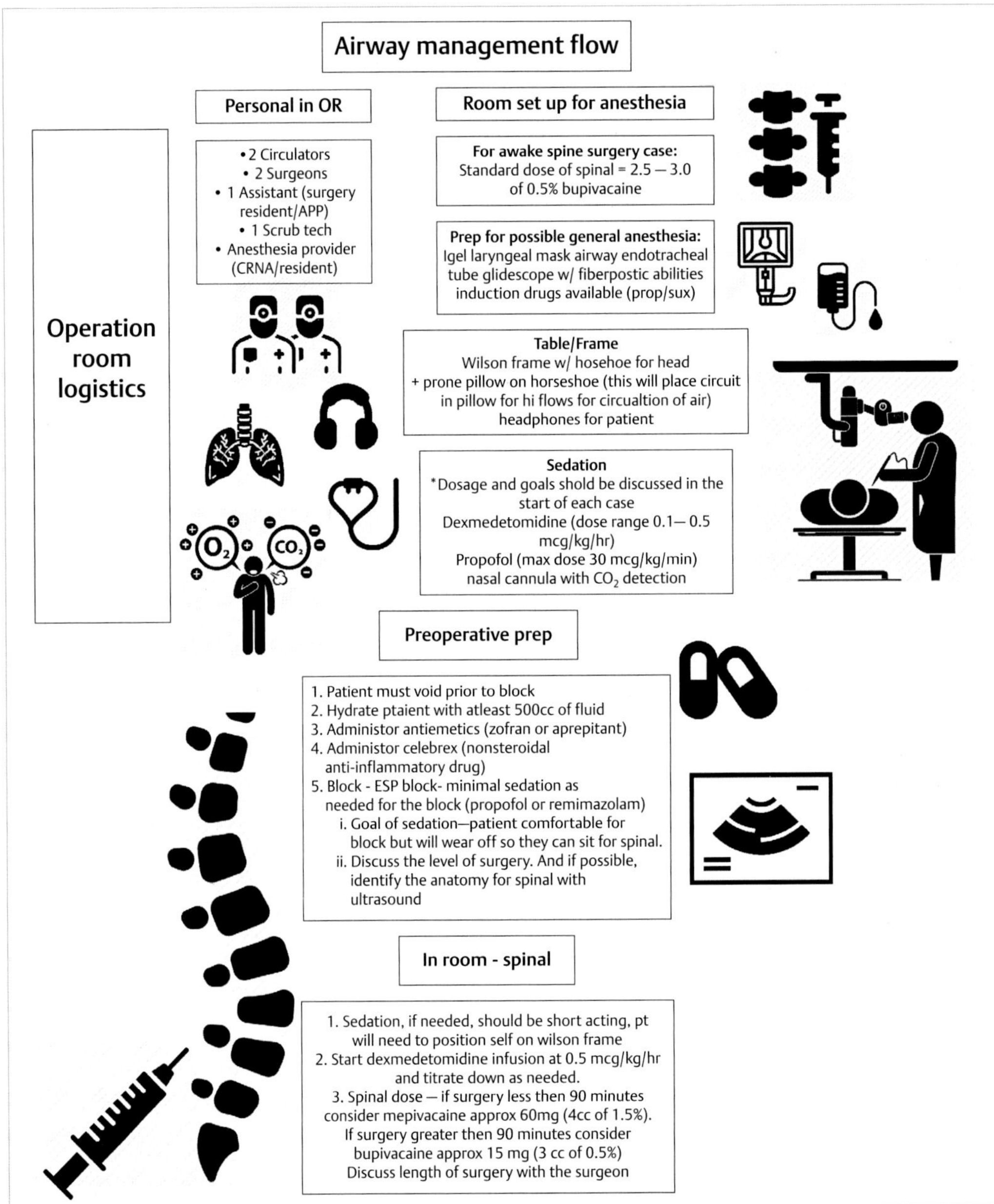

Fig. 22.2 Airway management during awake spine surgery. This figure outlines the key steps and team roles in managing airway emergencies during awake spine surgery. It includes anesthesia preparation, patient positioning, and coordinated response of the surgical team to ensure patient safety and effective intervention during airway complications.

(Continued)

- Should intubation fail, the American Society of Anesthesiologists' practice guidelines for managing a difficult airway are followed.
- The decision to proceed with surgery under GA with a secured airway depends on the patient's stability.

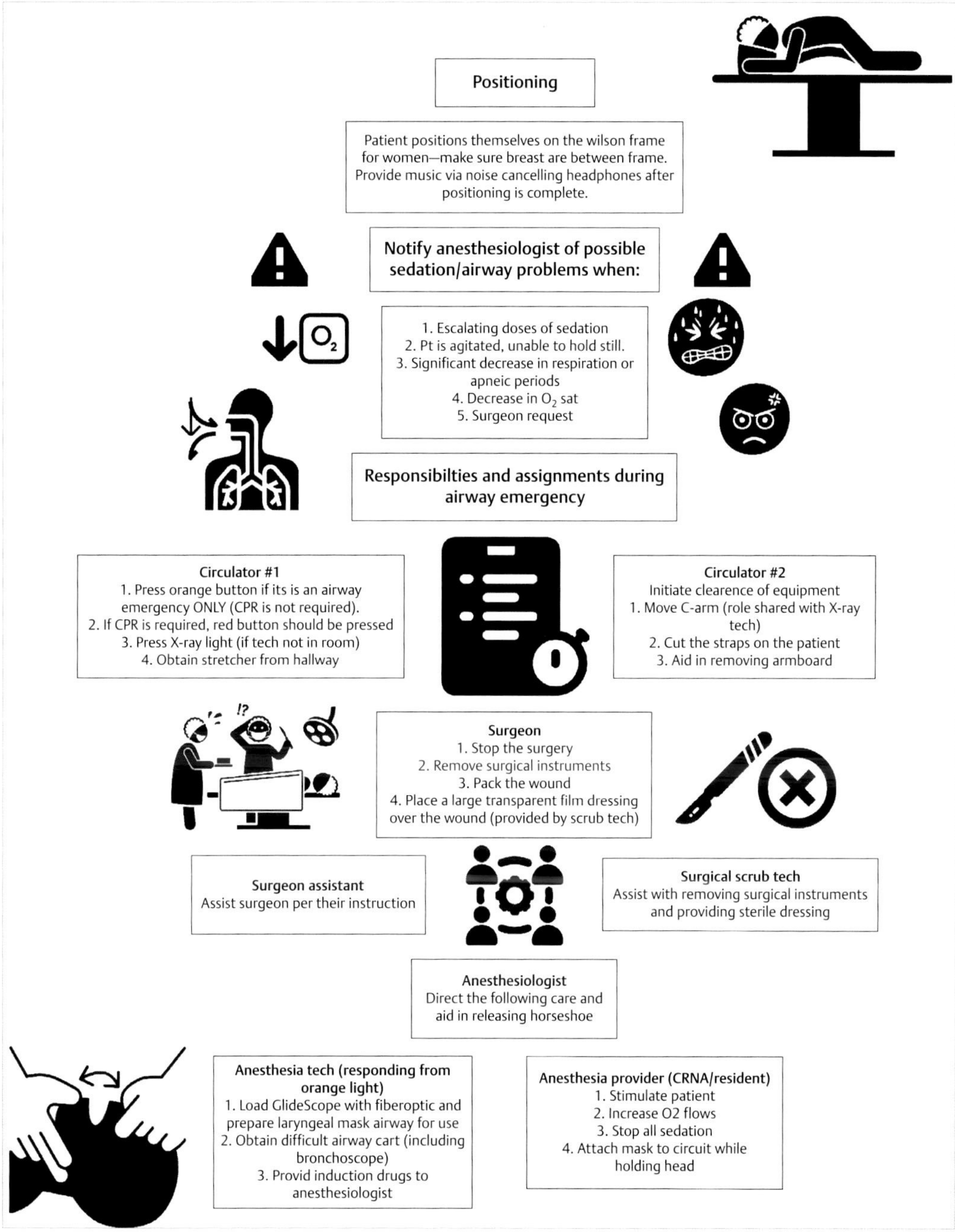

Fig. 22.2 *(Continued)*

(Continued)

Effective airway management in awake spine surgery is crucial to ensure the patient maintains spontaneous breathing and adequate oxygenation while minimizing the risk of carbon dioxide accumulation during the procedure, thereby enhancing safety and comfort.

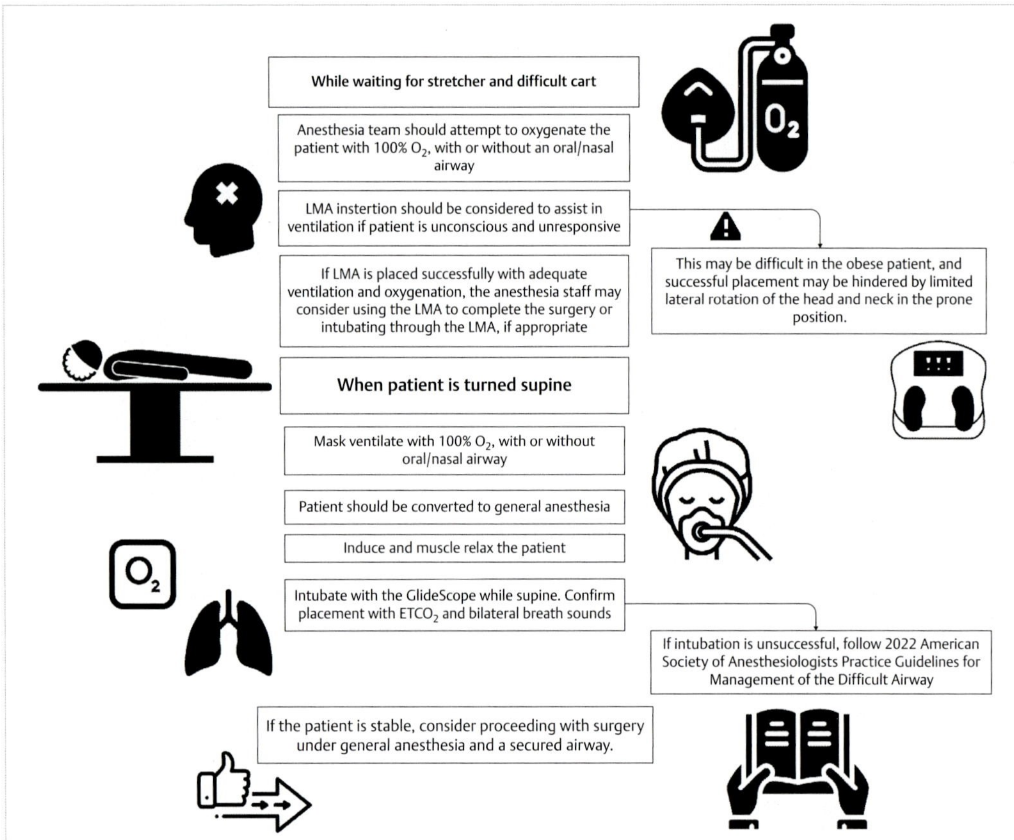

Fig. 22.2 (*Continued*)

22.6 Postoperative Course

22.6.1 Anesthesia Protocol: Postoperative

In terms of postoperative guidelines in anesthesia, protocols incorporate common and unique elements in managing patient care and comfort following surgery.

De Biase et al recommend the following[7]:

- Administration of acetaminophen as the SA begins to wear off at a dosage of 1,000 µg with adjustments made based on liver function.
- The use of scheduled muscle relaxants to aid in patient recovery postoperatively.

Waguia et al suggest the following[12]:

- A "soft landing" technique in the recovery room, which consists of the use of SA and ESP blocks. This approach contrasts with the experience of patients receiving GA without such blocks. They also advocated maximizing nonopioid analgesia to avoid opioid-related adverse effects such as nausea, vomiting, and respiratory depression.
- The regimen includes the following:
  - Acetaminophen and NSAIDs as standard, nonoptional medications, with gabapentinoids reserved for patients already on these medications.
  - Methocarbamol is suggested as an as-needed muscle relaxant for postoperative spasms.
  - Oxycodone (5–10 mg every 3–4 hours as needed) is prescribed for breakthrough pain, emphasizing its use following physical therapy or activity rather than routine administration.

Letchuman et al recommend the following[13]:

- A comprehensive analgesia strategy involving the following:

- Acetaminophen (1,000 mg every 4 hours around the clock).
- Gabapentin (3,000 mg three times a day).
- Oxycodone (5 mg every 3–4 hours as needed for moderate pain).
- For severe pain:
  - Hydromorphone (0.2–0.4 mg intravenously every 3–4 hours as needed) is recommended.
  - Advises against patient-controlled analgesia
  - Suggested managing postoperative nausea with Zofran (4 mg intravenously every 6 hours as needed).

Across the current guidelines for postoperative analgesic care, there is a shared consensus on the administration of acetaminophen and oxycodone for pain management, albeit with variations in administration strategies and additional medications.

22.6.2 Management

For postoperative management in patients who underwent awake spine surgery, a holistic approach to care including pain management, physical mobility, and careful monitoring to ensure a successful recovery is important.

Expert Tip

Early administration of oral pain medication and prompt ambulation are recommended for optimal patient recovery.

De Biase et al[7]:

- Note the importance of managing pain and muscle relaxation immediately after surgery.
- Patients should receive an intramuscular injection of long-acting local anesthetic prior to closure.
- Oral narcotics are to be administered once the effects of the spinal block begin to diminish.
- A scheduled muscle relaxant is prescribed postoperatively to alleviate discomfort.
- Patients are encouraged to ambulate as soon as the spinal block wears off to promote quicker recovery.
- Urinary retention must be carefully monitored during the recovery process.

Waguia et al[12]:

- Extend the focus on postoperative care to include comprehensive neurological assessment, mobilization, pain control, urination, and discharge planning.
- Neurological assessments prioritize evaluating lower extremity strength and sensation against preoperative baselines to detect any changes postsurgery.
- Physical therapy assistance is crucial in guiding patients through safe movements, minimizing pain by avoiding excessive twisting or bending.
- Pain management follows prescribed pharmacological regimens and supplementing with nonpharmaceutical measures like heat and cold therapy to ease muscle discomfort.
- In terms of urination, monitoring bladder function ensures patients' ability to urinate independently and postoperatively, a critical aspect of recovery.
- Discharge planning entails educating patients on physical limitations to prevent strain during the initial recovery phase, encouraging walking, and gradually increasing activity as advised by health care providers.

22.7 Conclusion

The protocol outlined in this chapter offers a comprehensive framework for conducting awake spine surgery, focusing on optimizing patient safety and improving surgical outcomes. By adhering to patient selection criteria, following anesthesia and airway protocols, and emphasizing postoperative care, this protocol ensures that awake spine surgery is both safe and effective. The collaborative efforts among surgeons, anesthesiologists, and nursing staff, supported by evidence-based guidelines, contribute to the success and growing adoption of this innovative approach.

References

[1] Fiani B, Reardon T, Selvage J, et al. Awake spine surgery: an eye-opening movement. Surg Neurol Int. 2021; 12:222

[2] Perez-Roman RJ, Govindarajan V, Bryant JP, Wang MY. Spinal anesthesia in awake surgical procedures of the lumbar spine: a systematic review and meta-analysis of 3709 patients. Neurosurg Focus. 2021; 51(6):E7

[3] Morris MT, Morris J, Wallace C, et al. An analysis of the cost-effectiveness of spinal versus general anesthesia for lumbar spine surgery in various hospital settings. Global Spine J. 2019; 9(4):368–374

[4] Deng H, Coumans JV, Anderson R, Houle TT, Peterfreund RA. Spinal anesthesia for lumbar spine surgery correlates with fewer total medications and less frequent use of vasoactive agents: a single center experience. PLoS One. 2019; 14(6): e0217939

[5] Walcott BP, Khanna A, Yanamadala V, Coumans JV, Peterfreund RA. Cost analysis of spinal and general anesthesia for the surgical treatment of lumbar spondylosis. J Clin Neurosci. 2015; 22(3):539–543

[6] Attari MA, Mirhosseini SA, Honarmand A, Safavi MR. Spinal anesthesia versus general anesthesia for elective lumbar spine surgery: a randomized clinical trial. J Res Med Sci. 2011; 16(4):524–529

[7] De Biase G, Bechtle P, Leone B, Quinones-Hinojosa A, Abode-Iyamah K. Awake minimally invasive transforaminal lumbar interbody fusion with a pedicle-based retraction system. Clin Neurol Neurosurg. 2021; 200:106313

[8] Abode-Iyamah K, Ghaith AK, Bhandarkar AR, et al. Single-level awake transforaminal lumbar interbody fusion: a Mayo Clinic institutional experience and national analysis. Neurosurg Focus. 2021; 51(6):E4

[9] De Biase G, Gruenbaum SE, West JL, et al. Spinal versus general anesthesia for minimally invasive transforaminal lumbar interbody fusion: implications on operating room time, pain, and ambulation. Neurosurg Focus. 2021; 51(6): E3

[10] Sykes DAW, Tabarestani TQ, Chaudhry NS, et al. Awake spinal fusion is associated with reduced length of stay, opioid use, and time to ambulation compared to general anesthesia: a matched cohort study. World Neurosurg. 2023; 176: e91–e100

[11] Azad TD, Alomari S, Khalifeh JM, et al. Adoption of awake spine surgery: trends from a national registry over 14 years. Spine J. 2022; 22(10):1601–1609

[12] Waguia R, Touko EK, Sykes DAW, et al. How to start an awake spine program: Protocol and illustrative cases. IBRO Neurosci Rep. 2022; 13:69–77

[13] Letchuman V, Agarwal N, Mummaneni VP, et al. Awake spinal surgery: simplifying the learning curve with a patient selection algorithm. Neurosurg Focus. 2021; 51(6):E2

[14] Collins LM, Vaghadia H. Regional anesthesia for laparoscopy. Anesthesiol Clin North America. 2001; 19(1):43–55

[15] Ames WA, Songhurst L, Gullan RW. Local anaesthesia for laminectomy surgery. Br J Neurosurg. 1999; 13(6):598–600

[16] Chan AK, Gnaedinger A, Ayoub C, Gupta DK, Abd-El-Barr MM. The "in-parallel" technique for awake, bilateral simultaneous minimally invasive transforaminal lumbar interbody fusion and multilevel lumbar decompression. Oper Neurosurg (Hagerstown). 2023; 24(3):e160–e169

[17] Ayoub CM, Rizk LB, Yaacoub CI, Gaal D, Kain ZN. Music and ambient operating room noise in patients undergoing spinal anesthesia. Anesth Analg. 2005; 100(5):1316–1319

[18] Soma Tech Intl. OSI Spinal Table—5943 Spinal Surgery Top—Jackson Table. 2023. Accessed May 2024 at: https://www.somatechnology.com/blog/products/osi-spinal-table-jackson-table/

[19] Park JH, Kwon JY, Lee SE, Kim YH, Kim SH. Sudden hemodynamic collapse after prone positioning on a Jackson spinal table for spinal surgery. Korean J Anesthesiol. 2020; 73(1):71–74

[20] Soma Tech Intl. Wilson Plus Radiolucent Frame – Wilson frame. 2024. Accessed May 2024 at: https://www.somatechnology.com/surgical-tables/wilson-plus-radiolucent-frame

[21] DePasse JM, Palumbo MA, Haque M, Eberson CP, Daniels AH. Complications associated with prone positioning in elective spinal surgery. World J Orthop. 2015; 6(3):351–359

[22] Schonauer C, Bocchetti A, Barbagallo G, Albanese V, Moraci A. Positioning on surgical table. Eur Spine J. 2004; 13 Suppl 1:S50–S55

Index

Note: Page numbers set **bold** or *italic* indicate headings or figures, respectively.

N

O

P

Q

R

S